Practical Occupational Medicine

Second edition

Raymond M. Agius MD, DM, FRCP, FRCPE, FFOM
Professor of Occupational and Environmental Medicine
Centre for Occupational and Environmental Health
The University of Manchester, UK
Honorary Consultant in Occupational Medicine, Manchester Royal Infirmary

Anthony Seaton CBE, MD, FRCP, FRCPE, FFOM, FMedSci
Emeritus Professor of Occupational and Environmental Medicine
University of Aberdeen
and Senior Consultant to the Institute of Occupational Medicine
Edinburgh, UK

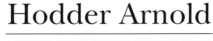

Hodder Arnold

A MEMBER OF THE HODDER HEADLINE GROUP

First published in Great Britain in 1994 by Hodder Arnold
This Second edition published in 2006 by
Hodder Arnold, an imprint of Hodder Education and a member of the
Hodder Headline Group,
338 Euston Road, London NW1 3BH

http://www.hoddereducation.com

Distributed in the United States of America by
Oxford University Press Inc.,
198 Madison Avenue, New York, NY10016
Oxford is a registered trademark of Oxford University Press

Whilst the advice and information in this book are believed to be true and
accurate at the date of going to press, neither the author[s] nor the
publisher can accept any legal responsibility or liability for any errors or
omissions that may be made. In particular (but without limiting the
generality of the preceding disclaimer) every effort has been made to check
drug dosages; however it is still possible that errors have been missed.
Furthermore, dosage schedules are constantly being revised and new side-
effects recognized. For these reasons the reader is strongly urged to consult
the drug companies' printed instructions before administering any of the
drugs recommended in this book.

British Library Cataloguing in Publication Data
A catalogue record for this book is available from the British Library

Library of Congress Cataloging-in-Publication Data
A catalog record for this book is available from the Library of Congress

ISBN-10   0 340 759 47 X
ISBN-13   978 0 340 759 47 9

1 2 3 4 5 6 7 8 9 10

Commissioning Editor: Joanna Koster
Project Editor: Heather Fyfe
Production Controller: Lindsay Smith
Cover Designer: Sarah Rees

Typeset in 10/12pt Minion by Phoenix Photosetting, Chatham, Kent
Printed and bound in Malta

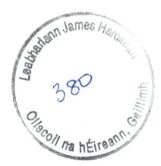

What do you think about this book? Or any other Hodder Arnold title?
Please send your comments to www.hoddereducation.com

Contents

Contributors

Dr Gillian Fletcher MB, ChB, FRCP, FFOM
Consultant in Occupational Medicine, Occupational Health and Safety Advisory Service and Honorary Senior Clinical Lecturer, University of Edinburgh, UK

Dr Elizabeth Wright MB, ChB, MSc, FFOM, MIOSH
Director of Occupational Health, Abermed Industrial Doctors Ltd, Aberdeen, and Honorary Senior Lecturer in the Department of Environmental and Occupational Medicine, University of Aberdeen, UK

Preface

The dual concerns of the influence of work on health, and of health on work are important issues to workers, to responsible employers and to society at large. More doctors are becoming involved in providing advice to employers and to workers on health in relation to the workplace. The need for this book can be restated in the following paragraph which is as true now as it was when written for the first edition.

'In our undergraduate and postgraduate teaching we have become aware of the need for an introductory textbook written in such a way as to bridge the gap between normal clinical practice, which is concerned mostly with diagnosis and treatment of disease, and occupational practice, which concerns itself with prevention of work-related disease and with non-pharmacological management of ill-health in relation to the workplace. Common to both types of practice is the ill or at-risk individual, and it is with such people and their management that this book is concerned. We have based the structure of the book on real examples of problems encountered in our practice, problems that may be familiar to our readers but that may nevertheless cause difficulties in management through unfamiliarity with occupational medical practice.'

In this second edition we have added a completely new chapter dealing with the effects of the wider environment on health. This is an area that many occupational physicians are beginning to contend with more often, by virtue of their training, experience or job. In any case it is an area of increasing public and professional concern. We have introduced 'new blood' by inviting guest authors who are both practising occupational physicians and teachers for two of the chapters. This second edition replaces many case studies by new ones. These permit more active learning by the reader, not merely through the guidance provided in the text, but perhaps equally importantly by allowing the reader to reflect on alternative management of the cases. Of necessity each case history may reveal many 'lessons' and therefore there is overlap between the chapters. However, this reflects practice in real life where few problems are demarcated by organ system or by hazard, or have strictly limited implications. The first edition was prompted in part by the realization that occupational medicine received little emphasis in the curricula of most UK medical schools, and doctors were often ill equipped to take on responsibilities in a specialty with which they have little familiarity. This concern remains, but in this new edition we have begun to introduce a wider, more European dimension, partly because of the influence of European legislation on practice throughout the European Union, but also in response to comments and needs from elsewhere in Europe.

The sentiments that concluded the preface to the first edition are equally apt for this edition: 'We hope this book will be of value to medical students as a complement to their studies of internal medicine, general practice and public health, and also to general practitioners and other postgraduates taking courses in occupational medicine. Increasingly, nurses are playing an important role in the provision of occupational health services, and we believe it will be of value to them when working for occupational health qualifications. Many established consultants who occasionally see patients suspected of having occupational disease will also find it contains useful, practical information and advice. If in writing it we have conveyed some of our own enthusiasm for a specialty that crosses traditional medical boundaries into other scientific fields and the world of industry, we shall be well satisfied.'

We have received a number of constructive comments following the first edition. In particular we wish to acknowledge the helpful suggestions and information from Dr Charles Veys, Dr Robbert Hermanns and Ms Kathy Jenkins. We are especially grateful to the many students and colleagues who have inspired us to continue with this work.

Raymond M. Agius and Anthony Seaton, 2005

The occupational history

SUMMARY

- The occupational history should serve two functions – to enable the doctor to detect influences of the patient's work on his or her health, and to allow sensible advice to be given on the effects of the patient's health on future working ability.

- This chapter describes the concepts of hazard and risk. It discusses the important questions to ask in a routine occupational history, about the name of the job, what it involves and what possible relevant hazards it entails.

- The chapter also describes how to take a more detailed history, especially of exposure, when work-related disease is suspected or when there is a need to give advice about return to work (or retirement from work) after illness.

INTRODUCTION

In an ideal world occupational diseases would be prevented. However, often in the real world they are not, and as many as one in five new patients presenting to a general practitioner may have an occupational component to his or her illness. Every medical student is taught the importance of taking an occupational history, the emphasis of this being on the need to think of occupational causes of disease. However, because in clinical practice such conditions are wrongly perceived as being relatively uncommon, the young doctor often forgets this early lesson and simply records the job title of the patient. Indeed, it is quite usual in reviewing hospital or general practice notes to find no reference at all to a patient's occupation. This lack of curiosity about what people spend half of their waking hours doing means that possible subtle influences of work on health are commonly missed by the doctor, and the perception that work-related ill-health is rare is thus reinforced. Furthermore, it results in the doctor being ill-equipped to answer the questions commonly asked by patients, such as, 'should I stay off work?', 'when can I go back to work?', 'is there anything I should avoid on going back to work?' and 'could my work have caused my problem?'.

The importance of occupation as a cause of disease was first systematically recorded by Bernardino Ramazzini, who was professor of medicine in Padua, Italy in the 18th century, in his book '*De morbis artificium diatriba*'. He taught physicians that illness in poor working people was just as worthy of their interest as were diseases of the rich, and was the first teacher of medicine after Hippocrates to extend the medical history-taking process by adding the question 'what is your work?'. The occupational history should be taken in such a way as to equip the doctor to judge whether the patient's health has been affected by their work and also to decide whether the illness will affect the patient's ability to continue working normally. Forming the basis of occupational medical practice are these two concepts:

- the effects of work on health; and
- the effects of health on work.

HAZARD AND RISK

The different but related concepts of hazard and risk are fundamental to occupational medicine, and will be discussed further in Chapter 5. The word 'hazard' derives from the Arabic for a gaming die, and means something with the potential to cause harm. 'Risk' describes a quantification of the likelihood of harm and its severity occurring with defined exposure to a hazard. Further problems may arise from confusing two different concepts of risk, relative and absolute. What concerns most people is the absolute risk – their own chance of running into trouble; for example, a smoker's chance of developing lung cancer is about one in eight and someone who has been heavily exposed to asbestos may have a one in ten lifetime risk of the pleural tumour mesothelioma. All of us have an approximately one in three chance of developing some form of cancer. Relative risk is a concept used in epidemiology to describe increases in risk when exposed to a particular environment; for example, a study may have shown a doubling of the risk of brain cancer in certain occupations, but the absolute risk of any individual in those occupations having this uncommon disease may remain clinically insignificant.

In the occupational history, a judgement as to whether a patient has developed an occupational disease, or the extent to which the patient may have an increased likelihood of developing it, depends on assessment of the hazards in the workplace and whether exposure to the hazard may be sufficient to constitute a significant risk of causing the disease in question. Hazards may conveniently be categorized as physical, chemical, biological and psychological.

TAKING THE HISTORY

This need not be a lengthy procedure, although in certain circumstances it may be. Nevertheless, it should involve more than merely recording the job title. Consider, for example, the range of activities covered by those with the title 'doctor': a surgeon rushing from a blood-spattered operation; the out-patient clinic; a fevered committee meeting; a community physician, who may spend much of the day planning provision of services, arguing in meetings and working at a computer. What is necessary is to obtain information on what the patient does at work. The key questions are:

- do you have a job?
- what is it?
- what do you do at work?

Additional questions, if thought to be relevant, may be:

- do you work with any chemical, dusts or fumes?
- do you have any problems at work?
- do you have any difficulty doing your work?
- do you think that your work is affecting your health?

The first of this latter group of questions may be adapted to the patient's complaint, asking for example about awkward postures, movements or loads in the case of someone with musculoskeletal complaints, or of relations with other workers, managers, etc., in the case of psychological illness.
Finally, it is often sensible to ask:

- do you have any other jobs?

Here there is overlap with hobbies and pastimes, which may also be relevant. It is important to know how long the patient has had the job. If it has been for a relatively short period, it is sensible to ask about the main work the patient had carried out previously. In certain circumstances, when a patient presents with a chronic disease or with a cancer, it may be useful to know about jobs many years before.

The job

Consider the following case histories.

Case history 1.1

A 30-year-old chemical process worker presented with an itchy red scaly rash affecting his right thumb. The appearance was of a severe irritant dermatitis. Careful history taking and a detailed assessment of his personal protective gloves and of his workplace did not reveal any potential cause.

Eventually the physician enquired about other activities. It transpired that he had purchased an acetoxysilane-based filler for a crack between his bath and the surrounding tiles, and had used his bare thumb as the grouting tool. The physician explained that this activity was equivalent to pickling his thumb in vinegar. He stayed off work for a week and applied aqueous cream to his skin while it healed.

Case history 1.2

A 30-year-old man presented with episodic wheeze and cough. He gave as his occupation 'panel beater', a trade involving the repair of the bodywork of crashed cars. Further questions were therefore directed at the possibility of exposure to sprayed paint and he said that this activity did take place in the garage, but by others and in a specially constructed booth; he was not exposed to the paint. By way of explanation, he was told that some two-part paints contain isocyanates and that these chemicals can cause asthma. He then admitted that he had a second job in which he repaired car bodywork in his own garage at home. He had been using an isocyanate-based paint spray without any exhaust ventilation or respiratory protection! This proved to be the cause of his asthma, and after he had purchased appropriate respiratory protection and ventilation equipment he was able to continue this work without symptoms. The outcome might not have been so satisfactory, as most such patients are so sensitive as to be unable to continue even the slightest exposure to isocyanates.

Case history 1.3

A 50-year-old lady presented with increasing and severe breathlessness over a period of about 5 years. She looked ill and her chest radiographs showed bilateral upper lobe fibrosis and lower zone emphysema. She had never smoked, and had worked for the same company as a clerical officer for 30 years. She was employed as a clerk but described her current task as operating an industrial camera. This involved a stage during which she dusted exposed plates with a special powder. The work was undertaken in a small room and the powder was dispersed everywhere; apparently the service engineer for another machine in the room had complained that the dust repeatedly jammed its works.

Upper lobe fibrosis has relatively few causes, the best known of which is tuberculosis. Accelerated silicosis is a rare cause, and examination of the powder she had been using showed it to be pure crystalline silicon dioxide. This information came too late to help the unfortunate patient, but did allow action to be taken to prevent others suffering the same fate.

These histories illustrate the importance of obtaining some detail about the work involved in someone's job, and also show the difficulties that may lead to an occupational cause being missed. In Chapter 2 we discuss the range of diseases that may have an occupational cause; there is almost no specialty in medicine in which possible occupational causes of ill-health can be disregarded.

As a doctor becomes more experienced, the process of history taking becomes more economical of time. In a busy practice it is usual to record the essentials of the occupational history initially, but to return for further elaboration if the medical history or examination reveals further clues. In taking a medical history, always be open-minded about the possibility of environmental causes of disease. Most illness is clearly not wholly genetically determined. Environment therefore must play a part in the aetiology of many diseases; if we do not know the cause of a disease, that does not mean that it cannot be discovered or that a cause does not exist.

In taking a history aimed at investigating the possibility of work-related disease, the temporal relationship between work and exposure is crucial. In acute conditions, such as pneumonitis and urticaria, a history of recent exposure to a gas or an allergen will be obtained. Variable conditions, such as asthma and some forms of dermatitis, may fluctuate as exposure fluctuates, improving during holidays and at weekends. Conditions such as pneumoconiosis and industrial deafness are usually the consequence of prolonged exposure over several years, although relatively short, high intensity exposure may sometimes be responsible. Most cancers are a response to exposure to carcinogens several decades previously, again usually over a prolonged period, although in some rare instances more recent exposure may be responsible. In all these instances, it is helpful to enquire in the history as to whether any of the patient's workmates are known to have suffered similar symptoms or illnesses.

A particular situation arises with respect to some asbestos-related diseases, when environmental rather than direct occupational exposure may lead to pleural plaques or even mesothelioma. If these conditions are suspected, the history should include enquiry about possible exposure from other tradesmen working nearby. Knowledge that such exposures occurred, especially in shipyards and during construction work, may lead to appropriate questions being asked.

Case history 1.4

A 55-year-old man presented with shortness of breath resulting from a pleural effusion, which proved, on investigation, to be caused by mesothelioma. His occupational history seemed innocuous in that he had worked in a paper mill all his life, where he denied exposure to asbestos. The only possible source might have been dust from brake linings on the machines, and doubt about this led to further questions. His relatively young age suggested exposure in childhood. It transpired that his father had worked in a factory making large diameter cement pipes and had always brought his overalls home for washing. Crocidolite asbestos was an important constituent of the cement for such pipes so this seemed a more likely cause of the disease.

Hazardous workplace environments

If occupational disease is suspected, the occupational history should include an attempt to assess the patient's exposure to risk. This is achieved by asking two questions:

- what has the patient been exposed to?
- to how much?

Of course, the provisional diagnosis of occupational disease will not have been made unless the occupational and medical histories have provided appropriate clues. These clues are then followed up by questions about likely causes of the syndrome and about the patient's working practices in relation to the suspect cause.

Case history 1.5

A 55-year-old man presented with progressive difficulty with arm and leg coordination over a period of some 4 years. This had eventually forced him to retire from his job, since when the symptoms had ceased to progress although they remained very disabling. He gave his job as an armaments fitter. Examination showed classical signs of cerebellar ataxia, without evidence of disease of other parts of the nervous system. Investigations led to the diagnosis of cerebellar degeneration, confirmed by computerized tomography.

The patient himself, puzzling about the cause of his disease, joined a self-help group and learned that the condition could sometimes be caused by the drug phenytoin. He told his doctor that this led him to consider the possibility that chemicals at his work might have been responsible. A detailed occupational history revealed that for 10 years he had worked in a relatively confined space, without exhaust ventilation, disassembling missiles. After stripping these down, he spent about 3 hours each day cleaning their parts with solvents, using a rag onto which he poured the solvent from an open tin. Much of this cleaning work took place at face level. He wore no protective gloves or respirator. Subsequent measurements of exposure levels showed them to be considerably in excess of the appropriate hygiene standards during this work. Although workplace exposure to the solvents in question, mainly methyl ethyl ketone, had not previously been shown to cause neurological damage, by analogy with neurological syndromes in glue-sniffers, it seemed very likely that his disease was in fact a result of his very high and prolonged workplace exposure. This opinion received some support from a small but definite subsequent clinical improvement after exposure had ceased for about a year.

The above case history illustrates an important point. From time to time patients may present with a disease that has not previously been described in relation to the substances they are exposed to at work. It is important to keep an open mind, because occasionally, as in this case, the occupational history reveals exposures very much in excess of what would normally have been expected – this patient used solvents for at least 15 hours each week and absorbed them both through his lungs and his skin. It should also be borne in mind that individuals differ in susceptibility to harmful substances; this is particularly true in the case of asthma and dermatitis and will be discussed later.

The sensible way to take a semi-quantitative occupational exposure history is to obtain the patient's account of a typical day: 'What time do you go to work?' 'What do you do when you get in?' 'How long do you do it for?' 'Do any dusts or fumes come off?' 'Do you handle chemicals?' ... and so on, until the end of the shift. Remember to ask for how long the patient has been in this job and about protective clothing and equipment. With respect to the latter, workers often wear quite inappropriate masks or gloves in the mistaken belief that they are protective as, for example, a doctor who sprays his roses with organophosphates wearing a cotton surgical mask. This sort of history, which is of course only necessary when an occupational disease is suspected, allows an estimate to be made of cumulative exposure, which can subsequently be enhanced by actual workplace measurements (see Chapter 3).

A careful structured occupational history may sometimes reveal a totally unexpected cause.

Case history 1.6

A patient was cleaning a heat exchanger in a potato crisp factory when he developed a severe attack of asthma, the first he had ever experienced. He had to go home, where he recovered after treatment by his doctor, but he suffered a similar attack, also when in the vicinity of the heat exchanger, the next day. Several subsequent attacks occurred at work and he arrived at the view that he had occupational asthma, attributing it to something in the heat exchanger and to chemicals used as fungicides on the potatoes he had to handle.

The original occupational history revealed that he had very little contact with the potatoes and that his work in the heat exchanger had involved exposure to dust which was almost certainly carbon. There seemed to be no plausible antigen. However, using the technique described above, it transpired that his first task on entering the factory was to sweep out the joiners' workshop. Thereafter he went on to other labouring jobs of a more or less innocuous nature, of which cleaning the heat exchanger had been one. The joiners had been using red cedar, a wood he had used in a previous job as a joiner himself with consequent exposure to dust from it. He proved to have red cedar allergy, and this knowledge allowed steps to be taken to prevent further trouble.

Case history 1.7

An 18-year-old male was admitted to a surgical ward from the casualty department with worsening abdominal pain, constipation and loss of appetite over a period of 4 weeks. His job was recorded as restoring old furniture in a family business. His abdomen was diffusely tender, more so in the right iliac fossa, but rectal examination was normal.

A diagnosis of probable appendicitis was made but it was decided to observe his condition overnight. That evening a call from the haematology technician reported a haemoglobin of 11.7 g/L and basophilic stippling of the red cells, diagnostic of lead poisoning. A more detailed history then showed that part of his work had involved sanding and burning off old paint from furniture. He was in the habit of both eating and smoking while at work and only used a handkerchief round his face as protection against particularly bad fumes!

His blood lead level was greatly raised at 4.8 μmol/l and he had elevated urinary 5-aminolaevulinic acid; moreover, his father's blood lead was found to be 5.2 μmol/L.

It is certainly unreasonable to expect surgical staff to take a detailed occupational history of everyone presenting with abdominal pain, but the clue in this case would have come from asking the question suggested earlier: 'Do you work with any dusts or fumes?'. This patient was one of two seen recently by the authors, who presented in the same way with lead poisoning.

Identifying the harmful substance – data sheets

The patient will often know only in rather general terms to what substances he or she has been exposed. If this knowledge is very unspecific, such as a paint, further questions should be asked to find out whether it was water- or oil-based, single part or two part, and what solvents were used with it. More commonly, the patient will be able to give a trade name and/or the manufacturer, and this should allow a data sheet to be found. The patient is often able to obtain this from the workplace, but it can also be obtained through the manufacturer or the relevant trade union. The data sheet ideally gives the manufacturer's trade name, the chemical ingredients (not always in as much detail as one would wish) and their approximate proportions, the physical properties, fire and explosion hazards, reactivity risks (for example with water), health hazards and protective measures/equipment necessary, together with precautions to be taken when handling, storing, disposing of and transporting the substance.

When reading a data sheet it is important to be aware that the harmful effects are likely to be described only in very general terms, such as 'irritating to skin'. Further information may then need to be obtained from a standard chemical/toxicological data source and from the medical and toxicological literature. Sometimes data sheets may also be positively misleading, and it is important to beware particularly of bland statements such as 'Contains no aldehydes'. What the substance does contain is clearly more relevant. In some cases, more specific investigation of the workplace will be thought desirable. This is discussed in Chapter 3.

Quantifying exposure

If there is a strong suspicion that workplace exposure has contributed to the patient's illness, an attempt may be made to quantify the exposure. This is rarely necessary in routine clinical practice, but becomes important in the workplace, where the occupational physician needs to give advice on risk reduction, and in medico-legal situations. It also has an important role in epidemiological investigations (see Chapter 3). Quantification of exposure ideally requires the estimation of the product of intensity and duration.

With respect to exposure to chemicals, the simplest and least accurate method is to identify the substances most likely to be the cause of the illness and to add up the years of probable exposure to them. Increasing accuracy may be obtained by estimating the number of hours of exposure per average week and multiplying this by an index of exposure intensity on a simple linear scale. Again, at its simplest this might be 1 for minimal, 2 for slight, 3 for moderate and 4 for heavy, while increasing accuracy may be obtained if information on workplace hygiene monitoring is available. In occasional cases, guesses can be made as to possible concentrations from known odour thresholds, although there are well-known traps: for example, hydrogen sulphide in high concentration can poison the olfactory nerves and achieve fatal levels unnoticed, whereas chlorine can be smelt at levels that are harmless.

With respect to exposure to musculoskeletal stressors, a good account of the method of working and frequency of the different movements made and loads imposed is useful. The patient is usually able to mimic the postures and movements adopted in the job, and this not infrequently leads to a diagnosis of the cause.

Case history 1.8

A 50-year-old man complained of a painful right hand. Examination showed tenderness in the palm over the finger flexor tendons and triggering of the right third and fourth fingers. His job included operation of a centrifuge used for drying a powdered chemical prior to bagging. The task was carried out about four times daily, two or three times a week. The chemical tended to stick inside the centrifuge, which was rather like a small cement mixer, and the patient needed to scrape it out. He used a chisel held in his left hand and knocked into the concretions of chemical with the palm of his right hand. Demonstration of this movement immediately gave the causal diagnosis.

The intensity of exposure to noise may be estimated very approximately by asking about the level with respect to hearing conversation, but taking account of any impairment the patient may have: for example, if people need to shout to be heard at work, the levels are likely to be over about 90 decibels (dB). Knowledge of the place in which noise is generated and the machines operating therein may also give clues to the experienced occupational physician. Some approximate noise levels for comparative purposes are given in Table 1.1.

Exposures to noise over about the 85 dB level imply risk of hearing loss if prolonged. In addition, impact noise, such as from shooting, may cause long-term loss of hearing. It is likely that some individuals are more susceptible to the effects of noise than others, and certain conditions, such as concurrent exposure to neurotoxic agents or cigarette smoke, may increase risk.

Protective measures taken

When occupational disease is suspected, the history is not complete without an assessment of the adequacy of any preventive measures. This is particularly so in medico-legal practice, where a patient may find the employer claiming that the worker's injury or illness was contributed to by a failure to protect him or herself. The principles

Table 1.1 *Noise levels in different situations*

Degree of loudness	Equivalent to:
Quiet (<60 dB)	Normal conversation
	Distant traffic
Moderately loud (60–80 dB)	Washing machine
	Vacuum cleaner
	Close traffic
Loud (80–100 dB)	Food mixer
	Shouting
	Motor mower
	Lathe
	Tractor
Very loud (>100 dB)	Disco
	Thunder
	Chainsaw
	Textile loom
	Rivet gun

of protection are discussed in Chapter 6, but essentially they are based on an understanding that risks to health should, as far as is reasonably practicable, be designed out. Thus, relatively safe substances should be preferred to harmful ones, harmful substances should not come into contact with individuals, and finally, personal protection should be provided when necessary. The occupational history should reveal whether these criteria were observed and also when. Remember that harmful substances may enter the body via the lungs, skin or the alimentary tract.

Sometimes a well-known occupational disease may occur despite adequate precautions being taken, because particular groups of workers or individuals escape the protective net.

Case history 1.9

Bladder cancer is a well-known hazard of workers exposed to certain organic dyes, and for this reason the manufacturers are particularly careful to protect their workers by enclosure of processes and provision of protective clothing and changing facilities. One patient with the disease, however, had spent many years working for an engineering company as a fitter. His company had a contract to service and repair the machinery at the dye factory. He therefore had to penetrate the protective barriers and became regularly soaked in the chemicals when undertaking his work. By an oversight, the company had not provided him, as an outside contract worker, with the protective clothing and facilities enjoyed by the company's employees, and consequently he was exposed through skin contact to hazardous amounts of bladder carcinogens.

Several lessons arise from this case history. First, the term 'fitter' covers a multitude of jobs and workplaces, but usually means the worker will be employed when something needs repairing. This is often a dangerous time, as the protective barriers are down and harmful substances may be present. Second, an employer is responsible for the health and safety of all on the work site, not just the direct employees, but also contractors and visitors. Third, old-fashioned occupational diseases still occur. The reason they are old-fashioned is that precautions have generally been taken to prevent them; if people forget about these precautions, the diseases come back.

In enquiring about protective measures in the occupational history, ask about:

- enclosure of the process and segregation from it
- local exhaust and general ventilation
- protective clothing, respirators, hearing protection, etc.
- what happens when the process is serviced or repaired
- information provided on hazards
- education given to workers on protecting themselves.

Assessing fitness for the job

The occupational history is often thought of solely in terms of diagnosis of the cause of ill-health. Equally important, however, is its role in assessing the fitness of a patient for return to work. It is never sufficient to assume the level of activity in a job; a lorry driver, for example, is usually responsible for loading and unloading his vehicle, whereas a miner may sometimes ride to the coalface and spend his day sitting on a cutting or drilling machine. Most workers learn the most physically economical method of carrying out their job, while some severely impaired individuals manage a demanding job by relying on the support of fitter colleagues. A great deal of time is lost from industry, and thus much money spent unproductively, as a result of sickness absence (see Chapter 8). A doctor has a responsibility both to the patient and to the employer in this respect, and should not keep patients off work needlessly. Knowledge of the demands of the job will often help in planning appropriate rehabilitative measures.

Case history 1.10

An auxiliary nurse had a car crash, causing a whiplash type of neck injury. She had no neurological problems, but developed stiffness and pains in her neck and shoulders. She worked on a geriatric assessment ward, and most of her day was spent assisting patients out of bed and encouraging their mobility. All of this work involved moderately vigorous arm activity. Knowledge of the specific activities involved in her work allowed a rehabilitation programme to be planned to encourage recovery of upper limb mobility. Within 2 weeks of starting the programme she was able to return to supervised but initially restricted duties on the ward.

In order to make a realistic assessment of the demands of a job when considering return to work, a similar occupational history to that for assessing exposure is required. However, there are some differences. The most notable of these is that for many people the problems of returning to work after illness are as much related to travel to and from work as to the demands of the job. Remember to ask what time the patient has to get up in the morning and how he or she gets to and from work. An hour or two each day in the rush hour of a large city is considerably more stressful, both physically and psychologically, than many jobs. In addition, for many low-paid workers a tiring shift pattern and regular overtime are an inescapable part of the job, making return to full-time work more difficult. Finally, ask whether the patient enjoys the job. The attentions of macho managers and bullying colleagues can make the lives of some workers miserable, while, equally, financial pressures and production targets can be strong factors in decisions about when managers should return to work.

The patient is usually the best judge of when he or she is ready to return to work. However, the doctor who has some knowledge of the implications of the diagnosis and its prognosis must provide guidance, based on the patient's job. Some large companies have rehabilitation programmes, while some small companies can often provide appropriate gradual reintroduction to work if asked. These matters are discussed further in Chapter 9.

CONCLUSION

It can be seen that there is more to the occupational history than simply recording someone's job title. From an understanding of what someone does at work it is possible not only to help diagnose the cause of ill-health and plan rehabilitation, but also prevent ill-health in other workers. It is thus the foundation stone upon which the practice of occupational medicine is built.

2

Work-related diseases

SUMMARY

- Whatever your specialty, you are likely to come across illnesses related to occupation. The most common of these are stress reactions presenting to the general practitioner, psychiatrist or physician, and orthopaedic complaints – overuse syndromes in the arm, and back problems. Almost as frequent is dermatitis presenting to the general practitioner and the dermatologist. The general surgeon may see Raynaud's syndrome caused by vibrating tools; the ear, nose and throat surgeon may treat tinnitus and deafness as a result of noise; the gynaecologist and endocrinologist may encounter reproductive problems caused by chemicals; the chest physician can expect to see occupational asthma and mesothelioma; less commonly, the neurologist may see brain problems caused by solvents; and the renal physician may find kidney and bladder problems caused by chemicals. Even the general surgeon may see a patient with lead colic. The general practitioner will see any of these, together with an array of non-specific symptoms that may be related to the workplace.

- This chapter describes the broad range of occupational diseases, as far as possible according to the features they present to the general practitioner or hospital doctor. Their diagnosis usually depends on the doctor being alert to the possibility of an occupational cause and being able to take an appropriate occupational history.

INTRODUCTION

The earliest interest in occupational diseases arose from the investigations of Bernardino Ramazzini (1633–1714), who was professor of medicine in Padua, Italy. His book '*De morbis artificium diatriba*' (Thesis on the diseases of workers) described for the first time a very wide range of disorders, which he attributed to work, but his most important observation was that doctors should enquire about their patients' occupations. The Industrial Revolution in Europe brought with it a great expansion of manufacturing industry, and the ensuing prosperity was associated with considerable increases in population and life expectancy, but paradoxically an increase also in illness as a result of poverty, overcrowding, infectious disease and hazardous working conditions. The entrepreneurial ethos that led to this was balanced by the development of the concept of professionalism, originally the disinterested desire to alleviate the suffering of those less fortunate, and the late 19th century was characterized by the development of legislation aimed at protection of workers from exploitation as well as by the growth of the public health movement. It was during this period that the first descriptions of the clinical features and pathology of occupational diseases were recorded. Several of the earliest to be recognized were cancers – scrotal and skin cancer in Scottish oil shale refiners (although scrotal cancer in chimney sweeps' apprentices – climbing boys – was first described by Percivall Pott in his *Surgical Works* in 1766), lung cancer in Bohemian metal miners, and bladder cancer in aniline dye workers. Other almost equally serious conditions were also common in the industrial world at the turn of the 20th century – silicosis, lead and arsenic poisoning, and the effects of radiation, for example. This pattern has now changed, metal poisonings and the classical occupational cancers having almost been eliminated in the developed world, pneumoconiosis being under partial control, and diseases caused by pesticides, asbestos and other chemicals having taken their place. Most of the classical conditions are relatively uncommon save in countries now passing through their own industrial revolutions. The type of work people do in the developed world has led to recognition of a different spectrum of less dramatic but often very troublesome and chronic conditions – dermatitis, vibration injury and deafness, subtle changes in neuropsychological function related to chronic chemical exposures, locomotor problems, especially related to the spine, and overuse injury such as tenosynovitis. Finally, psychological disease of the anxiety–depression type is commonly related, at least in part, to problems in the workplace. Interestingly, this pattern of work-related ill-health is much closer to that which Ramazzini described than to what has traditionally been taught to medical students for the large part of the last 50 years.

Whether occupational diseases are becoming more or less common is impossible to say in the absence of good statistics. Mortality from some serious diseases, such as bladder cancer in dye and rubber workers, has clearly declined, as has metal poisoning. Worldwide, pesticide poisoning remains an important cause of death and less severe episodes are not uncommon in the West. Chronic intoxication by solvents remains a largely underrecognized condition. Death rates from mesothelioma as a result of asbestos exposure in the period from the 1940s to the 1980s continue to rise, while newly described diseases, such as hepatic angiosarcoma in vinyl chloride workers, appear in a cluster and then decline as preventive action is taken. In Britain, official statistics are published by the Health and Safety Executive on notifications of occupational disease from various sources and by the Registrars General on causes of death. In addition, statistics on successful claims for Industrial Injuries Benefit give some indication of the incidence of certain recognized (or 'prescribed') diseases. This latter source, although limited to people who have felt it necessary to make a claim and have then been assessed as disabled, is currently the most useful source for studying trends over time. However, some data of increasing value are now available as a result of informal reporting schemes operated on behalf of specialists. These sources are summarized in Table 2.1, and some further information is given in Appendix 1.

Table 2.1 *Sources of information on occupational diseases in the United Kingdom*

Survey	Information available
Department of Social Security's Industrial injuries scheme	Numbers successfully claiming disability benefits for prescribed diseases
Voluntary reporting schemes	Numbers with organ-specific conditions reported by specialists
Health and Safety Executive's household surveys	Numbers self-reporting specific conditions
Registrar General's decennial supplement on occupational health	Mortality from occupational diseases, together with data on illness, injuries, cancer registration and sickness absence

THE SIZE OF THE PROBLEM

The data are patchy and incomplete so only a very rough estimate of the size of the problem may be arrived at, and that only for certain conditions. The following figures apply to the United Kingdom, a country with a population of about 55 million, of whom some 20 million are in employment. Just under 50% of the workforce is female, these jobs on average tending to be more poorly paid and to include a higher proportion of part-timers, who because of this are working in somewhat less skilled areas.

In terms of disability, approximately 8500 people were newly assessed as disabled by occupational diseases in 1993. Such figures are biased by fashions in making claims, thus providing a truer picture at present of the prevalence of deafness than, say, of vibration injury or upper limb strain disorders. They are also affected by additions to the list of prescribed diseases: for example, in 1993 chronic bronchitis and emphysema in coal miners were added to the list, resulting in an additional 1500 certifications. Pneumoconiosis caused by inhalation of coal dust (approximately 300–400 cases per annum) and quartz dust (approximately 20–30 cases per annum) has been declining slowly, although it should be noted that there has been a comparable reduction in the numbers of people at risk in the relevant industries. Asbestos-related diseases have continued to rise. Mesothelioma deaths, of which at least 90 per cent are attributable to occupational exposure, had reached 1300 in 1996, in which year 479 people received disablement benefit for asbestosis. Asbestos continued to be used and workers exposed through the 1980s, so these rates are likely to rise to between 2000 and 3000 per annum by 2010, declining thereafter. About half of all people with asbestosis die each year of lung cancer, although (as epidemiological studies of workforces consistently show similar excesses of lung cancer and mesothelioma) the actual incidence of asbestos-related lung cancer is probably higher than this. Other recognized occupational cancers account for some 80–100 disablement awards per annum, although estimates of the likely number of cases in which occupation has contributed to cancer deaths suggest that (including asbestos cancer and mesothelioma) perhaps 3000–12 000 occur each year.

Of the less dramatic conditions, it is estimated that approximately 1500 new cases of occupational asthma are occurring each year. Surveys suggest that some 66 000 patients with occupational dermatitis present to general practitioners annually, and approximately 3000–4000 of these seem to be sufficiently severe to be seen by a dermatologist or occupational physician each year. The numbers receiving new benefits for industrial deafness have fallen steadily from around 1500 in 1985 to about 400 currently. Hand–arm vibration syndrome accounts for around 3000 and upper limb strain disorders for about 800 awards each year. Again, those receiving benefit may be the tip of a large iceberg, and a survey of 60 000 households in 1995 (the Labour Force Survey) showed that the cumulative effect of self-reported work-related locomotor illnesses was a prevalence of over 1.1 million people in that year. A comparable prevalence figure for work-related psychological illness in that survey was around 0.5 million. Some updated figures are shown in Appendix 1.

CAUSES AND TARGETS

Hazards and risks

The concepts of hazard and risk have been discussed in Chapter 1. Consider a workplace environment with which all doctors and clinical students are familiar, the hospital. Most people working within it will not have thought of it as a particularly hazardous environment, at least to themselves (Figs 2.1, 2.2). The complementary meanings of hazard and risk, terms which are often used synonymously, are important in occupational medicine; a hazardous substance may need to be used, but this can often be achieved in a way that substantially reduces the risk to the individuals concerned. How might hazards in the hospital environment be classified? What are the risks, and to whom do they apply?

Table 2.2 gives a general classification of hazards that can be applied to any workplace. Let us consider these in relation to the job of, say, a nurse. First, let us deal

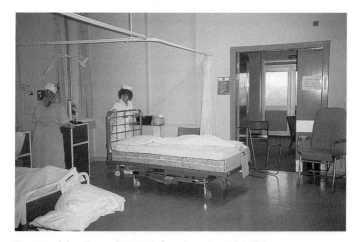

Fig. 2.1 *A familiar environment. See also colour plate 2.1.*

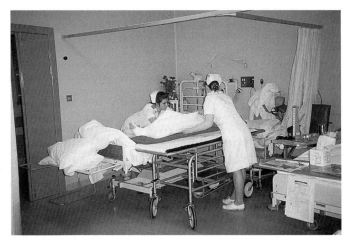

Fig. 2.2 *The risk of back injury in nurses can be measured. See also colour plate 2.2.*

Table 2.2 *Hazards in the workplace*

Hazard	Sources
Psychological	Other people, patterns of work, domestic problems
Physical	Materials, other people, noise, heat, radiation, vibration
Chemical	Fumes, gases, minerals, drugs, materials
Biological	Bacteria, viruses, allergens, other animals and plants

with psychological hazards. In this regard the demands of the job may be considerable: the anxiety of personal responsibility for the health of others, the stresses imposed by looking after seriously ill and dying people, the sense of loss when death occurs, and the difficulties of coping when the ward is understaffed. Such heavy psychological stresses may be compounded by difficult relationships with senior colleagues, who may appear not to appreciate the problems of the young nurse, and by poor pay. The environment may also be unsatisfactory, with poor recreational facilities, a bedroom close to a busy main road, poor catering, social pressures to smoke and drink to excess, and so on. It is clear that such hazards entail a high risk of psychological problems, and may be one reason for the high drop-out rate from the profession.

Next are the physical hazards. While many hospitals are noisy and overheated, these factors do not normally approach levels sufficient to cause deafness or heat stroke (although there are exceptions – the boiler room and laundry can be very noisy and heat stress may occur in certain operating theatres). There is, of course, a small risk if lasers are used or if the nurse is exposed to ionizing radiation, but such well-recognized hazards are normally controlled very carefully. The most important physical risk to the nurse is trauma, especially leading to back and shoulder injuries from lifting and assisting immobile patients. Assault by a confused or drunken patient is not uncommon, and accidental injury by a knife or needle still occurs regrettably frequently. Awkward postures, for example in assisting at operations, may also contribute to accident or injury.

Chemical hazards might be thought to be unimportant, but nevertheless some, such as potential dangers to reproduction from anaesthetic gases and cytotoxic drugs, are present. Nasobronchial and eye irritant reactions to glutaraldehyde used in sterilizing endoscopes may occur, as may bronchial sensitization to latex in rubber gloves. Skin allergies or irritant reactions to rubber gloves, to some drugs and to substances used for scrubbing up are all well recognized. Mineral hazards even exist; for example, nickel in surgical instruments may cause dermatitis. Asbestos in lagging in hospital ducts and boiler houses is only a threat to the engineering staff, who may be exposed frequently if the risk is not recognized.

Biological hazards are well known in hospitals. The classical examples, tuberculosis and streptococcal septicaemia, have now largely been prevented, but the emergence of multi-drug resistant *Mycobacterium tuberculosis* has caused us to cease to be complacent. Hepatitis B and C and HIV infection have now taken over as potential infective causes of death in hospital employees, although the risks are much smaller than was the pre-chemotherapy risk of tuberculosis. Preventive measures in hospitals should ensure that these risks are kept to a minimum. The other important infective hazard in modern hospitals is Legionnaire's disease, although this seems more inclined to afflict patients and visitors, perhaps because of pre-existing susceptibility, than nurses. Again, the risk may be reduced substantially by appropriate preventive action.

It is worth remembering that hazards and risks may not fall neatly into one or other category, and that physical illness is often accompanied by a psychological component, as the following case history illustrates.

Case history 2.1

A student nurse working on a chest ward developed a severe cough and purulent sputum. Several patients on the ward were currently suffering from infection with *Branhamella catarrhalis*, an organism not at the time generally recognized as a lung pathogen. Her general practitioner sent sputum to a laboratory, which reported the presence of *Neisseria catarrhalis*, an earlier name for the organism. Misinterpretation of the report led her doctor to question her about possible sexual contacts that could have led to pharyngeal gonorrhoea, resulting in considerable anxiety and distress. Fortunately, the registrar on the ward was currently researching infection by *Branhamella* spp. for his MD, discovered the nosocomial nature of the nurse's infection and retrieved the situation.

This analysis serves to illustrate the operation of hazard and risk in a familiar environment. In terms of risk, nurses may be expected to suffer periods of anxiety and depression, even despite the action taken to ameliorate working conditions. The more susceptible will suffer serious psychological illness. Many nurses will injure their back lifting a patient or catching one who is falling. Some will be assaulted by a drug addict or by a drunk in the Emergency Department. Risk of cuts and needlestick injury are high (Fig. 2.3), although fortunately most are minor; nevertheless, especially in poorer countries, the HIV epidemic and hepatitis B and C mean that in the future none will be able to be regarded as trivial even though the risk of infection from a single such injury remains low. Chemical risks may no longer be regarded as very low with the rise in latex and rubber allergies and the problems associated with careless use of glutaraldehyde. All these risks may be reduced by appropriate preventive action. Rather than accepting them as necessary accompaniments of the job, the occupational physician should take active steps to promote awareness of risk and to develop a strategy to reduce it. This is considered further in Chapter 6.

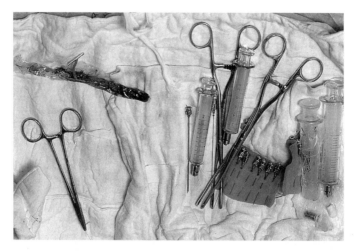

Fig. 2.3 *A day's collection of 'sharps' from the hospital laundry. See also colour plate 2.3.*

The targets of injury

The remainder of this chapter describes the main syndromes of occupational disease, considered as far as practicable from the point of view of the presenting features. These features are usually common to many different conditions, non-occupational as well as occupational, and the aim of the chapter is to alert the reader to the possibility of occupational causes. The diseases have been grouped generally according to organ systems, and reflect those systems that are most usually the target of occupational disease. Thus, the skin and the lung, both of which are in direct contact with the outside environment, feature prominently, as does the locomotor system, as the site of much traumatic injury and physical stress. The ear and eye may also quite commonly be affected at work by physical hazards. Less commonly, absorbed chemical substances may injure the brain and nervous system or the liver and urinary tract in the process of biotransformation and excretion.

Substances and physical hazards in the workplace may injure the body by any of the range of known mechanisms: inflammatory reactions as a result of trauma, infection; allergy and other cellular responses to foreign particles; interference with normal metabolism by chemicals; initiation or promotion of neoplastic change by carcinogens; other consequences of genotoxicity; and the subtle changes in neuroendocrine function associated with adverse psychological environments leading to stress reactions.

Skin disease

The main symptoms of occupational skin disease, as of other sorts, are soreness, itch, the appearance of a rash or lump, and occasionally pigmentary changes. Occupational causes can evoke a wide range of pathological responses, but the site of the lesion is of great importance in making the diagnosis, because in all cases it occurs, at least initially, at the site of contact with the offending agent. Equally important is a careful history of the evolution of the lesion and of chemicals and materials with which the patient comes into contact. Finally, it is essential to ask whether others in the workplace have similar problems – occupational skin disease often occurs in clusters. Simple itch may be a consequence of working in an excessively dry atmosphere, as is required in some industrial processes but which also occurs inadvertently in some offices with inadequate air conditioning systems. In such circumstances most of the workers develop the same symptom.

Contact dermatitis

Contact dermatitis is the most common occupational disease seen in practice, responsible for about 80% of all reported cases. It may be of irritant or allergic types (Fig. 2.4).

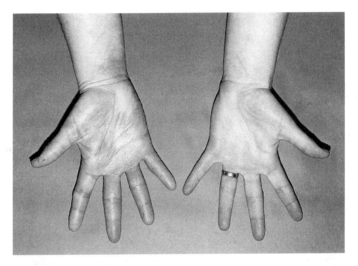

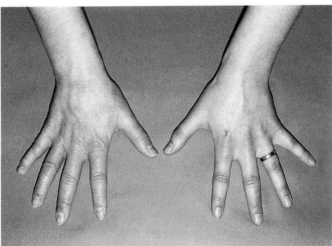

Fig. 2.4 *Dermatitis of the right hand in a nurse. The unilateral distribution resulted from her using a rubber surgical glove on her right hand for certain cleaning duties.*

Case history 2.2

Sore, itchy hands were reported by two technicians working in a medical school. In one, the backs and sides of the fingers were red and sore with some fissuring. In the other the fingers were red and swollen and itchy and the technician said that when the condition was bad her eyelids swelled up and itched also. Both had to wear rubber gloves frequently for their work with cell cultures and tissue slices. In the first case, the cause was frequent washing and scrubbing of the skin of the hands, an irritant dermatitis, while in the second case sensitization to the rubber gloves (or rather to one of the chemicals added to the latex in their manufacture) had occurred – an allergic dermatitis. The first was treated by modifying the washing procedure and the second by changing to non-allergenic vinyl gloves.

Both types of contact dermatitis may become chronic if the cause is not identified and eliminated. Allergic dermatitis is an example of a Type 4 immunological reaction involving sensitized T-lymphocytes. It commonly spreads to other parts of the skin and may even present as a widespread eczematous rash. It usually occurs after several weeks' exposure to the sensitizing agent, although faster responses to potent sensitizers do occur. Some of the important causes and occupations in which contact dermatitis occurs are shown in Table 2.3.

Table 2.3 *Common causes of contact dermatitis*

Cause	Some occupations at risk
Irritant	
Cement	Construction
Oils	Operating machinery
Solvents	Painting, cleaning, flooring
Detergents	Housework, hairdressing, cleaning
Fibre glass	Insulation, construction
Allergic	
Rubber gloves	Medicine, nursing, laboratory work
Epoxy resin hardeners	Joinery, painting, electrical manufacture
Colophony	Soldering, lacquering, electronics
Cobalt	Hard metal industry, pottery and glass
Nickel	Plating, use of metal tools
Formaldehyde, glutaraldehyde	Nursing, laboratory work
Dyes, perms	Hairdressing
Plants (e.g. primula)	Horticulture, florists
Wood (especially hardwoods)	Joinery, carpentry

Urticaria

Occasionally a Type 1, immunoglobulin E- (IgE) mediated urticarial reaction occurs in the skin as a consequence of workplace exposure. In the hospital service, the introduction of gloves made from cheaper, less well-washed, latex has caused not only an increase in contact dermatitis but also a number of cases of both asthma and urticaria. This may become a serious condition and anaphylactic reactions have occurred.

Skin infections and infestations

Itchy eruptions may be a reaction to the scabies mite or to flea bites. The first is a risk of healthcare workers, the second of people in contact with some animals, particularly cats. Mites from stored vegetable matter, especially grain, and from bird droppings may occasionally cause itchy lesions. All these reactions are caused by a sensitivity reaction to substances, usually intestinal or salivary proteins, excreted or injected by the arthropod.

Skin infections are less common, apart from fungal infections of the feet transmitted in communal shower facilities such as at coalmines. A few exotic infections may be seen.

Case history 2.3

A young surgical registrar presented at the Occupational Health Department with a non-tender lump on her finger (Fig. 2.5). She informed the doctor that she had orf, a pox virus lesion, which she had acquired the previous weekend during which she had helped her parents with the lambing. In particular she had hand-fed one lamb that had severe buccal ulceration. Care was taken to prevent her uncovered hand coming into contact with patients and she was prohibited from operating until the lesion had evolved through ulcerative and granulomatous stages to healing over the subsequent month.

Anthrax, which also presents with a boil-like lesion, though in this case associated with systemic illness, is now quite rare. Less rare is erysipeloid, an infection caused by *Erysipelothrix rhusiopathiae*, a Gram-positive bacillus. It causes a spreading, red, itchy patch around a skin scratch or laceration, and may produce systemic malaise, lymphadenopathy and even septicaemia and endocarditis. It afflicts people handling animals or their carcasses, most commonly fish, which gives it its common name of fish handlers' disease.

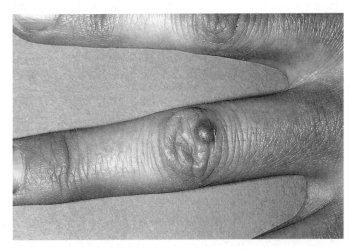

Fig. 2.5 *Early lesion of orf in a hospital registrar. See also colour plate 2.5.*

Pigmentary changes

Exposure to tar and similar substances, as in road work or roofing, and to certain plants, such as fennel and dill, can cause photosensitization and unexpected sunburn, as can inadvertent exposure to ultraviolet (UV) light.

Case history 2.4

A group of workers in a sausage factory came to the attention of the Health and Safety Executive's doctor because of complaints of sunburn on arms and faces at work. No chemical exposure was taking place but, in common with many food-processing factories, there were insect traps, which used UV light as an attractant. Examination of these lights showed that they had been fitted, by mistake, with bulbs emitting UV-C rather than UV-A. UV-C is used as a method of killing airborne bacteria and has high photon energy. It is absorbed by the superficial layers of the skin, where it causes burning.

Hyperpigmentation of the skin may be a consequence of prolonged exposure to tar products, dyes, heavy metals and chlorinated hydrocarbons. Loss of pigmentation, vitiligo, of a patchy sort is caused by exposure to certain chemicals used in adhesives and disinfectants, most notably hydroquinone and para-substituted phenols (Fig. 2.6).

Spots

Acne may occasionally be a consequence of workplace exposure. Oils and oil mists may cause such lesions, especially on the arms. A severe form, chloracne, with itchy cystic lesions that often progress to scarring and particularly affect the face, is caused by exposure to chlorinated biphenyls used in the electrical industry. Other chlorinated compounds may cause the same condition.

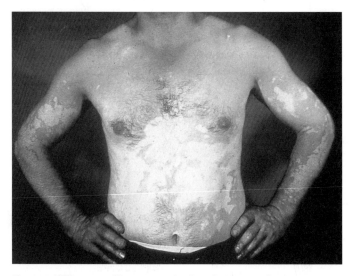

Fig. 2.6 *Vitiligo caused by exposure to phenolic compounds (photo courtesy of Dr C.J. Stevenson). See also colour plate 2.6.*

Scleroderma and related conditions

Occasionally sclerodermatous changes may be seen in patients as a result of occupational exposure. When confined to the hands and associated with Raynaud's syndrome and erosion of the terminal phalanges, a syndrome known as acro-osteolysis, it is caused by high levels of exposure to vinyl chloride in PVC production. It is unlikely to be seen nowadays, except possibly in developing countries, because control measures to prevent angiosarcoma should prevent workers being subjected to the high exposures required to cause the finger changes. Scleroderma, sometimes associated with systemic sclerosis, is also a risk of prolonged exposure to quartz and may accompany silicosis.

Lung disease

The usual presentation of patients with occupational lung disease is no different from that of patients with non-occupational disease, with one or more symptoms of breathlessness, persistent cough, chest pain, or the report of an abnormal chest radiograph. Occasionally they may present with anxiety that they are being harmed with something at work. Most of the well-known syndromes of lung disease have one or more occupational causes (Table 2.4). The key to the detection of these is the occupational history, as outlined in Chapter 1.

Table 2.4 *Some occupational causes of lung disease*

Syndrome	Main causes
Allergic asthma	Animals, including crustaceans, rats and mice; vegetables such as grains, flour, hardwoods; chemicals such as isocyanates, colophony, latex, acid anhydrides, vanadium and cobalt
Irritant asthma (RADS)	Any irritant gas or fume
Allergic alveolitis	Mouldy hay
Chronic airflow obstruction	Coal dust, cigarette smoke, cadmium
Bronchial carcinoma	Cigarette smoke, radiation, asbestos, *bis*-chloromethyl ether
Nodular fibrosis	Coal, quartz
Diffuse fibrosis	Asbestos
Sarcoidosis	Beryllium
Hilar lymph node enlargement	Quartz
Tuberculosis	*Mycobacterium tuberculosis* in healthcare workers
Pneumonitis, bronchiolitis	Irritant fumes and gases
Pneumonia	*Legionella* spp.
Pleural fibrosis	Asbestos, quartz
Mesothelioma	Asbestos

Occupational asthma

Occupational asthma is reported in about 500 people each year in Britain, but is estimated to occur up to three times as frequently as this. The diagnosis is easily missed unless the key questions are asked of all new asthmatic patients:

- does the wheeze change at weekends or on holiday?
- does anything at work affect your chest?

Case history 2.5

A 50-year-old man complained of episodic but increasing wheeze and shortness of breath over a period of about a year. The symptoms were typically asthmatic and he was instructed in appropriate treatment after he had denied knowledge of any provocative factors. His work as a labourer in a washing machine factory sounded innocuous. However, no sooner was he out of the clinic than his wife came in, insisting that his work was to blame. This uninvited intervention led to the discovery that isocyanates were being used in the factory to produce foam; serial peak flow recording showed falls on certain days when the process was running, and a challenge test proved him to be sensitized to toluene diisocyanate. His symptoms remitted when he was redeployed.

Onset of occupational asthma occurs after the patient has started the job, the interval being variable, sometimes after years but usually within 6 months. At first intermittent and mild, with continuing exposure it tends to become more persistent and severe. If the exposure is to protein allergens, there is often a preceding history of rhinitis. Sometimes there is worsening through the week, partial relief at weekends and more complete relief on holidays. After several months of symptoms, the asthma may become intractable. While it is still relatively mild, the usual diurnal pattern is of onset an hour or two into the shift, progressively worsening during the day and often with attacks in the night. If exposure to the sensitizing agent is intermittent, the asthma usually reflects this, although a single exposure may sometimes lead to recurrent attacks over several days.

If the condition has been diagnosed soon after onset and further exposure prevented, the asthma usually remits. If, however, it has become chronic, this remission may take months and may never be complete. Indeed, persistent chronic asthma is a not infrequent consequence. Once sensitized, the patient's future exposure should be controlled very carefully, as severe recurrence may occur. In general, workers sensitized to large molecular weight substances, such as flour and rat protein, may resume work with careful control of exposure, whereas those sensitized to small molecules, such as isocyanates or reactive dyes, need to be completely excluded from work entailing the possibility of exposure. Indeed, occasional deaths have been reported in relation to re-exposure to some chemical allergens after an interval away from work.

The main causes of occupational asthma are given in Table 2.5. They divide into classical protein antigens and low molecular weight chemicals. The former elicit an IgE-mediated allergic reaction, as do some of the chemicals by the formation of haptens. Other chemicals cause indistinguishable disease, but without the intervention of IgE, and the mechanisms of sensitization remain unknown. The pathophysiology of occupational asthma, with mediator-induced bronchial mucosal eosinophilic inflammation and oedema, and airway smooth muscle constriction, does not differ from that of classical asthma.

Table 2.5 *Some important causes of allergic occupational asthma*

Cause	Typical jobs
Animal	
Cats, dogs, horses	Veterinary work
Rodents, insects	Laboratory research
Prawns, crabs, salmon	Sea food processing
Grain mites	Farming
Vegetable	
Flour, grains	Farming, milling, baking
Henna	Hairdressing
Pine resin (colophony)	Soldering, especially electronics
Wood, especially hardwoods	Carpentry, joinery
Latex	Hospital, laboratory work
Gums, beans	Food production
Microbial	
Bacterium subtilis proteases	Detergent manufacture
Other enzymes (glucose oxidase, lipases)	Food production, enzyme production
Fungi	Biotechnology, farming, laboratory work
Pharmaceutical	
Antibiotics, ipecacuanha, piperazine	Pharmaceutical industry
Other chemicals	
Acid anhydrides	
Epoxy resin use	
Aluminium fumes	Smelting
Azodicarbonamide	Plastics, foam manufacture
Chromates	Plating, metallurgy
Cobalt	Hard metal work
Chloramines	Swimming pool attendants
Diisocyanates	Plastics production, painting, varnishing
Formaldehyde, glutaraldehyde	Hospital, laboratory work
Nickel salts	Plating, metallurgy
Organic dyes	Dyeing (fabrics, fibres)
Perchlorates	Hairdressing
Platinum salts	Refining, metallurgy
Vanadium	Industrial boiler cleaning

Certain people may be predisposed to occupational asthma. Atopy, an inherited tendency to produce excessive levels of IgE in response to exposure to organic allergen, makes an individual more liable to develop symptoms if exposed to protein allergens. Cigarette smoking also increases the likelihood of sensitization to allergen, perhaps through increasing the permeability of airway mucosa to inhaled allergen and thus allowing it greater access to submucosal T-lymphocytes. The extent to which these two factors should be taken into account in preventing occupational asthma will vary from individual to individual and from industry to industry. Clearly, the first principle is to reduce exposures as far as practicable, but in many circumstances the total prevention of exposure and sensitization is impracticable: for example, in bakery. Where the sensitizing agent is potent, it may be sensible to screen out smokers and people with clinical manifestations of atopy. However, it is rarely necessary or desirable to exclude people from work simply on the basis of positive skin tests (see Chapter 5).

Reactive airways dysfunction syndrome

It is now recognized that a syndrome indistinguishable from asthma may occur after acute exposure to relatively high concentrations of irritant chemicals, as illustrated by the following case history.

Case history 2.6

A 30-year-old non-smoking man, who had no previous history of chest illness, was instructed, while working for a local authority, to kill algae on steps leading from a sea wall with a strong chlorine-releasing disinfectant. He sprayed this over the steps for 10 minutes in windy conditions and was aware of a strong irritating fume that made him cough and his eyes stream. Within an hour he had started to wheeze, and was disturbed that night by cough and wheezy breathlessness. He saw his doctor, who diagnosed asthma and prescribed inhaled bronchodilators and steroids. Three months later the man still experienced recurrent wheezy attacks and required occasional courses of oral steroids. Over the next 2 years his asthma gradually improved but he continued to require regular inhaled steroids.

The usual history of asthma following acute exposures to irritant chemicals is of slow resolution, but permanent disease can result. A similar syndrome, not so well recognized, may occur in people exposed to irritants at lower concentrations over a more prolonged period.

Bronchial carcinoma

Lung cancer has become such a common disease, killing some 37 000 people each year in the UK, and is so clearly associated with smoking that we rarely consider other causes. It is worth remembering that the first cause, described in 1879, was associated with work in metal mines, subsequently shown to be the result of ionizing radiation.

Case history 2.7

In 1961 a man aged 34 years presented to his doctor with haemoptysis. He had never smoked. Nevertheless, he proved to have an oat cell carcinoma of the bronchus. Over the next 20 years, 11 other men, aged between 41 and 67 years, also died of rapidly progressive, undifferentiated carcinomas of the bronchus. Only seven of them had been smokers but all had worked for the same chemical company making ion-exchange resins, a notoriously dirty and smelly outfit. No doctors made the connection, but the trade union at the factory found out that one of the chemicals used was *bis*-chloromethyl ether, a substance chemically analogous to mustard gas. This had been found in 1967 to be one of the most potent causes of bronchial carcinoma in rats, and shortly thereafter in humans. Ultimately some 16 men from this small factory died of anaplastic lung cancer.

Table 2.6 *Occupational causes of lung cancer*

Cause	Some occupations
Arsenic trioxide, arsenites	Smelting, pesticide use
Asbestos	Insulation, construction, ship repair
Dichromates	Manufacture from ore
Bis-chloromethyl ether	Ion exchange resin manufacture
Mustard gas	Weapons manufacture
Nickel subsulphide	Nickel refining
Polycyclic aromatic hydrocarbons	Coke, tar work, aluminium smelting
Radon daughters	Metal mining

This sad story illustrates an important general point. If a patient presents with a rare cancer, or a common cancer in unusual circumstances (in this case, oat cell carcinoma in a young non-smoker), always suspect an environmental or occupational cause. Moreover, if someone with cancer has worked in the 'chemical' industry, make further enquiries. Known occupational causes of lung cancer are listed in Table 2.6. In addition to these, there is some evidence that patients with silicosis have an elevated risk of developing the disease.

There are no features that distinguish occupational lung cancer from the same disease associated with cigarette smoking (Case history 2.7). If an asbestos worker develops lung cancer, the disease is normally assumed to be related to his asbestos exposure if he also has asbestosis or bilateral pleural fibrosis. If not, the likelihood of it being caused by asbestos depends on the severity of exposure (cumulative exposure or duration × concentration); asbestos exposure and smoking interact to increase risk of the disease. Radiation, exposure to polycyclic aromatic hydrocarbons and other occupational causes probably add to the risks from smoking. Whereas smokers generally develop lung cancer relatively late in life, those who have been exposed to chemical carcinogens often develop the disease rather earlier. In the case of exposure to chloromethyl ethers, the peak incidence has been about 10 years after the start of the exposure.

Case history 2.8

A 70-year-old man presented with cough and haemoptysis, which he had been experiencing for the previous 2 weeks. Chest film showed a lesion in the left upper lobe, which was a squamous tumour on bronchoscopic biopsy. He was a lifelong non-smoker, but had worked all his career on the roads, operating a tar boiler. Had he been a smoker, it is likely that the significance of his prolonged exposure to polycyclic aromatic hydrocarbons might have been missed or discounted. As it was, he was able to claim Industrial Injuries Benefit and, by good fortune, radiation therapy induced a prolonged remission in which to enjoy it.

Acute attacks of breathlessness

An acute attack of breathlessness is most commonly the result of asthma or left ventricular failure. Occasionally, however, a patient presents with a similar clinical picture without signs of cardiac disease or severe airflow obstruction. The presence of repetitive crackles on inspiration and a tachycardia will often mislead the doctor into thinking, in spite of a normal cardiograph, that left ventricular disease is the cause, and sometimes the chest radiograph may support this diagnosis by showing the appearances of pulmonary oedema (but without Kerley B lines). Two occupational diseases may cause this syndrome – acute allergic alveolitis and inhalation of toxic gas.

Case history 2.9

A 30-year-old farmer was admitted to hospital during the autumn with severe breathlessness of 4 hours' duration. He was cyanosed, tachypnoeic and had a pulse rate of 120 beats per minute. Repetitive inspiratory crackles were audible through both lungs. The cardiograph was normal, chest film showed bilateral pulmonary oedema, and peak flow rate was normal at 500 L/min. Blood gases showed hypoxaemia and a low pCO_2. His doctor had given him intravenous diuretics without improvement. From his history it was found that he had spent the previous day ploughing a very dusty field and making silage. The silage had been stacked in a shallow pit in an open-sided barn rather than in a tower (Fig. 2.7). A clinical diagnosis of silo-fillers' lung (acute nitrogen dioxide poisoning) was made and he was treated with steroids, with slow improvement over 2 weeks. Over the course of this period, serology for *Mycoplasma pneumoniae* and farmer's lung organisms was negative, but a needle lung biopsy showed a granulomatous centriacinar inflammation diagnostic of acute allergic alveolitis. Investigation of his farm showed no nitrogen dioxide being given off by the silage, but large numbers of spores of *Micropolyspora faeni* in the soil of the ploughed field. Serology to this organism subsequently became positive.

This very unusual case illustrates the diagnostic difficulty that may arise with acute non-cardiac breathlessness. Acute allergic alveolitis and pulmonary oedema as a result of gas inhalation often present in the same way several hours after exposure to spores or gas, causing similar symptoms and clinical and radiological signs. They also mimic severe viral, mycoplasmal or similar pneumonias. Once again, the history of work undertaken several hours before onset should give the clue. Acute exposure to irritant gas, such as chlorine or sulphur dioxide, is of course always noticed by the patient. However, less

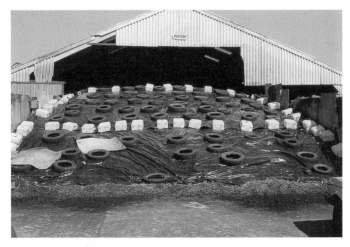

Fig. 2.7 *An open-air silage heap. Any gas given off will be rapidly dispersed. See also colour plate 2.7.*

irritant gas, such as nitrogen dioxide or high concentrations of hydrogen sulphide (which is a chemical asphyxiant), may not be appreciated as possible causes of subsequent breathlessness.

Farmers are usually aware of the dangers from mouldy hay, but other workers exposed to high concentrations of fungal spores may not appreciate the risk. Acute allergic alveolitis has been described most frequently in farmers feeding cattle with hay, but also in workers turning barley in whisky production, mushroom workers, and people exposed to fungal-containing dusts in sawmills. In addition, several episodes of allergic alveolitis have been described following exposure to isocyanates. Although many other causes of allergic alveolitis have been described, individual episodes seem to be relatively uncommon, only about 100 cases being reported in Britain each year. On the other hand, acute episodes of toxic gas inhalation occur relatively frequently, although, fortunately, few cause serious illness. Approximately 300 incidents are reported in Britain annually.

It should be noted that allergic alveolitis may present in a more insidious form and may progress to chronic pulmonary fibrosis (see next section). Breathlessness secondary to toxic gas inhalation usually resolves spontaneously. However, a number of different syndromes are recognized. Acute exposure to a toxic gas may cause airway irritation or even fatal laryngeal oedema, pulmonary oedema or acute bronchiolitis. The latter may resolve or progress to a chronic form causing permanent airflow obstruction, characterized pathologically by obliterative bronchiolitis. The occurrence of reactive airways dysfunction syndrome has been described above. To date, it is impossible to predict the outcome of an acute episode, nor is the value of initial treatment with steroids established.

Case history 2.10

A team of sewer workers, well used to unpleasant smells, was called out to investigate an odour of 'gas' coming from a city sewer in a residential area. Previous investigation by the gas company had found no escape of domestic gas. Note that North Sea gas is odourless but has traces of dimethyl disulphide added to it to give it the characteristic warning smell. In this case the smell was found to come from a sewer; this was entered, but no obvious source was found. Later investigation suggested that heavy rains had washed sulphide-containing chemicals, including dimethyl disulphide, out of an old landfill site. The workers complained of acute irritant symptoms affecting eyes and throats, and over the next week developed cough and shortness of breath, together with an array of autonomic nervous system symptoms and, in two cases, transient diabetes insipidus. Their lung function deteriorated in a manner consistent with obliterative bronchiolitis and several were left with sufficient impairment to force their retirement.

An interesting aspect of this unfortunate episode was that workers were allowed into the sewer without breathing apparatus, having first ensured that there was sufficient oxygen and that methane was absent. Subsequently the employers were advised on a change in working practices when investigating strange smells.

Case history 2.11

A 28-year-old previously fit and active 20 cigarettes a day smoker was supervising the addition of dimethyl disulphide into a oil pipe when the hose broke and he was sprayed with the chemical. He showered and changed within 15 minutes and went home. That night he had an acute attack of breathlessness requiring admission to hospital. He was treated with steroids and improved sufficiently to be discharged 2 days later. Over the next month he became increasingly breathless in spite of oral steroids and was referred to a specialist. He was found to have severe airflow obstruction, unresponsive to steroids or bronchodilators. He had an FEV$_1$ of 0.8l, 23% of predicted. He never recovered and remained permanently disabled by obliterative bronchiolitis.

Chronic breathlessness

Chronic, steadily worsening breathlessness is usually caused by irreversible or partly reversible airflow obstruction, cigarette smoking being the main cause. Less commonly, restrictive lung disease, usually the result of pulmonary fibrosis, is responsible. Occupational factors may be involved in either of these syndromes.

Non-asthmatic chronic airflow obstruction is usually caused pathologically by emphysema, although occasionally narrowing of small airways (as in the examples above) may be responsible. There is evidence that prolonged exposure to high levels of dust in workplaces, especially coalmines, may contribute to the development of emphysema and airflow obstruction, and it is plausible that many dusts and gases, inhaled in excessive amounts over years, could add to the harmful effects of cigarettes in this respect. However, in individual cases it is nearly always impossible to attribute such disease to factors other than smoking. Restrictive disease, with reduced vital capacity as well as FEV$_1$, however, is often more easily attributed to occupational causes, as smoking does not lead to this pattern of dysfunction.

Reduced lung volumes and transfer factor for carbon monoxide are the physiological manifestations of pulmonary fibrosis. Table 2.7 shows the main occupational causes of pulmonary fibrosis and of the acinar inflammation that leads to it.

Asbestosis is a progressive disease in which lower zone fibrosis gradually spreads up the lungs. It occurs in people with prolonged and heavy exposure to asbestos (ship repair, insulation, building work, asbestos textiles) and may sometimes present after exposure has ceased. Almost half of all victims eventually also develop lung cancer.

Table 2.7 *Occupational causes of pulmonary fibrosis*

Cause	Clinical features	Radiograph
Asbestos	Breathlessness, clubbing, basal crackles	Progressive lower zone and peripheral fibrosis, pleural plaques
Coal dust	Breathlessness, no physical signs	Nodular lesions with conglomeration into large masses
Quartz	Breathlessness, no physical signs	As above, with eggshell hilar calcification often
Beryllium	Breathlessness, crackles, responds to steroids	Diffuse, coarse, irregular fibrosis
Cobalt	Wheeze, breathlessness, sometimes crackles	Fine nodular change or sometimes none, reduced lung volumes
Mouldy hay dust	History of previous acute attacks with breathlessness, increasing breathlessness, crackles, some response to steroids	Upper lobe fibrosis

Silicosis is also progressive. It presents with asymptomatic nodules in the upper zones, which become more profuse and enlarge. Eventually they aggregate into large masses, causing a mixed restrictive and obstructive pattern of lung function. Miners, stonemasons and quarrymen, tunnellers and fettlers are at risk if exposed to quartz (crystalline silicon dioxide). Rapidly progressive acute and accelerated forms may occur in response to massive exposures.

Berylliosis is a granulomatous Type 4 immunological reaction to inhaled beryllium fume, mainly in refining and occasionally in electronics and the nuclear industry. It may mimic sarcoidosis, causing diffuse irregular fibrosis, but unlike other pneumoconioses responds partially to steroids.

Mixed patterns

One particular industrial disease may cause a confusing mixed pattern of lung responses (see Case history 2.12).

Case history 2.12

A 45-year-old man had recently been employed as a machine operator making drilling tools for oil exploration. He operated a grinding machine, sharpening the drill bits, using a cooling oil that was recirculated and that generated a fine mist. Extraction was inadequate. After several weeks at work he repeatedly experienced febrile episodes associated with shortness of breath and cough. His occupational physician diagnosed metal fume fever and advised him to take aspirin and if his symptoms were bad to take a day or two off work. Over a year he needed to take over 50 days off and nevertheless became progressively ill and more breathless. There were no signs in his chest, but his radiograph showed lung shrinkage and lung function showed a restrictive pattern.

This was clearly more than metal fume fever, particularly as the man was not exposed to fumes but to a mist. The clue is in the purpose for the metal parts being ground, rock drilling. These are made of hard metal, tungsten carbide, which contains cobalt as a binder. The cobalt dissolves in the coolant and causes a mixed allergic and irritant reaction that may present as asthma, allergic alveolitis, progressive fibrosis, or any combination of the three, a condition known as hard metal disease. This may progress to fatal fibrosis, so it is important to detect it early, at a reversible stage, and to prevent further exposure both of the patient and of other workers.

No symptoms, but abnormal chest film

Some occupational lung diseases cause abnormalities of the chest radiograph but no associated symptoms or functional abnormality. Pleural plaques, which often calcify, may be quite extensive as a result of asbestos exposure, and when they are found on a routine film may cause the patient much anxiety. They are harmless, the only potential future problems being related to the level of exposure to asbestos and not to the presence of plaques. Coalworkers' pneumoconiosis also may cause a heavy profusion of spots on the film without any functional impairment. Here the risk is of future development of massive fibrosis, a risk related to the profusion of small nodules. However, if a miner has no massive fibrosis, any symptoms should not be attributed to the pneumoconiosis.

Case history 2.13

A 60-year-old coalminer presented to his doctor with increasing shortness of breath over a period of 2 years. He had never smoked, but had extensive nodular shadowing on his chest film. The radiologist reported Category 3 simple pneumoconiosis. His doctor told him he was suffering from dust on his lungs and that nothing could be done. The specialist took a more detailed history, noted the initial episodic nature of the breathlessness and the important feature of nocturnal attacks, found him to have severe airflow obstruction and diagnosed asthma. His symptoms were relieved completely by bronchodilators and inhaled steroids. His pneumoconiosis remained unchanged.

Other pneumoconioses resulting from inhalation of tin refining fumes, iron oxide in welding and metal polishing, and barium sulphate in its production cause dramatic radiological abnormalities and no harm. Note, however, that tin and barium **mining** and polishing of metal castings (fettling) may cause silicosis, a progressive and disabling disease.

Chest pain

Work-related chest pain is a common, and commonly unrecognized, symptom resulting from inappropriate or unusual muscular activity. It is often associated with anxiety about possible myocardial infarction or angina, and recognition of its musculoskeletal origins is important in management. Two asbestos-related diseases may present with chest pain, usually associated with breathlessness. Mesothelioma is a malignant disease of the pleura (rarely the peritoneum) caused mainly by exposure to asbestos in shipyards, construction and insulation work several decades previously. Joiners and electricians are among many tradespeople who are likely to have been exposed in the past. It causes progressive obliteration of a hemithorax by tumour and effusion, spreads mainly locally within the thorax, and is usually fatal within a year or two of diagnosis. It occurs in about 1000 people annually in Britain. Rarely, acute pleural effusion occurs in asbestos workers. This resolves spontaneously, leaving pleural thickening by fibrosis. Such pleural thickening may also occur without prior effusion and may cause a mild restrictive pattern of lung function, usually without symptoms.

Pneumonia

Pneumonia must be an unusual occupational lung disease, but very occasional outbreaks have been traced to a source in the workplace. The use of biological agents may be one such, although contaminated water is more usually to blame.

Case history 2.14

Over the course of 10 years, three men, aged between 25 and 35 years, from one factory were admitted to the local hospital with fulminating bilateral bronchopneumonia. Bacteriological examination of sputum was negative, white cell counts were below 12 000 in each case, and all had high fever. Two had a prior history of diarrhoea and malaise over a 1-week period. All were treated with broad-spectrum antibiotics, oxygen and ventilatory support, but died of progressive respiratory failure. Post-mortem examination showed the pathology of adult respiratory distress syndrome in their lungs, but bacteriology was again unhelpful. In no case was the workplace suspected as a cause of the disease.

This coincidence was of course more striking to workers and management in the factory, who initiated investigations. The factory produced chemicals by a biotechnological process, using *Aspergillus niger*. The three men had all worked in the same part of the factory, and all had been doing the same job at the time of the annual shutdown for cleaning and repairs. All had been exposed to aerosols from water sprayed into contaminated areas. Extensive investigations failed to find a bacterial cause, and *Legionella* spp. were excluded. However, it was concluded that the workplace was the likely source of infection, and appropriate steps were taken to sterilize contaminated areas and protect workers from aerosols in future.

This case illustrates the often forgotten fact that pneumonia is acquired from the environment. With unusual types of pneumonia it is sensible to enquire about the workplace, and especially about the possibility of aerosols of recirculated or contaminated water. The best known case is Legionnaires' disease, spread by circulation of droplets from contaminated air-conditioning and cooling systems. Not only workers, but also visitors to hotels and hospitals and even people living in the local community have been infected by this organism spread from contaminated cooling towers. It originally acquired its name when the organism was discovered as a cause of an outbreak of pneumonia among members of the American Legion (military veterans) attending a conference in Philadelphia.

The hand, arm and back

Raynaud's syndrome

Case history 2.15

An offshore oil worker complained to his general practitioner of numbness and pain in the fingers of his right hand, especially in cold weather. He was a painter and was employed in renewing paintwork on the platform. Prior to painting he had to remove the old coating using an electric buffer and chisel. He had done this intermittently, with other jobs, until 6 months previously, but recently had been working on it full-time, 12-hour shifts for repeated 2-week stretches. Initially symptoms of numbness and tingling came on towards the end of the shift, but they had then started progressively earlier and pain had become prominent. At the time he was seen he was unable to work for more than about an hour. There were no neurological signs, but immersion of his hand in water at 10°C for 3 minutes reproduced his symptoms and caused blanching of the fingers. His employers were given advice on preventive measures.

This condition, known as hand–arm vibration syndrome (HAVS), previously termed vibration white finger, is primarily the result of vascular spasm induced by using tools vibrating mainly in the range 20–400 Hz (Fig. 2.8). It has both vascular and

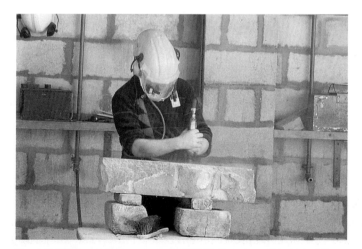

Fig. 2.8 *Buffing sandstone, a cause of HAVS. See also colour plate 2.8.*

neurological features and may be associated with sensory loss, muscle wasting and clumsiness with fine movements. In the early stages it is reversible, but neurological effects are unlikely to improve and may cause permanent disability even after use of the tools ceases. It is thus particularly important to arrange appropriate surveillance of workers who may be at risk. Any manual worker presenting with the features of Raynaud's disease should be questioned about the use of such tools. Occasionally, gangrene of finger tips or permanent loss of finger sensation may occur. Heavy percussive instruments may cause chronic damage to bones and joints in the hands, a different syndrome, which may be associated with radiological evidence of bone cysts.

Upper limb strain disorders

Pain on movement of the arm or hands is a very commonly seen syndrome in general practice and orthopaedic clinics. Whether the pain comes from the shoulder (frozen shoulder, rotator cuff syndrome), elbow (tennis elbow, golfer's elbow), forearm (tenosynovitis) or hand (trigger finger, de Quervain's syndrome), the patient's occupation may be an aetiological factor. In such cases, details of the work performed must always be sought. Frequently repetitive movements, often in awkward positions of the joints, are the usual cause. People most at risk are keyboard and visual display unit operators, assembly line workers, hairdressers, cleaners, musicians and music teachers. Carpal tunnel syndrome, typically presenting with paraesthesiae in the median nerve distribution, may also occur as a response to repeated pressure on the palmar aspect of the hand and wrist at work.

While such conditions are very common, according to the Labour Force Survey symptoms being attributed to their work by up to 60 000 people in the UK, an occupational cause is often missed. They may then become chronic and eventually the sufferer will be unable to continue the job. On the other hand, if they are diagnosed early, steps can usually be taken to redesign or modify the tasks and the condition may then remit (and be prevented in others). Most of these syndromes may be prevented by proper ergonomic design of jobs (see Chapter 5).

Case history 2.16

A process worker in a chemical plant was responsible for drying the product in an industrial centrifuge. He then had to remove it for further drying in an oven, and used a chisel to break the concretions in the centrifuge, hitting the end of the handle with the palm of his right hand. He developed tenosynovitis and triggering in the tendon sheaths of his right 3rd and 4th fingers. He was taken off the job temporarily, given clerical work and his trigger fingers settled spontaneously over a period of 2 months. An electric chisel was provided for his substitute.

Such syndromes may occur apparently spontaneously, but when a cause is apparent it is particularly important to ensure that the patient avoids the tasks that precipitated them if resolution is to take place. This will often take several months, and the job should be redesigned to avoid other workers developing the same problem.

The painful back

It is likely that most orthopaedic conditions related to wear and tear are contributed to by heavy physical work. The most problematical of these from an occupational point of view are those causing low back pain. It is important to recognize two syndromes, the management of which is discussed in Chapters 4 and 8.

The first is acute disc prolapse, which is usually provoked by a sudden strain on the lumbar spine and which is associated with sciatic pain, limitation of spinal flexion and straight leg raising and, often, neurological signs. This condition occurs frequently as a result of awkward lifting or sudden back strains in the workplace and is a major cause of loss of work. In large hospitals, as many as one nurse every week may be expected to present with an acute back injury caused by lifting or catching a patient. The incidence of the condition may be reduced by proper design of the workplace and of the tasks, provision of appropriate aids, and training in lifting techniques.

The other syndrome is the chronically painful back with limitation of movement, usually occurring in older male workers, and associated with degenerative changes in the spinal joints. Sometimes pain in the legs on walking and evidence of nerve root compression indicate stenosis of the spinal canal and compression of nerves as they pass out through the neural foramina. It is likely that this condition, which progressively disables people from physical work, is largely contributed to by repeated trauma to the back.

Apart from these two conditions, both of which have at least the potential to be alleviated surgically, there are many other syndromes of back pain that are seen frequently in occupational practice. Most commonly, patients present with lumbar ache, usually associated with uncomfortable postures or repeated bending and twisting. Similar complaints are often related to the neck and thoracic spine. Other patients complain of stiffness or lack of mobility, impairing their ability to perform their job. These syndromes have in common a lack of physical signs and a tendency to improve with rest. In all, redesign of the job will be more likely to alleviate the condition than the attention of an orthopaedic surgeon.

Back problems are important in occupational medicine for two reasons. First, care in the design of the job can play a large part in preventing them and, second, they are responsible for a considerable amount of sickness absence, causes being attributed to their work, according to recent figures, by about 700 000 people in the UK. The two groups of workers most at risk are those unused to physical exercise, with weak back musculature, and those working in very heavy physical jobs. It is important to recognize that regular physical exercise aids prevention.

The good occupational physician will become expert at examination of the back. The history of the occurrence is particularly important, and the author still recalls the case when he was a neurological registrar of a 25-year-old woman who presented with sciatica, progressively worsening over a period of 2 months. She had some L5/S1 sensory loss and an absent ankle jerk, but the history of progressive symptoms and no acute episode led the consultant to diagnose the rare malignant tumour, chordoma of the sacrum. Regrettably, he was right. An important step in diagnosis is to be aware that there are many causes of back pain, and the abdomen and pelvis should be considered as well as the back. In terms of examination, having excluded neurological features requiring further investigation, the occupational physician should make a functional assessment of the back in relation to the tasks expected of the employee.

Case history 2.17

A 55-year-old physician, with a long history of chronic back pain following sporting injuries and previous laminectomy for spinal stenosis, woke one morning with intense lumbar pain spreading into both buttocks. He was unable to stand and had to crawl to the toilet. However, he felt no numbness or weakness in his legs and he was relieved to be able to pass urine. Encouraged by a paper in the *British Medical Journal* that he had just read, which had shown 90% of such severe episodes would recover spontaneously within a couple of weeks, he took some anti-inflammatory pills and crossed his fingers. He was walking within 2 days and back at work within the week. Subsequent magnetic resonance imaging (MRI) investigation showed a large central disc prolapse, but surgery was not necessary and symptoms slowly settled over the subsequent 2 months.

In this case the main physical demand of the job was simply the effort required to travel to work, and once the patient was able to drive his car there was nothing about the job that he felt unable to do. In many jobs nowadays this is the case, and physical assessment needs only to take account of the individual's ability to get from home to work. Management of uncomplicated back pain should aim to return the sufferer to gainful employment as soon as possible. Assessment should indicate what aspects of the job can and cannot be done, in order to devise an appropriate rehabilitation programme.

The hip and other major joints

Osteoarthritis of the hip and knee, very common conditions in the elderly, may be contributed to by occupational factors. Workers such as farmers, who spend much of their lives in physical activity, have an increased risk of these diseases.

The ear

Hearing loss and tinnitus

The first symptom of noise-induced hearing loss is usually difficulty hearing a conversation against a noisy background. The patient comes to dislike parties where everyone is apparently chattering away happily, yet he or she hears just a jumble of noise. Consonants seem to be lost first. Often patients will mention intermittent high-pitched ringing in the ears, although this is rarely sufficient to be more than an irritant. By the time these symptoms have become sufficient to force medical consultation, the damage, as measured by audiometry, will be severe and, even with cessation of noise exposure, progressive. Workers at special risk of hearing damage are usually those in heavy productive industry, such as metal work, drilling and quarrying, stone cutting, or those using noisy machinery, as in textiles, printing, wood-cutting, transportation and agriculture. Noises above 90 dB, as measured with special instruments that are electronically weighted to mimic the loudness functions of the human ear, are likely to cause damage to a proportion of the exposed population with continued exposure. Very high levels may cause damage after relatively short periods, even when the noise is intermittent. This may be illustrated by the frequent finding of hearing loss in people who have fired guns as an occasional hobby, as well as in people who are exposed to noise of lower levels but more constantly, such as those working on construction sites. High noise levels damage the hair cells of the organ of Corti, affecting first those in the basal part of the cochlea concerned with reception of the highest frequency sounds and progressing through to those receiving lower frequencies. This is reflected in audiometric changes, which show loss of sound perception first in the 4–5 kHz range, progressing both in severity and into lower frequency ranges (Fig. 2.9). When hearing is reduced at 3 kHz and below, conversation is interfered with.

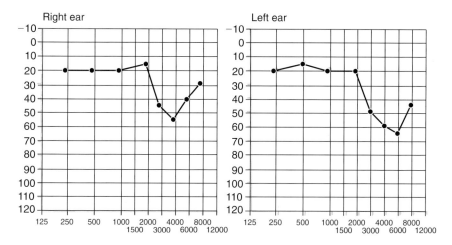

Fig. 2.9 *Bilateral noise-induced hearing loss in audiogram of a papermill worker.*

The harmful effects of noise are cumulative and not, of course, confined to the workplace. The use of personal stereos and frequenting of discos has resulted in young people having some early damage to hearing before they even start work. As well as attempting to protect workers from noise, many companies now carry out pre-employment audiometry.

The eye

Sore eyes

Complaints about sore or aching eyes are among the most common symptoms encountered by occupational physicians in organizations that use visual display units. They are rarely serious or even accompanied by evidence of a defect of refraction, but usually indicate poor design of the workplace in terms of lighting, screen reflectance or even posture at the desk. In contrast, eye injuries by foreign body or burns are potentially very serious and common, although easily preventable, problems in manufacturing industry.

Eye injury may also occur as a result of exposure to light – keratitis or conjunctivitis may be caused by inadequate eye protection in arc welding, while accidental exposure of the eye to laser beams (sometimes reflected inadvertently off a polished surface) may cause serious corneal or retinal burns. Protection from lasers depends critically on the wavelength of the light, and goggles must be specific to the lasers being used.

Itchy eyes

Itchy eyes are a frequent complaint in workers exposed to organic antigen, such as flour, rodent protein and grain dusts. This symptom is often a herald of occupational asthma, and the combination of itchy eyes and runny nose should always draw attention to this possibility. Non-allergic eye irritation by, for example, chlorine or formaldehyde, is also a common complaint.

The nose

Rhinitis

Allergic rhinitis is a common herald of occupational asthma, usually in association with exposure to organic antigen from vegetable matter or from animals, and it is not uncommon to see patients in whom the rhinitis is the sole manifestation of such allergy. The author has seen a number of patients in whom workplace exposure to animal allergen appeared to be the only cause of nasal polyposis.

Septal ulceration

Ulceration of the nasal septum, often painless, has been described following uncontrolled exposure to metal fume or dust; chromates (in metal plating and sometimes in cement) are the best known cause, although in earlier times arsenic and mercury were recognized causes.

Carcinoma

Carcinoma of the nasal sinuses has been described as a consequence of exposure to hardwood dust in woodwork and to an unknown carcinogen in leather goods manufacture, where the otherwise rare adenocarcinoma seems to be the usual histological type. Highly malignant undifferentiated nasal carcinomas have also occurred following exposure to nickel subsulphide and *bis*-chloromethyl ether.

Case history 2.18

A 50-year-old man presented to his doctor with left-sided nasal obstruction and facial pain. He failed to respond to treatment for sinusitis, and a radiograph showed probable maxillary carcinoma. Major surgery, followed by radiotherapy, eradicated the tumour and he was fitted with a facial prosthesis. The tumour proved to be an epidermoid carcinoma. He had worked all his life as a carpenter, using primarily hardwoods. His workplace had only used general ventilation and no local extraction was fitted to saws or sanders. He took civil action against his employer, who admitted liability but challenged the association between hardwood and epidermoid cancer of the sinuses. The judge found for the plaintiff, being persuaded that the epidemiological evidence made it more likely than not that heavy exposure to hardwood dust could cause nasal sinus carcinoma of any histological type. The settlement was substantial.

When a clear association between exposure to toxic substances at work and disease has been shown, the wise employer will take all reasonably practicable measures to prevent it. This should particularly be the case with known causes of cancer.

The nervous system

A wide range of neurological syndromes have been described in relation to occupational exposures; some are shown in Table 2.8.

Case history 2.19

A 58-year-old man presented to a neurologist with muscular weakness and unsteadiness, affecting mainly his legs and fine movements of his hands. The condition had developed insidiously over about 4 years but had been brought to medical attention when he was referred to an occupational physician

Table 2.8 *Some neurotoxic effects of occupational exposures*

Syndrome	Toxic agents	Occupations
Narcosis	Solvents	Degreasing, tank cleaning, painting
	Vinyl chloride	PVC manufacture
Organic psychosis	Carbon disulphide	Viscose rayon manufacture
	Mercury	Seed production, laboratories
Behavioural disorders	Solvents	Painting, floor tiling, degreasing
	Styrene	Boat building
Pyramidal tract disease	Solvents	As above
Parkinsonism	Carbon disulphide	Viscose rayon manufacture
	Carbon monoxide	Combustion exposure
	Manganese	Battery and alloy work
	Organophosphates	Agriculture, horticulture
Cerebellar disease	Solvents	As above
	Alcohol	Bar work, catering
Diffuse neurological disease	Gas embolism	Diving, caisson work
Autonomic hyperreactivity	Anticholinesterases	Agriculture, horticulture
Bladder neuropathy	Dimethyl aminoproprionitrile	Polyurethane production
Peripheral neuropathy	Lead	Smelting, painting
	Acrylamide	Polymerization
	n-hexane, methyl butyl ketone	Solvent use as above

on suspicion of drunkenness at work. The physician found that he was a teetotaller but that he had bilateral brisk reflexes and some hand–nose incoordination. The neurologist found signs of neurological disease affecting cerebellar and pyramidal tracts, with no sensory involvement. Routine tests, including computerized tomography scan, were unhelpful but electromyograms showed some evidence of denervation. No firm diagnosis was made, but arrangements were made to follow his case up and assess the progress of the condition.

The patient himself wondered whether his work was responsible and, after consulting his trade union, took a civil action against his employer. His work had involved 12 years of painting within the hulls of ships, often in very confined spaces. He had always used spray paints, solvent-based but of several different sorts. He had never used respiratory protection and had undertaken paint spraying for at least 4 hours every day, 5 days per week.

His illness forced him to retire from work. Over the course of the next 18 months he showed a slow improvement in his ability to perform physical tasks. Review by the neurologist confirmed that a previously progressive condition had ceased to deteriorate but that the pattern of symptoms and signs did not fit with any recognized neurological syndrome. Further investigation showed that, of the patient's eight colleagues in the dockyard paint shop, one had died with cerebellar degeneration and respiratory failure and two others had serious neurological disease.

Very many workers in Britain are exposed to organic solvents, chemicals that by their nature are themselves lipid-soluble and therefore capable of retention in nervous tissue. Painting, cleaning, carpet-tile laying, laboratory and chemical work, degreasing operations and exposure to petroleum are just a few of the situations in which high exposures may occur. Moreover, exposure in hobbies, such as model making or DIY, may add to that at work. Solvent exposure may also occur as a form of substance abuse – the best known types being alcoholism and glue-sniffing.

Physicians should be alert to the possibility of solvent exposure contributing to or causing neuropsychiatric disease. This ranges from a syndrome of headache, loss of concentration and short-term memory, and depression, to full-blown dementia or neurological disease, such as peripheral neuropathy, cerebellar ataxia, Parkinsonism or motor neurone disease. In particular, if the presentation is in any way clinically unusual or atypical of the well-known syndromes of neurological disease, the possibility of occupational causation should be borne in mind.

Peripheral neuropathy

A motor neuropathy, characteristically with wrist drop, is a classical feature of lead poisoning, now rarely seen. Mixed sensorimotor neuropathy may occur after exposure to acrylamide, *n*-hexane, methyl butyl ketone and some mercury compounds. Recently, concern has been expressed about possible neurotoxic effects of organophosphate insecticides, and the author has seen a number of patients with a syndrome consistent with this.

Case history 2.20

A previously healthy 45-year-old man was bothered by insects in the Spanish villa in which he was on holiday. He purchased three cans of a spray insecticide in the local pharmacy and spent several hours emptying them around the ground floor rooms that evening. The next day he noticed pains in his muscles associated with some weakness. Over a week the symptoms worsened, causing him considerable difficulty with walking and any movements of his limbs. On return home he was admitted to a neurological unit where he was found to have non-specific impairment of peripheral nerve conduction. His condition progressed for several months and then stabilized, leaving him with constant muscle pains, particularly in legs and back, that made it difficult for him to walk. He was never able to return to his job and was permanently incapacitated.

Parkinsonism and other neurological syndromes

Chronic manganese poisoning, prolonged exposure to carbon disulphide and acute carbon monoxide poisoning may all lead to the development of a Parkinsonian syndrome, as well as to other central nervous system damage. There is also evidence that the risk of Parkinsonism may be increased by exposure to organophosphates. There is much current interest in the possibility that some people are predisposed to react adversely to a range of chemicals, owing to an inability to detoxify them because of a genetic lack of certain enzymes, thus explaining why reports of neurotoxic effects in individuals appear to be sporadic in exposed populations.

Stress reactions

The majority of patients seen in occupational medical practice with neuropsychiatric symptoms are suffering from psychological rather than physical or chemical stressors. Such patients commonly present with a picture of anxiety and depression, and an array of minor physical symptoms. A history of adverse reaction to stress at previous times is often present, and the causes are usually multiple, involving home and family as well as work. Women with two jobs, one at home and one at work, are particularly vulnerable, especially when their jobs, as is often the case, are poorly paid and offer little prospect of satisfaction or promotion. People promoted beyond their capabilities or switched to new technology are also at risk. Physical ill-health is often the last straw in an otherwise marginally adjusted individual. In addition to this, stress-related problems are often precipitated or complicated by alcohol abuse. Some factors to look out for in the workplace are shown in Table 2.9.

Personal factors are, of course, important, some people thriving on what would grind others into the ground. Such individuals often obtain management posts and expect others to behave as they do, putting unreasonable pressure on them. Their inability to understand that different people are motivated in different ways often causes great problems in the workplace, reflected in decreased productivity. Poor training in management techniques lies behind this and poses considerable challenges to occupational physicians, who are often faced with the problem in terms of a pattern of excessive sickness absence.

Psychological problems, often of a relatively minor nature, are commonplace in occupational health practice, usually presenting through management referral for repeated or prolonged sickness absence. The spectrum of these conditions is wide, from frankly psychotic illness, through serious depression with suicide risk, to mild anxiety and simple dislike of work. Assessment of provocative workplace factors, potentially amenable to intervention, requires time and patience, especially when (as is often the case) the patient presents with somatic symptoms.

Case history 2.21

A 55-year-old consultant community physician was referred to occupational health because of prolonged sickness absence. He was severely depressed and somewhat hostile, suspecting (probably rightly) that the referral was motivated by a desire to terminate his employment on grounds of ill-health. Some personal and domestic factors were put forward as an explanation of his mood change, but changes at work connected with Health Service reorganization had been dramatic. These had involved a considerable increase in workload, the introduction of unrealistic targets and the expectation that he

Table 2.9 *Common adverse factors in the workplace leading to psychological breakdown*

Recent promotion beyond capabilities
Conflicts resulting from multiple responsibilities
Too many demands on time
Tiring shift pattern, excess overtime
Too little or boring work
New technology, inadequate training for changed role
A new or unreasonable boss, macho management
Increased, unrealistic productivity targets
Threat of redundancy
Sexual harassment or bullying
High sickness absence in colleagues
Lazy colleagues

would always take work home with him. Pressures of the same nature on his superiors were being passed down and there was little sympathy in the department for those who were unable to keep up.

After a series of discussions with the patient, his general practitioner and (respecting medical confidentiality) his superior, it proved possible to plan a course of rehabilitation to work that took account of the patient's illness and likely response to various stresses in the workplace, and of the effects of the patient's drug therapy. In due course, however, he took the opportunity of early retirement.

This case had a moderately successful outcome, as it was possible to modify the patient's workload and to persuade his seniors to be a little more tolerant of someone who clearly had a rather difficult personality. However, in the medium term, the prospect of leaving his job became irresistible and his pension rights happily allowed him to do this without major financial loss. Most people are not in such a fortunate situation. Such cases are often complicated by alcohol abuse and marital difficulties, and management is correspondingly less easy or successful. Nevertheless, clinical skills in eliciting the various provocative factors leading to breakdown are the key to successful intervention. Further discussion of the management of such problems is to be found in Chapters 4 and 7.

Disease of the liver and gastrointestinal tract

Several liver diseases have occupational causes, but all are rare. In contrast, the gastrointestinal tract is almost untouched by occupational disease, with the notable exception of lead poisoning (see below). However, oesophageal and stomach cancers occur to excess in rubber vulcanizers and coalminers, respectively.

The liver has a key role in transformation of lipid-soluble into water-soluble chemicals. While this usually results in a less toxic metabolite, occasionally the reverse occurs. The classic example is acute hepatic necrosis caused by carbon tetrachloride, a condition that used to occur in dry cleaning workers, where free radical formation causes peroxidation of cell membrane lipids. Polychlorinated biphenyls may cause a similar syndrome, and both chemicals may also lead to cirrhosis. Cholestasis has been described following exposure to methylene dianiline in the use of epoxy resins, and portal cirrhosis and haemangiosarcoma may occur as a result of exposure to high levels of vinyl chloride monomer in PVC production. However, even in a worker in the chemical industry, abnormalities of liver function are more likely to be related to alcohol or other causes than to occupational factors.

Urinary tract diseases

Acute renal failure may occur following high-level exposure to cadmium dust or fumes produced by cutting metal alloys, making pigments or battery manufacture. Mercury exposure in, for example, barometer repair or accidental spillage and vaporization of the metal, and carbon tetrachloride exposure may also cause this syndrome. These agents, carbon disulphide and a wide range of solvents may also cause damage to the nephron and chronic renal failure. Bladder cancer has been a well-authenticated risk in workers in the rubber tyre industry and in the manufacture of organic dyes. Benzidine and 2-naphthylamine are the chemicals that have been shown to have this effect, being converted in the liver into carcinogens, which then exert their effect on the bladder through excretion in the urine.

Disorders of the reproductive system

Infertility, miscarriage and fetal abnormality may sometimes be blamed on factors at work, and the gynaecologist should always take such a possibility seriously. There is some evidence that heavy physical work during pregnancy may have a harmful effect on the outcome, and there are plenty of opportunities during the process of gametogenesis, fertilization and pregnancy for toxic substances to exert an effect. The effects of ionizing radiation are well known, as are those of handling cytotoxic drugs. Less well known are the effects of chlorinated biphenyls on microsomal enzymes in the liver, increasing their ability to metabolize oral contraceptives and thus cause pill failure, or the adverse effects on male fertility of work in oestrogen production or of handling dibromo-chloropropane in nematocide manufacture or application. Lead, in males and females, and organic mercury, in females, are potent reproductive poisons, causing infertility, miscarriage and fetal abnormality. Solvents used in the manufacture of electrical and electronic apparatus, and ethylene oxide used in sterilization procedures have also been shown to increase risks of miscarriage. However, suggestions that anaesthetic gases, in levels normally found in operating theatres, and non-ionizing radiation from visual display units are harmful have not been supported by scientific investigation.

Blood disorders

While all are rare, toxic effects of workplace substances have been described in the past as causing a wide range of haematological disorders (Table 2.10).

Case history 2.22

A 25-year-old man spent 3 months training in college as a welder. He then obtained employment in a company making pipelines for the North Sea oil industry. After about a month working in the shop with no local exhaust ventilation he complained of stomach pains, loss of appetite, malaise and constipation. He was admitted to a surgical ward as an abdominal emergency, but his symptoms settled while he was being investigated. No cause was found and he made a slow recovery over a month. Within 2 days of return to work his symptoms had returned and he noticed increasing weakness of his arms and legs. He was again admitted for investigation, and himself raised the

Table 2.10 *Occupational blood disorders*

Disorder	Features	Causes
Marrow aplasia	Normocytic anaemia, neutropenia	Benzene, gamma radiation
Anaemia	Impaired haem synthesis, stippled red cells	Lead
Methaemoglobinaemia	Cyanosis reversed by methylene blue	Aniline and analogues, nitrites
Haemolysis	Intravascular haemolysis, haemoglobinuria	Arsine, trimellitic anhydride
Leukaemia	Usually chronic myeloid, occasionally acute	Benzene

possibility of fumes at work being the cause. He was referred to the author with the possible diagnosis of metal fume fever. The pipes he had been welding were coated with red lead paint, and he had a pot of this to apply to the hot weld.

In spite of careful regulation, such episodes of lead poisoning still occur in industry in the developed world. In less well regulated places they remain common, and the author has seen many such patients in a lead refinery in India where no controls were exerted over who worked in the place. Even young women were found exposed to very high levels of lead oxide dust (Fig. 2.10). The classical features of abdominal colic, motor nerve paralysis and anaemia are fortunately rare, but evidence of excessive exposure in terms of blood levels over 40 µg/100 mL are not infrequent. Above this level, inhibition of haem synthesis, related to inhibition of δaminolaevulinic acid dehydratase (δALA-D) and ferrochelatase may be expected and some interference with central or peripheral nervous function may occur. Reproductive hazards have already been mentioned.

Adverse effects of chronic benzene and radiation exposure have largely been prevented by regulation. Arsine poisoning does, however, occur sporadically. This gas (hydrogen arsenide) is used in the microelectronics industry, where it is usually handled with great care. It is also given off inadvertently when metal containing traces of arsenic is burnt or treated with acid, or when hot metal is cooled with water. Cases occur in the scrap metal industry.

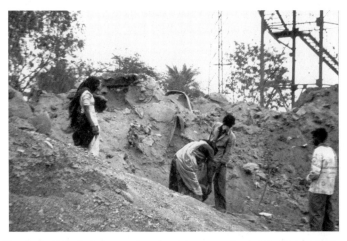

Fig. 2.10 *Unprotected young female workers recycling lead oxide in an Indian lead refinery; a dramatic example of what not to do. See also colour plate 2.10.*

Cardiac disease

There is strong evidence of association between risk of heart disease and specific occupation in the following three circumstances.

- Workers exposed to carbon disulphide in manufacture of viscose rayon have an increased likelihood of death from coronary artery disease.
- People exposed to nitrates, such as glyceryl trinitrate and ethylene glycol dinitrate, in the manufacture of explosives and of pharmaceuticals have an increased risk of angina and infarction.

- Those exposed to high levels of halogenated organic solvents such as trichloroethylene may suffer sudden death, probably related to ventricular fibrillation.

Carbon monoxide exposures of the levels to which some workers may be subjected in industry, for example working by blast furnaces in steel production, probably do not reach those generated by cigarette smoking, and have not convincingly been shown to increase risk of heart attack. However, the author has come across a case of unexplained death in a young man found lying by a defective furnace in a lead refinery in India, where the cause was almost certainly carbon monoxide poisoning.

General ill-health and infection

The most difficult patients to investigate and manage in medical practice are often those with non-specific symptoms of malaise and general ill-health. As with all other symptom complexes, the occupational history may lead to diagnosis and appropriate management. The most important occupational factors are psychological problems and physical problems associated with the building in which the person works, the two not infrequently interacting. Less commonly, chronic poisoning or occupational infection may occur.

Case history 2.23

A 38-year-old lady presented with complaints of tiredness, headaches and blurred vision, which she attributed to the use of a visual display unit (VDU) in a hospital switchboard. There were no physical abnormalities and testing of her vision was normal. Inspection of the workplace showed good ergonomic design of the workstation, appropriate positioning and anti-reflective screening of the VDU, and adequate temperature and humidity control of the room. Further investigation, however, showed a high sickness absence rate among the operators, many complaints of bad temperature control and general dissatisfaction with the job. An alcohol problem was found in one operator and a long-term health problem in another, leading to a requirement on the others to do excessive overtime. In addition, the staff was entirely female, all of whom combined their jobs with domestic responsibilities. The patient herself had worked 7 days a week for the past 3 weeks!

Almost everyone in that workplace had symptoms related to the pressures of the job. These were relieved when the long-term problems were dealt with, extra staff were taken on and overtime reduced. The temperature complaints were solved by asking the staff to decide on what temperature they preferred, and setting it at that.

This history illustrates one of the many ways in which workplace stress may present with somatic symptoms. Often the full story only comes out when the workplace is visited, giving the occupational physician an advantage over the general practitioner.

Vague physical symptoms occur not infrequently in workers in modern buildings, especially those built to conserve energy with recirculating air and in which individuals have little or no control over their environment. The symptoms include headaches, pain in the face, sore or dry throats, loss of voice, wheeziness, cough and general malaise. They are typically better at weekends and on holiday. Sometimes investigation of the building shows a contaminated air-conditioning system, spreading amoebal antigen and Gram-negative bacterial endotoxin around the building. Often, however, nothing is found other than recirculated air and windows that do not open. This condition has acquired the inapt name of 'sick building syndrome', but is better called 'building-related sickness'.

Case history 2.24

Several radiographers reported cough and wheeze when working in their department, which was situated in a basement and ventilated artificially. Investigation of the workforce showed widespread complaints of malaise, itchy skins, sore eyes, cough and, in two dramatic cases, loss of voice within an hour of entering the department. The air-conditioning system was uncontaminated and the temperature and humidity control adequate (excessive dryness is an important cause of itchy skins in workplaces). However, the ceiling tiles were perforated and covered with loose glass wool. These tiles were being disturbed frequently by building work. When the glass wool was removed and replaced by insulation in bags all the complaints ceased, suggesting strongly that they had been the result of an irritant reaction to the mineral fibres. But there was also little doubt that uninformed anxieties about possible long-term serious consequences and perceived management inaction had been responsible for exacerbating the symptoms.

Occupational infections may sometimes be severe, as when *Legionella* spp. contaminate an air conditioner and cause outbreaks of pneumonia, or when a farmer is infected by *Leptospira* spp. and dies of hepatorenal failure. Occasionally chronic debilitating infections cause diagnostic problems – the two best known are infection by *Brucella* spp., a now uncommon hazard of farmers and veterinary surgeons, and Lyme disease, caused by *Borrelia burgdorferi* infection acquired by tick bite in deer country and therefore a hazard of forestry workers. This latter condition often starts with a spreading erythematous lesion at the site of the bite (usually the lower leg), accompanied by influenza-like symptoms and enlarged lymph nodes. Subsequently the patient may develop meningitis and radiculopathies, polyarthritis and myopericarditis. These manifestations are very variable and may occur up to 2 years after initial infection. Transmission of the bacterium across the placenta may cause abortion or fetal abnormality. Early diagnosis, achieved by suspecting the disease in those exposed to deer country, and antibiotic treatment are very important.

Chronic poisoning in the workplace is relatively uncommon in the developed world, although episodes of lead and mercury poisoning still occur. More commonly, recurrent overdosage with pesticides and solvents may be seen, often leading to non-specific symptoms. Farmers and fruit growers may easily spray themselves with carbamate or organophosphorous insecticides and manifest symptoms of anticholinesterase poisoning – headache, blurred vision, weakness, sweating and tremor. Recurrent exposure to solvents is particularly liable to occur in the self-employed or in people employed in small companies involving painting and floor covering with flexible vinyl materials. Headaches and a feeling of drunkenness are the usual features, with the threat of long-term neurological damage as discussed above.

CONCLUSION

Doctors who in the past have remembered to ask their patients about their work and its relationship to their symptoms have made many important contributions to the understanding of disease. This chapter illustrates, from the personal experience of the authors, the variety of ways in which occupational disease may present and thus give the alert doctor the opportunity of helping both the patient and the workforce.

3

Investigation of occupational disease

SUMMARY

- In the investigation of occupational disease, there are three complementary methods: the clinical, workplace and epidemiological approaches. The clinical approach uses history, examination and special tests to reach a diagnosis of the disease and its cause. This is often sufficient for the patient's purposes, so long as the cause may be avoided in the future. However, it does not take account of the need to eliminate the cause in order to prevent similar disease in others.

- The workplace visit is best made by someone such as an occupational physician, who is familiar with the necessary methods, and it is this familiarity that defines the specialty of occupational medicine. Full investigation of a workplace requires knowledge of occupational hygiene, toxicology and ergonomics. The objective of the investigation is to find hazards and define and reduce the risks from them; this chapter describes the means of making such an investigation.

- The epidemiological approach may be used to investigate possible causes of disease and their effects, to measure risks from exposure to harmful environments or substances, and to test the effectiveness of preventive measures. In designing such a study many practical matters need to be considered, including time, costs, validity of tests and methods of selecting, sampling and ensuring maximal attendance of the subjects. Care has to be taken to design a study appropriate to the hypothesis to be tested, and the main types of such studies are described.

- Finally two notes of caution are sounded with respect to problems arising from screening for disease and jumping too readily to conclusions about environmental factors and disease causation.

INTRODUCTION

Doctors may encounter great difficulty in investigating occupational disease. Consider the following case history.

Case history 3.1

A 40-year-old man had developed progressive shortness of breath over 12 months. There were no physical signs of respiratory disease other than breathlessness at rest, and a chest film showed diffuse hazy shadowing in both lungs with some irregular fibrosis in the upper zones. Lung function showed a severe restrictive pattern, with gas transfer reduced to 30 per cent of the predicted value.

He had been a stonemason for 24 years, and for the previous four had been working on a mediaeval cathedral, renovating the window tracery with newly quarried sandstone, and using pneumatic chisels and saws. The physician made a diagnosis of silicosis and referred the patient to the doctors of the Department of Social Security's Respiratory Diseases Board for consideration for Industrial Injuries Benefit. These doctors disagreed with the diagnosis, saying that the radiological appearances were inconsistent with silicosis.

There was therefore a conflict of opinion. Does the patient have silicosis or some other disease? How may this be resolved? The immediate reaction of the doctor is the clinical approach – to carry out further diagnostic tests.

It was decided to carry out open lung biopsy. The surgeon commented on a nodular feel to the lungs and removed two pieces, one from a part that felt fibrosed and one from a more normal area. The pathologist reported diffuse interstitial fibrosis with desquamation of alveolar cells and no nodular change. Relatively little doubly refractile material was seen and it was concluded that the changes were not attributable to silicosis but to cryptogenic fibrosis. The patient did not improve with steroid treatment and died of respiratory failure a year later. The death certificate recorded cryptogenic pulmonary fibrosis.

At this stage the physician has accepted what seemed to be expert opinion, although he remained uncertain as the radiological appearances were quite unlike those of crypto-genic pulmonary fibrosis. Is there any other step that you would have taken at this stage? Unfortunately, a necropsy was not carried out when the patient died at home.

Two years later, a second mason from the same workplace presented to the consultant chest physician with similar symptoms and radiological changes. Again, Industrial Injuries Benefits were refused on the grounds of inconsistent radiological appearances. On this occasion, an urgent visit to the workplace was arranged (Fig. 3.1). The stonemasons were found to be working in primitive conditions, respirable quartz dust levels often reaching 100 times the 8-hour exposure limit. The diagnosis of accelerated silicosis was made and mineralogical analysis of the first patient's lung biopsies showed them to contain massive amounts of quartz, generally of a particle size too small to show up with polarized light. An epidemiological survey of all 350 masons employed by the same company was arranged and four other men were discovered to have less severe stages of silicosis.

This episode illustrates the three complementary methods used in the investigation of occupational disease – clinical, workplace and epidemiological. A clinician often finds difficulty with workplace and epidemiological investigation, and it is with these that this chapter is particularly concerned. An appropriate answer to the question posed above, 'Is there any other step that you would have taken at this stage?' would have been, 'Yes, I would arrange a visit to the workplace'. Doctors, whose training has largely been confined to purely clinical matters, rarely consider this. We are conditioned to look further and further inside a patient to discover the cause of disease; the main lesson of this book is that the seat of disease is inside the patient but the cause is usually outside, in the environment.

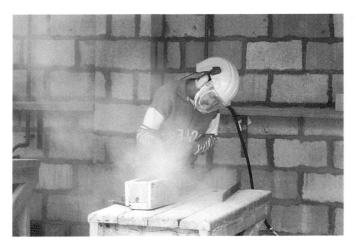

Fig. 3.1 *Stonemason generating cloud of quartz dust in cutting sandstone. See also colour plate 3.1.*

STRATEGY OF INVESTIGATION

The starting point of investigation is the realization by a doctor that the patient may have an occupational disease. This leads to a more detailed occupational history, as described in Chapter 1, and this in itself may be sufficient to confirm the diagnosis. More usually, however, other tests may be necessary; for example, serial measurements of peak flow rate in occupational asthma, audiograms in hearing loss or patch testing in dermatitis. This is the clinical investigation. If an occupational cause seems likely, the clinician is then faced with a twofold problem. First, the patient may not be able to return to work unless the workplace is modified and, second, if the patient does have an occupational disease, there may well be others in the same workplace exposed to the same risk; indeed, some may already have the same disease. Thus, some form of workplace investigation becomes mandatory, perhaps allied to an epidemiological study of the exposed workforce. In this respect, the doctor's role becomes wider than that of simply diagnosing and treating the patient; there is an obligation also to take on a preventive role.

The clinical investigation

The most important component of the clinical investigation is a careful occupational history, as detailed in Chapter 1. Thereafter, investigation depends on the type of disease and the organ or systems affected. The aims of investigation are first to establish the pathological and functional diagnosis and, second, to establish the cause. The former step will only be briefly alluded to here. The latter may require more than clinical skills, and may involve workplace and epidemiological investigation. This is not to say that clinical skills are unimportant in occupational practice; on the contrary, they are an essential foundation on which to build, and lack of such skills can be very much to the patient's disadvantage.

Case history 3.2

A general practitioner was employed on a sessional basis at a local chemical factory. As part of his duties, he was asked to make an annual health examination of workers exposed to formaldehyde. One such worker with symptoms of asthma consulted him in his role as general practitioner. The doctor prescribed treatment and, because he had seen him in the surgery, excused him from attending his workplace check-up. In doing so he forgot his workplace role of ensuring protection of the employees and failed to make a connection between the patient's work and his job. The asthma became progressively worse and the patient eventually asked for a second opinion. The consultant confirmed the diagnosis of formaldehyde asthma, but by this time the patient's illness had become severe and persistent, causing him to be obliged to retire on the grounds of ill-health. The doctor was sued for negligence.

This case illustrates the dangers of practising in a field of medicine in which you have no training, and also shows what may happen if basic clinical history-taking skills are neglected. Another point, to which we shall return later in this chapter and again in Chapter 5, concerns the rationale for screening or 'routine' surveillance. The objectives of such a procedure must be clear, as must the action to be taken on finding a positive result.

Skin diseases

Of the conditions mentioned in Chapter 2, contact dermatitis is by far the most common. The diagnosis of all these conditions depends mainly on a careful history and clinical examination, and often also on obtaining samples of the material to which the patient has been exposed.

The site of the lesion is of primary importance, although it should be remembered that allergic contact dermatitis may spread to other parts of the body, especially the eyelids. The condition may also be mimicked by non-occupational dermatitis, for example to nickel, spreading to the hands. The time course of the condition and its development in relation to exposure to possible allergens or irritants are also essential details to obtain.

Case history 3.3

A 53-year-old man was referred to a consultant dermatologist with recent onset of an itchy rash on hands and face. He had worked processing film in a photographer's shop for 3 years and was aware that developer solution would splash on his skin and that he would sometimes rub his hand over his face when tired. The dermatologist diagnosed contact dermatitis but also noticed patches of vitiligo over his right hand. Patch testing showed allergy to p-phenylenediamine, a constituent of the colour developers he was using and a likely explanation of his dermatitis. In addition he reacted to hydroquinone, which is present in black and white developers, indicating past exposure to this substance, which causes vitiligo owing to its chemical similarity to the melanin precursor tyrosine.

This patient was unusual in having two separate skin diseases, one allergic and one toxic, resulting from exposure to chemicals in his work. The most usual problem in occupational skin disease is differentiation of allergic and irritant contact dermatitis (Table 3.1). For this, the use of patch testing is often essential.

Table 3.1 *Clues to differentiating allergic and irritant dermatitis**

	Irritant	Allergic
Common causes	Detergents, cleaning materials, oils, dusts	Low molecular weight chemicals (nickel, cobalt, colophony, epoxy resin precursors, formaldehyde)
Onset	May be acute or subacute	Days, or weeks after first exposure
Distribution	Backs of hands then palms, sometimes under rings where cleaning agents, for example, may be trapped	Site of contact, plus eyelids frequently
Progression	Tendency to local worsening	Spreads to other areas of skin
Patch tests	Negative	Positive

*It is often impossible to differentiate the two conditions clinically.

Patch testing

Patch tests are used to diagnose allergic contact dermatitis. The suspected antigens, or more commonly a battery of antigens including those suspected, are placed on absorbent material in small aluminium strips or chambers and applied by permeable tape to an area of unaffected skin, usually the back (Fig. 3.2). They are left in place for 48 hours, removed and the area is inspected for evidence of a reaction about 30 minutes later, and then at intervals over the next week. Care is necessary to avoid using irritant concentrations of chemicals, which may give a spuriously positive result. A true allergic reaction usually shows erythema and induration, but vesiculation and blistering may occur in severe reactions. The reaction, being one of delayed hypersensitivity, may occur up to 5 days after application of the antigen. It typically increases in size and severity over a few days, and this is one feature that helps to distinguish it from an irritant dermatitis (Table 3.2).

The choice of antigen for patch testing depends on the suspected cause. Details of one battery commonly used and available commercially are given in Table 3.3. However, the choice should be guided primarily by the history of likely exposures, and in some cases, where the patient appears to have reacted to some material not known to be a sensitizing agent, dilutions of that substance may be used as a first stage to identification of the chemical concerned. In general, patch testing is best undertaken in a special clinic by staff with appropriate experience.

Table 3.2 *Differentiating irritant and allergic dermatitis on patch testing*

Irritant	Allergic
High concentrations required to cause reaction	Reaction with low concentrations
Affects most people exposed	Affects relatively few people
Reaction comes and goes quickly	Develops late and gets worse

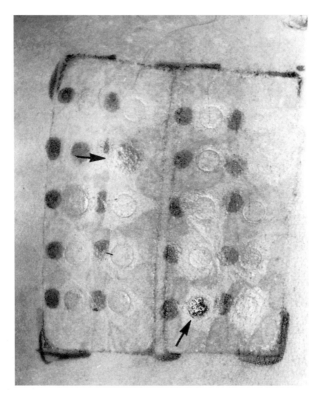

Fig. 3.2 *Patch testing on a nurse with allergy to surgical gloves. Positive results to thiuram mix (upper arrow) and nickel sulphate (lower arrow).*

Table 3.3 *Useful occupational contact dermatitis patch tests*

Sensitizer	Some workplace sources
Potassium dichromate	Cement, paints, tannery
Cobalt chloride	Cement, coolant oils
Nickel sulphate	Plating, metal tools
Colophony	Glues, solder flux, adhesive tape
Wool alcohols	Handling woollens
Formaldehyde	Disinfectants
Thiurams	Rubber, adhesives, pesticides
Mercaptones	Rubber
Mercaptobenzthiazoles	Rubber
Paraphenylene diamine	Dyes, hairdressing, printing
Epoxy resins	Adhesives, paints
Primin	Primulas

Other diagnostic aids

Occasionally skin biopsy and appropriate staining may be necessary to make a diagnosis in obscure cases of occupational skin disease. In patients exposed to hydroquinone and *p*-tertiary butylphenol at risk of vitiligo, a Wood's lamp may be helpful for medical surveillance and detection of early cases.

Lung diseases

As with skin disease, the diagnosis of occupational lung disease depends critically on a history that takes account of the development and evolution of symptoms in relation to exposure to suspected causes. In contrast, physical examination is much less useful and the diagnosis is usually clinched by relatively simple investigations. Some conditions may not be diagnosed with the usually accepted degree of clinical confidence; for example, it is rarely possible to be sure that emphysema or lung cancer are occupational in aetiology. The most useful tests are described briefly below.

Chest radiography

The main use of radiography is in the diagnosis of the pneumoconioses, and an outline of typical appearances is given in Fig. 3.3. Amorphous particles, such as quartz and coal, cause small, discrete, nodular lesions that may aggregate together to form large masses [known as progressive massive fibrosis (PMF)]. Asbestosis causes diffuse fine irregular shadows, predominantly peripherally and in the lower zones. Berylliosis causes coarser irregular shadows through the lungs, while chronic allergic alveolitis may cause irregular streaky shadows in the upper zones. Appearances mimicking cardiac pulmonary oedema may occur in acute allergic alveolitis and toxic pneumonitis.

Lung function testing

Lung function tests measure the pathophysiological effects of the disease, and are therefore usually only complementary to other procedures in reaching a diagnosis. The main changes found in occupational lung diseases are given in Table 3.4 – note the important negative findings in simple pneumoconiosis. The most useful tests in a diagnostic sense are those used in monitoring changes in relation either to exposure in the workplace or to challenge testing.

In suspected occupational asthma, it is usual to carry out serial recordings of peak flow rate, the readings being made by the patient several times daily over a month (Fig. 3.4).

At least 2 weeks of recordings should be made when the patient is off work, and the record inspected for differences in level when exposed and not exposed. If clear reduction in flow rates occurs while at work, occupational asthma is likely and a sensitizing agent is usually easily identified. If one is not obvious from the history, inspection of the workplace (see later) and subsequent challenge testing may be necessary. Challenge testing may also be helpful when serial peak flow recordings are equivocal. It is a specialized procedure that needs to be carried out in hospital under medical supervision.

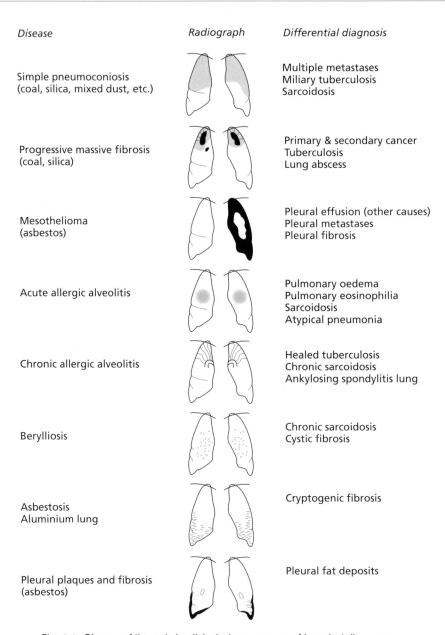

Disease	Radiograph	Differential diagnosis
Simple pneumoconiosis (coal, silica, mixed dust, etc.)		Multiple metastases Miliary tuberculosis Sarcoidosis
Progressive massive fibrosis (coal, silica)		Primary & secondary cancer Tuberculosis Lung abscess
Mesothelioma (asbestos)		Pleural effusion (other causes) Pleural metastases Pleural fibrosis
Acute allergic alveolitis		Pulmonary oedema Pulmonary eosinophilia Sarcoidosis Atypical pneumonia
Chronic allergic alveolitis		Healed tuberculosis Chronic sarcoidosis Ankylosing spondylitis lung
Berylliosis		Chronic sarcoidosis Cystic fibrosis
Asbestosis Aluminium lung		Cryptogenic fibrosis
Pleural plaques and fibrosis (asbestos)		Pleural fat deposits

Fig. 3.3 *Diagram of the varied radiological appearances of lung dust diseases*

Case history 3.4

A 30-year-old man was referred to a chest physician with a suspected diagnosis of work-related asthma. He gave a history of occasional wheezy episodes over the previous 2 months and was working in a company where powdered enzymes were handled in the production of washing powders. The history suggested that the process was enclosed appropriately and that any exposure to airborne chemical was likely to be very limited. Serial peak flows showed variability consistent with asthma and

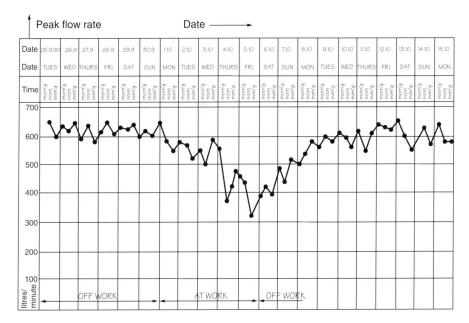

Fig. 3.4 *Peak flow rate recorded in a man working unloading grain at an animal foodstuff manufacturer. Note fall in flow rate during period at work.*

Table 3.4 *Functional changes in occupational lung disease*

Disease	Changes
Simple pneumoconiosis	Usually none
PMF	Mixed restriction and obstruction
Asbestosis	Restriction and low diffusing capacity
Allergic alveolitis	Low diffusing capacity
Toxic pneumonitis	Low diffusing capacity
Berylliosis	Restriction, low diffusing capacity
Asthma, reactive airways dysfunction syndrome (RADS)	Variable airflow obstruction

PMF, progressive massive fibrosis.

a suggestion of worsening while at work. In view of the importance of a firm diagnosis from the point of view of his future employment, challenge testing with the enzyme was carried out, using increasing exposure times over 3 days. No reaction occurred, his asthma was treated along routine lines and he continued at work under medical supervision.

The implications of occupational asthma in terms of future employment are considerable, and a negative challenge test may be of great benefit to the patient, as well as reassuring to the employer that the control measures are working. Challenge testing should only be undertaken in a hospital setting because delayed and severe reactions may occur. This said, it is a relatively simple procedure whereby dilutions of the

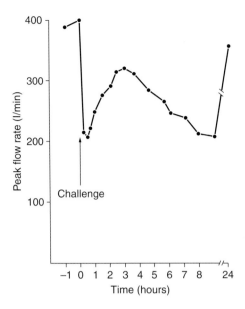

Fig. 3.5 *Immediate and delayed responses to challenge testing with isocyanates.*

suspected causative agent are either nebulized or put into the air by tipping from dish to dish or other straightforward manner so that the patient can inhale it and the functional effect can be measured. The closer the challenge mimics the actual workplace exposure, the better (Fig. 3.5).

In allergic asthma, both an immediate and a delayed fall in peak flow may occur, the latter lasting up to 48 hours. In allergic alveolitis, the response is a rise in temperature, a feeling of malaise and a fall in gas transfer at about 3 hours, lasting up to 48 hours.

Other tests

In asthma, positive results to skin prick testing would be expected to protein antigens and to some chemicals such as complex salts of platinum, although not to colophony or isocyanates. This test is performed by lifting the epidermis (without drawing blood) with a fine needle through a drop of antigen. Similarly, positive radioallergosorbent (RAST) tests may be helpful in diagnosis if an antigen is available, and are useful in monitoring successful prevention of exposure as concentrations decline with time. In allergic alveolitis intradermal skin tests have been used but are not advisable because of possible systemic reactions. However, precipitating antibodies to the common antigens may be found in the blood. These are useful in the presence of disease, but do not of themselves indicate that lung disease is present.

Lung biopsy and study of bronchoalveolar lavage fluid are occasionally helpful in the investigation of obscure cases, usually to differentiate between occupational and non-occupational disease.

Occupational poisonings

A wide variety of syndromes, discussed in Chapter 2, may be caused by occupational exposure to toxic substances. Again, the diagnosis rests largely on the occupational history and awareness that exposure to gases, fumes and chemicals may lead to disease. In the early 20th century such episodes were frequent in the UK and were easily recognized by physicians, but nowadays episodes occur sporadically, usually in small, poorly regulated workplaces and the diagnosis is often missed. They do, however, remain common in poor countries.

Case history 3.5

A 54-year-old man was employed by an industrial cleaning company. The company obtained a contract to assist the annual maintenance in a factory producing seeds. He was required to clean a hopper that had become encrusted with a rind of biological material, and spent 2 days working in this space with powered tools, coming out covered with dust. By midday on the second day he felt unwell, with a cough and tremulous hands. He became agitated and seemed confused, and the factory nurse sent him to see his general practitioner. No diagnosis was made, but an anxiolytic was prescribed. He continued with tremor, but his agitation improved over the next 2 weeks. Because he had previously been quite fit, his doctor referred him to a physician, who took a detailed history, found albuminuria and suspected acute heavy metal poisoning. Investigation through the Health and Safety Executive showed that the hopper was used for dressing the seeds with a mercurial powder. Fortunately the patient recovered without serious sequelae.

In general, toxic gases and fumes attack the lung, metals damage internal organs, solvents may cause damage to the skin, liver and nervous system, and a number of insecticides cause symptoms of parasympathetic overactivity. There are some investigations that are of value in establishing a diagnosis and monitoring exposure or response to treatment in some of these poisonings; the more important ones are summarized in Table 3.5.

In general, inorganic chemicals may be measured in either blood or urine and some (such as mercury and arsenic which accumulate in the tissues) in hair and nail parings. The metabolites of organic substances, which are rapidly biotransformed into water-soluble chemicals, may be measured in urine, while poorly biotransformed organics are measured in blood. Volatile organics (of which the best known example is ethyl alcohol) may be measured in alveolar air. In cases of suspected chronic poisoning by metals such as lead, mercury or cadmium, *in-vivo* methods using neutron activation or X-ray fluorescence are being developed. There is further discussion of biological monitoring in Chapter 7.

Investigation of the workplace

Investigation of the workplace is the aspect of occupational medicine with which doctors are least familiar; almost no doctor thinks to visit a patient's workplace and those few who do rarely know how to proceed once there.

Why should one wish to visit the workplace? Three reasons, related to the investigation of illness are:

Table 3.5 *Some occupational poisons*

Poison	Clinical features	Investigations
Metals		
Inorganic lead	Lethargy, fatigue, abdominal pain, constipation, vomiting, anaemia, neuropathy	Blood lead, urinary δ-amino laevulinic acid, red cell protoporphyrin
Organic lead	Sleep disturbance, nausea, anorexia	Urine lead
Mercury	*Acute*: fever, tremor, pneumonitis, renal tubular necrosis	Blood and urine mercury – may be misleading because of irregular excretion
	Chronic: gingivitis, tremor, cerebellar signs, psychosis	
Cadmium	*Acute*: fever, pneumonitis, renal cortical necrosis	Urine cadmium
	Chronic: renal tubular dysfunction, emphysema	Urine β2-microglobulin, *n*-acetyl glucosaminidase
Beryllium	*Acute*: pneumonitis, dermatitis	Urine beryllium
	Chronic: pulmonary fibrosis	Beryllium lymphocyte transformation
Pesticides		
Organophosphates	Headache, nausea, abdominal pain, twitching, small pupils, convulsions	Low blood cholinesterase
Carbamates	As organophosphates	Low blood cholinesterase
Organochlorines	Headache, abdominal pain, ataxia, tremor	Specific agent in blood
Pyrethroids	Allergies, rarely paraesthesiae	Urine pyrethroids
Herbicides		
Dinitro-orthocresol	Hyperpyrexia	Blood dinitro-orthocresol
Paraquat	Pulmonary fibrosis	Plasma paraquat
Organic solvents		
Benzene	Marrow suppression, acute leukaemia	Blood count, blood benzene, urine phenol, muconic acid
Toluene	Narcosis, neurological syndromes	Blood toluene, urine hippuric acid or ortho cresol
Carbon tetrachloride	Nausea, narcosis, arrhythmias, liver and kidney failure	Breath CCl_4
Trichloroethylene	Narcosis, alcohol flush, arrhythmias	Breath trichloroethyene, urine trichloroacetic acid
Carbon disulphide	Peripheral neuropathy, psychoses, cardiotoxicity	Urine 2-thiothiazolidine
Methyl butyl ketone (2-hexanone), *n*-hexane	Peripheral neuropathy	Urine 2,5-hexanedione

- to seek a cause of the patient's illness
- to see whether the cause can be eliminated
- to see whether others are affected.

In addition, regular workplace visits to assess hazards and to plan to reduce risks are part of the bread-and-butter work of an occupational physician acting in his or her preventive role.

There are, however, serious problems that make it difficult for the doctor to make a workplace visit:

- ethical issues
- unfamiliarity with the approach to management
- industrial relations problems
- lack of time
- ignorance of how to carry out the investigation.

Usually a combination of these factors results in no visit being made, and an opportunity to prevent disease in others is lost.

When should the workplace be visited?

Occupational physicians should see regular workplace visits as much a part of the job as clinical examinations, with a view to spotting hazards and reducing risks before injury occurs. But what about the doctor who happens to see a patient with a suspected occupational disease? When should the extra, time-consuming step to visit the workplace be taken?

The short answer is whenever possible (but the visit does not have to be made by the doctor who is looking after the patient – see below, page 60). Usually the reason for the visit is not to investigate the cause – this is only necessary when the cause is suspected but not known – but to help in rehabilitation of the patient and to prevent disease in others. Of course, there are many circumstances when a visit is neither practicable nor necessary; for example, in the case of diagnosis of a well-known disease such as coal worker's pneumoconiosis when the industry concerned is already aware of and is addressing the problem, or in the case of an occupational cancer as a result of work many years previously. However, in many cases of obvious occupational disease, such as dermatitis or back injury, failure to make any contact with the workplace means that the chance to prevent the same problems in others is missed. Indeed, in such circumstances, the medical management of the problem in the individual patient is of little effect if the underlying cause is not corrected.

How to make contact with the workplace

Case history 3.6

In a lecture to 25 general practitioners, one of the authors discussed a local health problem: allergies in the fish-processing industry. During the discussion period, a member of the audience said that it was commonplace to see patients in his surgery with rhinitis and wheeze attributed to work in one of the prawn-processing factories. These cases rarely responded satisfactorily to treatment and the patients usually ended up leaving their jobs. The general practitioner appreciated the problem, but did not know how to do anything about it.

What would have been the appropriate action? This was the question that the lecturer put back to the class.

Two hands went up. The first doctor suggested a visit to the factory, but when asked how he would approach it, he was unsure. The other doctor suggested contacting a local specialist in occupational medicine. In the UK, a nationwide network of such specialists is maintained by the Health and Safety Executive. However, few members of the class were aware of this.

This event was one of the factors in the decision to write this book. In all other areas of medicine, if a doctor does not know how to handle a situation, the way out is clear – seek the advice of a colleague more expert in the area. But when it comes to occupational problems, this simple lesson is forgotten. In the UK, occupational medicine, because of its traditional separation from the mainstream of the National Health Service, is not looked upon as an accessible resource. And yet since the mid-1970s, there has been a UK-wide group of doctors and nurses trained in occupational health and specifically available for advice on such matters. In addition, there are now increasing numbers of specialist consultants employed within the NHS.

Sources of advice

The most important source of advice in Britain is the Employment Medical Advisory Service of the Health and Safety Executive (EMAS), described more fully in Chapter 5. A telephone call to the local branch of the Health and Safety Executive, asking for the Medical Inspector, is all that is necessary. In doing this, it is of course important to obtain the patient's agreement to this confidential medical referral. The EMAS doctor may wish to see the patient and will take all necessary subsequent steps, including visiting the workplace, examining other workers at risk and, if necessary, arranging a visit by the Factory Inspector.

There are alternative approaches that a doctor might wish to take. If the workplace already has its own occupational health service, the doctor should approach the physician in charge, who could then make the investigation. That doctor, in turn, should advise his employer to make a report to EMAS if the condition is a reportable one under the RIDDOR regulations (see Chapter 4 and Appendix 1). Or the doctor might wish to consult a university department of occupational medicine, a National Health Service consultant in occupational medicine, or an independent consultant. Finally, the doctor may wish personally to visit the workplace.

In some parts of Europe, a workplace visit may result from a compulsory reporting of occupational disease. Thus every physician in Germany is required by law to report a suspected case of occupational disease, this being one of the few exceptions to the physician's duty to protect the medical information of a patient. The report is sent to the 'Berufsgenossenschaft', a semi-governmental institution that is responsible for insuring companies against occupational accidents and diseases. The 'Berufsgenossenschaft' has a legal obligation to investigate every report, but the investigation may be carried out by technical people with limited knowledge in the health field.

Problems in arranging a workplace visit

Ethics (see also Chapter 11)

The relationship between a doctor and patient is confidential, and it is not acceptable to disclose information obtained from that relationship to a third party without the patient's permission. There may be particular dangers, perceived or real, to disclosure of clinical information to an agent of the employer, in that the worker may fear loss of job or some other form of discrimination. Even disclosure to another doctor, as to one in EMAS, may allow identification of individuals and their complaints by management. However, on the other side is the doctor's duty to do everything reasonably practicable for the health of the patient and to prevent disease in others.

The solution to this conundrum lies in clear explanation of the care to be taken to preserve confidentiality and to protect the patient from possible discriminatory action prior to seeking permission for referral or agreement to make a visit. Two points can be made here – in almost all cases, if the patient desires confidentiality it can be maintained (and if it cannot, the patient will withhold agreement) and, in general, managers are anxious not to cause injury to their employees and will be extremely cooperative in acting to prevent further trouble. Furthermore, if they are not, their legal obligations such as those in the UK under the Health and Safety at Work, etc., Act (see Chapter 6) can be pointed out to them.

Ethical problems are avoided by clear explanation to the patient of the doctor's desire to help by preventing further harm and of the confidential nature of communications between doctors. With the patient's permission, it is then possible to refer the problem to a specialist, who will discuss with the patient further approaches to the workplace and to the management. Only if the patient's permission is given can management be informed of the clinical problem, and then only in general terms. This should not of course hinder the doctor in the workplace from giving explicit advice to managers on preventive measures to protect workers.

The approach to management

If the company employs a doctor, the best approach is directly to him or her. If not, it is usual to speak to the most senior person on the site, normally the managing director or factory manager. The reasons for requesting a visit should be clearly explained, namely an anxiety that something in the workplace may be causing illness among the workers, and an eagerness to help in preventing future problems. It is both sensible and good medicine to stress this positive objective, because the management may have fears about an approach from outside – fears of litigation and trade union disputes, and fears of unrealistic demands on the budget in order to put things right. Responsibility for safety in a workplace is usually delegated by the managing director to a safety manager or safety officer. Such individuals should be trained in safety and the relevant legislation, but their knowledge varies considerably with regard to more strictly medical matters. Nevertheless, they have a detailed understanding of the workplace and its hazards and are the most useful people with whom to liaise over a visit.

Workers' representatives

In general, and in contrast to their popular image, trade unionists are helpful and cooperative when it comes to dealing with possible health hazards in the workplace. There is, however, a risk that individuals may take the opportunity of fomenting industrial unrest if they suspect such a problem but have not been fully informed. For this reason, as also for ethical reasons, it is advisable that the workforce's representatives should be made aware of the visit and be taken into the management's confidence about the reasons, the arrangements, and the means of reporting the outcome. In most workplaces, the employees will have appointed safety representatives, who sit on the factory safety committee with managers and the safety officer. This is often a useful forum for discussion of possible hazards to health, although again care has to be taken to preserve the confidentiality of individuals. Lay people are often ignorant of the ethical responsibilities of doctors, and may ask inappropriate questions.

The visit

Arrangements

The initial approach should lead to a meeting with appropriate managers to discuss the purpose of the visit and the anticipated outcome. The advisability of discussion with unions or workers' representatives should be brought up and normally a joint meeting is arranged. This gives an opportunity to allay fears and suspicions and to make clear that the purpose of a medical visit is to help prevent possible health problems.

The initial meeting with the management should also be used to learn about the factory or workplace – in the case of the manufacturing industry, about the raw materials, the processes, the products and by-products, waste and pollutants and the workforce. A brief checklist is given in Table 3.6.

Table 3.6 *The workplace visit – important information*

What raw materials are used?
How are they processed?
What are the products?
What by-products are there?
How are waste and pollutants removed?
What happens during maintenance and shutdown?
How large is the workforce?
What is the shift pattern?
Which workers work in the different areas/processes?
Who comes into contact with hazards?
Who carries out repair/maintenance?
What use is made of contract workers, and how do their safety precautions differ from those of the regular workforce?
What evidence is there of compliance with health and safety law?

In service industries, this matter is simplified as complex questions about processes are unnecessary and the emphasis is on environmental hazards, usually related to the building, and on methods of work organization.

In many industries, the process is complex and difficult for a non-specialist to understand. All such organizations have a flow diagram, often in the control room, which allows an outsider to obtain an overview of what goes on.

Looking around

Looking around, the vital part of the visit, is best undertaken in a structured way. It varies in complexity, from a short look at the particular process thought to be responsible for trouble, to a detailed examination of a whole industry. The former is more usual for the clinical doctor, the latter for the epidemiologist and occupational physician. The visit should, of course, be made in the company of someone who understands the workplace and the processes. The factory general manager usually has overall knowledge, although the production manager will often have more detailed knowledge of processes. The safety manager or safety officer has a particular responsibility for health and safety matters and the personnel manager (to whom the safety officer commonly reports) is most knowledgeable about the workforce, sickness absence and welfare matters. In service industries, personnel and safety managers and, often, engineers and building officers are useful contacts.

The simplest method of making a visit, having learnt about the process, is to follow it through from the entry of raw materials to the dispatch of the final product. It is important to watch what people actually do and to ask what happens when the process breaks down or shuts down. Particular attention should be paid to the handling of materials and chemicals and to possible exposure to airborne hazards. Of course, the doctor making a visit will be influenced by the condition of the patient or patients that provoked the visit, and here special attention would be paid to the particular job in question. If the likely cause is found, an assessment should be made of whether other workers are at risk (and not necessarily only on the shift during which the visit took place).

Watching the patient, or a colleague of the patient, do the job is an extension of the occupational history (Fig. 3.6). Workers vary in the care they take, just as organizations

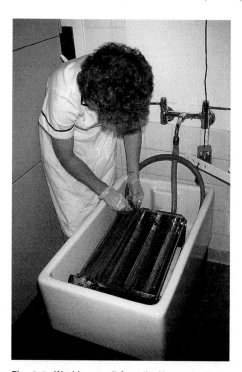

Fig. 3.6 *Washing a unit from the X-ray processor. Normally this is enclosed but has to be removed on a regular basis for cleaning, allowing exposure to chemical vapours. See also colour plate 3.6.*

vary in their protective measures. In the investigation of dermatitis, for example, a very fastidious worker may be found to be at greater risk because of repeated washing of the hands, while some less hygienic people may become sensitized as a consequence of contaminating their cigarettes with allergenic chemicals. In some instances, quite unexpected procedures come to light on a workplace visit.

Case history 3.7

A doctor was asked to advise an organization about safety in its animal laboratories. A careful examination of the workplace showed a number of areas in which there was a risk of skin and lung sensitization to people working on rodents. Appropriate recommendations were made. Some months later, the same doctor was asked to investigate an outbreak of skin disease in a biochemical laboratory in the same organization. While the technicians were showing him the way they carried out their work, one of their colleagues brought a live rat into the laboratory and proceeded to anaesthetize it on the bench. At the time five other people in the laboratory were working in the small laboratory; all were therefore at risk of developing occupational asthma, even though only one actually worked with rats.

The doctor dealt with the dermatitis problem and went back, a chastened man, to rewrite the animal house codes of practice. He had assumed that all work with rodents took place in the designated part of the animal laboratory and had forgotten that human beings often put convenience before safety!

The investigation of workplaces may bring to light the use of substances, often chemicals, that are not known to the doctor. Frequently their identity is concealed by trade names or by their presence in complex mixtures. However, all chemicals used in industry should be subject to a data sheet provided by the maker or supplier, which gives appropriate physical, chemical and toxicological data, together with advice on any precautions to be taken and action when accidental exposure occurs. Furthermore, in the UK, regulations on the Control of Substances Hazardous to Health (COSHH, see Chapter 6) require employers to have made an assessment of risk from the use of any hazardous substances, and to have made a written record of the assessment. These documents should be available for inspection. If further information on such substances is required, a list of readily accessible sources is given in Appendix 3.

The outcome of the visit

The visit should lead to three outcomes:

- confirmation of the hazard and assessment of risk
- action to reduce risk
- identification of others affected or at risk.

Once a hazard has been identified, it may be necessary to study it in more detail prior to planning preventive measures. This requires the use of the techniques of occupational hygiene and ergonomics.

Occupational hygiene is a discipline that applies scientific methods to investigation and measurement of hazards in the workplace and to control of risks from those hazards.

Ergonomics is a discipline devoted to the study of people in relation to their work and workplace.

These disciplines are discussed further in Chapter 5. All occupational physicians learn something of them – essentially an occupational hygienist is concerned with chemical, noise and radiation hazards and with their measurement and control, while an ergonomist is concerned with workplace, machinery and system design so as to ensure that a person's work is as well suited to his or her capabilities as possible. An occupational hygienist might be consulted, for example, for advice on control of airborne hazards from laboratory animals, an ergonomist for assistance in design of manual work so as to reduce risk of backache.

The measures taken to reduce risk and to manage individuals with occupational disease are discussed in Chapter 4. The workplace visit should allow these measures to be planned so that, ideally, the patient can return to the job and others will not be affected. In some cases, the visit may point to the need for a more extensive study of the workforce – this requires the epidemiological approach.

Epidemiological investigation

In a fascinating book, *The Rise and Fall of Modern Medicine*, Dr James le Fanu has argued, *inter alia* and tongue only half in cheek, that the public interest would be served by the abolition of all university departments of epidemiology. In doing this he takes what might be regarded as the popular view that epidemiology consists in demonstrating weak relationships between ill-health and environmental factors and thus adds spurious weight to campaigns for unrealistic changes to the environment. Many industrialists would endorse this view, and it has to be admitted that, particularly in North America, epidemiologists have sometimes confused their roles of objective scientist and of concerned citizen. On the other hand, it may be argued that epidemiology is the principal means of determining quantitative relationships between risk of disease in humans and environmental exposure, and that its achievements have been considerable. Led by the pioneering work, a century apart, of Snow on cholera and Doll and Hill on smoking and lung cancer, epidemiological studies have produced evidence that has led to the control of many occupational diseases – think, for example, of cancers in nickel refining; polyvinyl chloride (PVC) and ion exchange resin manufacture; those working with shale oil, polycyclic aromatic hydrocarbons, chrome and asbestos; and of silicosis, coal workers' pneumoconiosis and occupational asthma. In view of popular misconceptions about epidemiology, it is worth explaining its practical applications in occupational medicine.

Epidemiology involves the study of groups of people in order to determine patterns of health and ill-health within these groups. Analysis of the data derived from such studies may show relationships between disease (or health) and the environment, and lead to action to modify these relationships in order to improve health. This important outcome is often not considered by many doctors, whose curiosity is satisfied when a probable causative relationship is demonstrated. As can be seen from the best known example of epidemiology – the demonstration of a relationship between smoking and lung cancer – this is because the action required to prevent disease is usually largely out of the hands of doctors and depends more on politicians and other policy makers.

The epidemiological process is in fact analogous to the clinical process, as shown in Fig. 3.7. The clinician studies a patient and makes an examination, the synthesis of which leads to a diagnosis. In turn, this should lead to decisions about treatment and

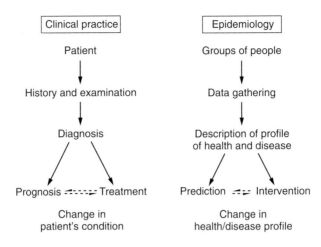

Fig. 3.7 *The epidemiological investigation.*

prognosis, each of which may modify the other. The epidemiologist studies groups of people, gathers data and makes analyses that lead to description of health/disease profiles in the group. This information may then lead to predictions of likely outcome of certain environmental changes and to interventions to make these outcomes more favourable. The clinician uses deductive logic in the diagnostic process, arguing from general medical knowledge to the particular circumstances of the patient, while the epidemiologist uses inductive logic, arguing from the particular findings in the group studied in order to make more general predictions.

In occupational medicine, there are several situations where an epidemiological study should be considered:

- investigation of a suspected health hazard in a well-established industry
- determination of quantitative relationships between hazard and risk of disease or injury
- measurement of the functional effects of occupational disease
- assessment of the effectiveness of preventive measures.

Whatever the reason, the investigator should bear in mind that the objective of the study is neither to reassure nor to attribute blame, but to find facts on which to plan possible preventive action.

The doctor involved in occupational medicine must be prepared to think broadly about the investigation of problems. Much may be learned from the investigation of individual patients – the clinical approach. Often epidemiological study is necessary to answer questions raised by the clinician, although for epidemiology to be of immediate value a workforce must have been exposed to an adverse environment for long enough for measurable effects to have occurred. If this is not the case, it may be necessary to apply toxicological methods to the investigation of suspect substances. Often, a combination of methods may be required and in occupational epidemiology it is always important that some assessment or measurement of the workplace or exposure is included in addition to measurement of effects on people. This is so for two reasons:

first, the demonstration of an exposure–response relationship is important evidence of causation; and second, because many hazards cannot be eliminated quantitative information can be used in setting standards to reduce the risk to a level acceptable to those concerned.

Case history 3.8

A worker in a factory making PVC (poly vinyl chloride) had a chest radiograph that was reported as showing fine diffuse nodularity. At the time there was much anxiety in the industry after the discovery of the association of hepatic angiosarcoma with exposure to vinyl chloride monomer in the retorts prior to polymerization, and it was feared that there might also be harmful effects on the lung. The factory doctor therefore arranged for chest X-rays to be carried out on the entire workforce and invited a specialist to report on the films. A proportion were said to show minor abnormalities. Anxiety was increased further, so a second expert was asked to read the films. This doctor found fewer abnormalities, and showed little agreement with the first reader, of whose results he was unaware.

The factory doctor now had a problem! What did he tell the workforce, and what did he do about the individuals whose films were reported abnormal by one or other reader? What would you have done?

In fact, the factory doctor decided to ask a third doctor, an 'even bigger expert', to read the films. Fortunately, this doctor asked the vital question, 'What do you want to know?' The factory doctor was encouraged to formulate a question in terms that could be answered epidemiologically. The first response was 'Does exposure to PVC cause pneumoconiosis?' This question could be answered experimentally by studies on rats, for example, but not convincingly epidemiologically. It would, however, be possible to demonstrate whether or not there was a relationship between exposures in the workplace to PVC dust and presence of radiographic change. If such a relationship existed, then it might be possible to make recommendations on levels of dust that would reduce the risk. It would also be possible to compare other measures of ill-health, such as lung function, in people with and without such radiographic change and thus comment on the physiological consequences of the abnormalities.

A cross-sectional chest X-ray survey was carried out of the current workforce and of a sample of those who had left the factory over the previous decade. Measurements of current exposures to dust were made by personal dust samplers, and estimates of the workers' total dust exposures were calculated from these, together with detailed individual job histories. Chest radiographs were categorized, according to a standardized format, by several readers independently, and the results were used to describe relationships between dust exposure and prevalence of radiographic change (Fig. 3.8). The company and the investigators were then able to discuss the findings with the workforce and with government authorities, and agree on appropriate occupational exposure standards to protect people from possible harm.

This case history illustrates the essentially practical nature of occupational epidemiology, and also points out the essential steps in such a study. These include:

- definition of the question in terms that can be addressed epidemiologically
- definition of the population to be studied
- choosing an appropriate study design
- standardizing the methods of measurement
- obtaining a good participation rate.

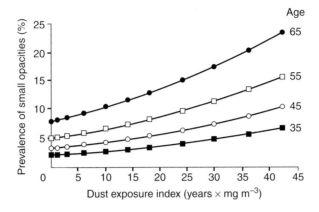

Fig. 3.8 *Exposure–response relationship derived from cross-sectional study of workers in a PVC factory, showing estimated increases in risk of early X-ray changes in relation to increasing current exposure to PVC dust.*

Defining the question

Research starts with a hypothesis to be tested, an idea or a question to which the answer is not known. Such questions arise commonly in clinical practice, if the doctor is of an inquisitive turn of mind. Often the answer may be found by searching the medical literature, but sometimes this is unsuccessful – the answer is not known. In occupational medicine, such problems fall into two groups: those in which people have been exposed to an agent for a sufficient period for measurable effects to have appeared and those in which they have not (yet). In the latter case, toxicological research may provide answers, while in the former epidemiological techniques are appropriate.

The question is usually a clinical one, such as, 'What has caused nasal cancers in these patients?', or, 'Why have I seen so many cases of tremor among painters?' These questions need to be changed into a format that allows an epidemiological approach, and this requires a hypothesis. In the case of the nasal cancer, for example, an ear, nose and throat surgeon noticed several such cases among workers in the furniture trade, and this led to the hypothesis that exposure to dust in that trade was responsible for the tumour. It was then possible to plan studies of groups of such workers to test this hypothesis and ultimately to show clear evidence of a relationship between such work and nasal cancer. The question about tremor in painters might be reframed as a hypothesis that exposure to paint solvents causes the condition. This then could be tested by appropriate studies, either of cases (people presenting with tremor) and controls (people without tremor), or of populations of painters or solvent-exposed workers.

Epidemiology is rarely able to establish a definite cause so questions are normally framed in terms of relationships and probabilities and the answers stated in terms of statistical likelihood. Thus the question will usually be of the form, 'Is there a relationship between disease and hypothetical cause and, if so, what is the likelihood of that relationship having occurred by chance?' or, 'What are the odds of people with a certain disease having been exposed to a particular agent, relative to controls?'.

Defining the population

All epidemiological studies are studies of groups of people, of populations. Many badly designed studies are inconclusive because of a failure to define the population at risk; it is clearly not possible to know the prevalence of a condition without knowing how many people are at risk of it.

The total population at risk may be called the **target population**. In the case of painters with tremor, this might be all painters in Britain. In practical terms, this would not be a group that could be studied, so a subgroup, such as all painters employed by a representative group of companies or working in a particular area, may be chosen as the **study population**. This, in turn, may prove impracticable to study, so a sample is taken, the **study sample**.

It is important to realize that any conclusions derived from the study ultimately refer only to those people studied, and can only be generalized after taking account of any biases that may have arisen in this selection process. In an infamous example, which reinforced the prejudices of those who decry the value of epidemiology, calculations of the likely contribution of occupational causes to the size of the cancer problem in the USA were based on prevalence data in specific studies of workers at high risk and were then extrapolated to all workers in the relevant occupations without regard to likely variations in exposure in different situations. This understandably gave rise to spuriously high estimates, great political argument and ultimately a general scepticism about the worth of epidemiology. But it was not the epidemiology that was at fault; rather it was its misinterpretation in arguing from the particular to the general.

In choosing the population, it is necessary to bear in mind the necessity of obtaining a good participation rate. Ideally, all those chosen as the study population should be seen, and it is generally held that a response of below 90 per cent of this considerably weakens any conclusions drawn. This is because it becomes less and less easy to estimate bias arising from non-participation – is it because the ill did not attend or because the well could not be bothered? The most challenging and time-consuming aspect of epidemiology is that concerned with ensuring a complete response. Nevertheless, it is accepted that many surveys, particularly those using questionnaires, elicit lower response rates and some means are available for estimating bias; for example, a sample of non-responders may be contacted by telephone or their health records may be available.

Designing the study

Few things are more disappointing than to have undertaken a great deal of work only to find out that it is valueless. This, regrettably, is the fate of many who rush into an epidemiological study without adequate thought and statistical advice. The study must clearly address the question or questions being asked and must be planned in such a way as to have a reasonable chance of obtaining a positive answer or a meaningful negative one. This latter concept, the probability of rejecting the null hypothesis when it is wrong, is known as the **statistical power** of the study. It depends on the sample size, the frequency of the characteristic sought in the population and the level of statistical significance chosen. The simplest type of study, conceptually, might set out to determine the **prevalence** of a certain condition in the defined population, that is the number of people with a predefined condition expressed as a proportion of the numbers in the population. This is analogous to a survey of voting intentions and similarly can only be taken to be true at the time of the study. Whether the prevalence of a particular disease or finding is abnormal requires reference to a control population or to a variable, usually exposure to a hazard, within the study population. Thus it may be possible to show that the prevalence of skin disease is greater in hairdressers than in shop assistants, leading to further hypotheses about possible causes of this problem in hairdressers. In turn, this may be addressed by investigating the relationship within a group of hairdressers between prevalence of the disease and exposure to agents thought to be responsible. Note that such studies are never quite as simple as they seem at first sight – are shop assistants an appropriate control population? How is skin disease defined for the purpose of the study? How may exposure to skin-damaging agents be quantified? Are there any **confounding factors**, such as age, use of make-up or exposure to sunlight or ultraviolet light, that could be associated both with the risk of skin disease and being a hairdresser, that might influence the results, and should therefore be taken into account in the design?

A **prevalence (or cross-sectional) study** therefore examines a population in a cross-sectional manner at a given time or over a short defined period. It is usually desirable to choose a population defined retrospectively, say all workers employed in the industry between certain dates, and this is especially necessary when studying conditions that develop only after a period of exposure. This method of selection allows one to avoid the trap of missing workers who have left the industry **because** they developed the condition in question, thus producing a spuriously low prevalence in the current population. Such cross-sectional studies should therefore attempt to include at least a sample of retired workers from the defined population. Prevalence studies are useful for defining relationships between disease and proposed cause, where the disease or abnormality being sought is a relatively common one. If the results of such a study are to be of real value, not only in contributing to understanding of cause but also in planning preventive measures, they need to incorporate measurements of hypothetical causative factors as well as response variables; for example, in Case study 3.8, exposures of workers to PVC dust were measured and this allowed the derivation of an index of exposure for each subject in the study. This was calculated from the occupational histories recorded, multiplying the concentration of dust in each job (mg/m^3) by the number of years spent in each job, and adding up these increments of dust exposure for all the jobs each individual worker had performed in the factory. This gave an index in $mg.years/m^3$ for each worker, and a wide range of such exposures in the workforce, from almost nil in secretaries up to very high levels in some long-serving process workers. This allowed the plotting of a relationship between exposure and risk of exhibiting changes at X-ray (Fig. 3.8). Such an **exposure–response relationship** is strong evidence of causality and, as happened in this case, provides information upon the basis of which an exposure standard may be negotiated.

Where the condition is relatively rare, or where one wishes to determine the effect of a particular condition on health, a **case–control (or retrospective) study** is often more appropriate. Here, **cases** are defined as individuals with the disease or abnormality in question, while **controls** are people from the same population but who do not have the disease. The two groups are then investigated in an identical manner, preferably by someone who does not know the case–control status of individuals. Differences between the two groups may then be expressed in terms of the **odds ratio** of one group having a particular exposure or functional abnormality compared to the other. This often gives a similar value to the **relative risk**, that is the risk of occurrence of disease in those exposed compared to those unexposed. Note the difference between controls in case–control studies and those in prevalence studies – in the former they are individuals without the condition being investigated, while in the latter they are a group without the hypothetically causative exposure.

Case history 3.9

A hospital registrar had read the suggestion that proliferative glomerulonephritis might be associated with exposure to solvents. A review of the literature showed that this hypothesis, although plausible (excretion through the kidneys could damage the nephron), was still in dispute. He had access, through the records of renal biopsy, to a reasonable number of patients with this clearly defined condition, and sought advice on an appropriate study.

If he came to you, what would you suggest, a cross-sectional study of people exposed to solvents or a case–control study?

The problem was discussed. A cross-sectional study would require identification of an appropriate population of people exposed to solvents, and a survey to determine whether or not they had evidence of renal disease, perhaps by examination of their urine. It would require either estimates of exposure to solvents or identification of an otherwise comparable unexposed population. Clearly this would be a time-consuming and expensive study. Moreover, calculations based on the likely prevalence of renal disease in the population suggested that, unless solvent exposure was an important cause of the disease, a very large study would be required to find an effect.

In contrast, a case–control study seemed straightforward. Cases could be defined histologically and controls could be drawn from the same population – patients referred to the hospital at the same time as cases, but who did not have glomerulonephritis. Precautions were taken to match cases and controls for two important factors that could influence the development of glomerulonephritis, age and sex, and a questionnaire on exposure to solvents and occupations was administered to cases and controls by a clerk who was unaware of the diagnosis. The results showed that the group with glomerulonephritis were much more likely to have worked with or have been exposed to solvents than were the controls, and that this difference was unlikely to have been the result of chance.

A major problem in case–control studies is the choice of controls. In order to avoid bias, they should be drawn from the same original population and, were it not for the factor under investigation, should have had an equal chance of contracting the disease. The cases have the disease, the controls do not and the study seeks to determine risk factors associated with having the disease. Any factor that independently influences the chances of having the disease and the risk factor being investigated is called a **confounder**, and cases and controls should be matched for this. In the example above, age and sex were regarded as confounders. Other matching is best avoided, as overmatching can result in possible risk factors being eliminated; for example, matching on area of residence will eliminate the possibility of finding a geographical factor. In hospital-based studies, other patients attending the clinic or clinics may be suitable controls, but care should be taken to allow for differing referral patterns to different doctors. Other studies may use relatives, neighbours or random samples from the same general practice or electoral roll as controls. In planning case–control studies, as in all epidemiology, the involvement of a statistician is crucial.

The other common use of a case–control study is to investigate the functional effects of a disease. The same problems of control selection obtain, but the comparison is here made in terms of measured function, be it physical abnormality, liver or lung function, or whatever.

A particularly economical and useful study design is to base a case–control study on a cross-sectional study carried out previously. This is known as a **nested** case–control study. Such a design allows the initial cross-sectional study to be confined to aspects related to determination of case–control status, leaving the more detailed investigations to be confined to the smaller numbers thus identified. Thus the initial survey may identify asthmatic symptoms in a workforce by questionnaire while detailed estimates of exposure or functional consequences can be made in cases and controls rather than in the whole workforce.

A third type of study is the **longitudinal (or cohort) study**. This measures the **incidence or attack rate** of a disease or abnormality over a defined period of time. In one form it may measure mortality.

Case history 3.10

During a period of crisis in the world oil market, the United States government decided to investigate the possibility of exploiting its reserves of oil shale in the Rocky Mountains. Because shale oil had been known from the days of the late Industrial Revolution to be carcinogenic, it was considered advisable to take precautions to protect the workers, both miners and process workers. But what risks would these people run, and from what substances?

How might risks be assessed in a new, or fairly new industry? What options can you think of?

The US risk assessment team considered animal experiments and cytotoxicity tests of substances likely to be produced in the industry. They also considered analogy with other similar industries. But what they really needed to know was the effects of previous oil shale industries on the health of their workforce. Fortunately, it was possible to identify a cohort of several thousand men who had been working in the Scottish oil shale industry in 1950, prior to its final closure in 1962. It proved possible to identify which of these men were alive and which dead and, in the case of the latter, to identify the cause of death. After appropriate corrections for age, it was then possible to relate the risk of mortality from different conditions in these workers to the risk of members of the general population of Scotland. The results of such analyses, expressed as age-standardized mortality ratios and their 95% confidence intervals, showed that the Scottish workers had an increased risk of premature death from skin cancer but from no other disease. In particular, lung cancer was shown not to have occurred more frequently than expected.

The results of this study were useful in that they did not reveal any risks of major diseases and the power of the study made it very unlikely that a real risk had been missed. Similar mortality studies have been completed with measurements or estimates of exposure, for example to asbestos, in order to predict excess risk of death associated with different levels of exposure to harmful substances. Clearly such studies are of considerable value in planning preventive strategies. They do, however, have several disadvantages:

- they are expensive and time-consuming
- they require a population to have been exposed for many years
- they rarely are able to obtain accurate information on exposure.

Two other applications of longitudinal studies are in investigation of the incidence of disease and in measuring changes in function over time. Both require the same criteria for identification of population together with choice of an appropriate control, be it an unexposed population or measurement of a possible causative variable within the study population. It is also possible to nest a case–control study in a longitudinal one.

Case history 3.11

Several workers in a factory producing citric acid developed asthma, and this was shown to be caused by *Aspergillus niger*, a fungus used in the process. A cross-sectional survey was carried out and identified work-related asthma in 5 per cent of the workforce, of whom half had skin prick test evidence of allergy to *A. niger*. Extensive precautions were taken thereafter to reduce the exposure of workers to the antigen, and annual surveillance of the workforce by questionnaire and skin prick testing was carried out. Over the next 5 years it was shown that no new cases of asthma had occurred in the original cohort, nor had any new positive skin tests been found.

This example illustrates a simple use of a longitudinal survey in order to ensure that preventive measures are effective. If coupled to appropriate measurements of exposure, the results may be used to modify any exposure standards previously set. If the study design includes, in addition, measurements of function (in this example, lung function might have been appropriate), it may be possible to investigate the relative contributions to functional deterioration of age, smoking and exposure to antigen.

Standardizing methods of measurement

In epidemiology, as in clinical and laboratory medicine, the measurements made should be capable of producing the same result when repeated by the same or by another observer; in other words, intra-observer and inter-observer error must be small. Thus, when making observations on large numbers of people in an epidemiological population, the tests to be used should be carefully standardized in order to minimize variability. The same applies to methods used in the measurement of the workplace environment. Furthermore, methods should have been, or should be able to be, validated, so that the results derived should show some relationship to other standard measurement. Table 3.7 shows some of the methods and terms used in such validation.

Table 3.7 *validation of a test*

| | Standard method | | Study method |
	Positive	Negative	Totals
Study method			
Positive	True positives (a)	False positives (b)	Positives (a + b)
Negative	False negatives (c)	True negatives (d)	Negatives (c + d)
True totals	Positive (a + c)	Negative (b + d)	

From this table: the sensitivity of the study method is a/(a + c); the specificity of the study method is d/(b + d); the systematic error (study method positives to true positives) is (a + b)/(a + c); and the positive predictive value (proportion of study method positives that are true positives) is a/(a + b).

For many tests, the 'true' value is not directly measurable and the test may have to be validated indirectly; for example (a well-known one), the rather arbitrary classification of X-ray changes of pneumoconiosis, based on comparison of films of workers with standard films selected by a panel of experts, has been validated more effectively by relating results of epidemiological surveys to indices of dust exposure in the populations than by direct comparison of films with pathological changes in the lungs of individuals after death. The logic of this is illustrated below.

Case history 3.12

It had long been known that workers in certain dusty trades were at risk of developing pneumoconiosis, a condition characterized by small, and sometimes large, opacities on the chest radiograph. Various methods of classifying such shadows had been developed in different countries so that epidemiological studies of prevalence, incidence, progression and influence of preventive measures could be made. In order that results could be extrapolated, standardized methods were necessary for use in different industries worldwide.

After several international discussions, it was decided that standard films would be selected that illustrated different stages and types of pneumoconiosis, each being selected as an individual point on a continuum of change, from normal to extremely abnormal. Consensus was reached on the choice of films, which were then used in many international studies of dust-exposed workers. The films were validated by their use in studies on, for example, coalminers and asbestos workers, where it was shown that the higher exposure a worker had suffered, the greater the risk of the film showing more advanced changes. Thus it can now be stated that profusion of radiological change is an indirect measure of dust exposure.

These studies have also shown that the standard films are far from perfect, with low sensitivity and specificity, and must be used with great caution as a **diagnostic**, as opposed to an **epidemiological**, tool. Inter-reader and intra-reader variability is often considerable, and small opacities are related to factors other than dust exposure, age and smoking habits, for example. Further discussions are regularly convened to improve these methods of categorizing radiological changes.

The most frequent epidemiological tool in occupational medicine is the questionnaire. The design of a questionnaire is complex, and as far as possible investigators are encouraged to use one that has already been used and has been shown to produce reproducible answers and to be valid. If a new one needs to be designed, a few points should be borne in mind.

- The questions should be:
  - short
  - comprehensible by the group to be studied
  - unambiguous.
- The questions should not:
  - suggest an answer
  - combine two or more questions in one.
- The questionnaire:
  - should have a logical order
  - should include clear routing instructions.

Examples of bad questions are:

Do you ever suffer from an itch or redness of the skin?

These two questions should be asked separately, as subsequent questions could refer to either or both symptoms.

Have you ever suffered from hypertension?

Many people will not understand terms that are familiar to doctors – high blood pressure is better here.

Is your cough worse when you are at work?

This suggests a cause of the cough and introduces a bias into the study. It is better to ask:

Does your cough vary during the week?

If yes:

On which day or days is it worse? and
On which day or days is it better?

This can be achieved simply by providing a box for each day of the week and asking the subject to tick the boxes for the days on which the symptom is most troublesome.

In designing a questionnaire, after the questions have been decided upon (and they should generally be the smallest number consistent with achieving the aims of the study), the logic of the routing instructions should be checked. The rule is to have the subject answer only relevant questions, so if a 'No' is recorded to presence of a symptom, supplementary questions are avoided and the subject or questioner is directed to the next relevant one. The usual method of checking is to administer the draft questionnaire to a friend or relative. Mistakes will be found, and after these have been corrected, a pilot study should be made of a group of people from similar social backgrounds to the intended study population, to pick up ambiguities and incomprehensible terms.

Administration of a questionnaire may be by a trained clerk (who should know not to explain, elaborate or prompt) or by the subjects themselves. Many practical difficulties attend such surveys, chief of which is obtaining an adequate response rate.

Obtaining a good participation rate

No matter how good the methods and design, an epidemiological study is easily rendered valueless by a poor rate of participation by the subjects, just as a poll of voting intentions is rendered uncertain by a high proportion of 'Don't know' or 'Mind your own business'. The key to success is hard work: in designing a study that will be acceptable to the subjects; in publicizing the study and obtaining agreement and support from key people (such as union representatives) in the study population; and in tracing individuals and politely inviting their participation. In occupational epidemiology, where there is often a readily definable workplace population, the most important steps are those taken in explaining the purpose of the survey to the subjects beforehand and in telling them how and when the results will be communicated to them. Any hint of secrecy and the study is doomed to failure. Problems arise with tracing and follow-up of retired workers, and here the help of older workers and union or personnel/pension records is invaluable.

Screening for disease

The surveillance of workers for the presence of disease is considered further in Chapter 5. At this point, it is worth noting a few principles relating to the value of and justification for screening. The following questions should be asked before embarking on a screening programme.

- Is the condition important for individuals or the community?
- Are there effective means for management of the condition?
- Is the condition's natural history, especially its evolution from latent to overt, understood?
- Is there a recognizable latent or early stage?
- Is there a valid and reproducible screening test?
- Are facilities available for management of the positive findings, both true and false?
- Is there an agreed management policy?
- Does this management favourably influence the course of the disease?
- Is the cost of case-finding and management acceptable in relation to the overall costs of healthcare?
- Do the potential benefits to true positives outweigh the potential disadvantages for the false positives?

It is clear that any thoughtful person would pause before introducing general health screening in a workforce if such questions were considered. The chief disadvantage of 'health checks', apart from their grossly inefficient use of resources, is the harm done to individuals when insignificant findings lead to a series of unnecessary and sometimes dangerous investigations. When screening a healthy workforce, such false positives are likely greatly to outnumber true positives, for which useful intervention is possible.

Determining the cause of disease

As outlined at the start of this chapter, the cause of disease in an individual may be determined clinically by, for example, patch testing or bronchial challenge. In epidemiology, studies point to relationships between ill-health and possibly causative or contributory environmental factors. It is, however, ultimately possible to accumulate sufficient evidence to make a causal relationship extremely likely. The late Sir Austin Bradford Hill proposed widely accepted viewpoints from which the evidence should be assessed.

1. How **strong** is the association, or how unlikely is it to have occurred by chance?
2. How **consistent** are all the studies that have investigated the association?
3. Is the condition apparently **specific** to a group exposed to a particular agent?
4. Is there a **temporal relationship** between the proposed cause and the effect?
5. Is there an **exposure–response relationship** between cause and effect?

6. Is the relationship **biologically plausible?**
7. Is the evidence **coherent**, in that it does not conflict with known facts about the condition's natural history?
8. Is the evidence supported by **experimental evidence** in laboratories?
9. Does the evidence accord, by **analogy**, with that derived from other fields?

Two examples serve to illustrate the value of these tests; hepatic angiosarcoma in vinyl chloride workers and lung cancer in silica-exposed workers. In the case of the former, the first five are fully satisfied, the sixth was originally uncertain (was a simple anaesthetic agent likely to cause liver cancer?) but was settled with inhalation studies in rats (number 8), and 7 and 9 are unimportant in the face of all the other evidence. In the case of silica and lung cancer, the evidence of association is becoming stronger and more consistent, although the disease is certainly not specific to silica workers; increasing evidence is being produced in support of 4 to 7, and there is now some, weak, experimental evidence of causation. It may be concluded that vinyl chloride causes angiosarcoma, but that the case against silica remains unproved – if it has a role in causing lung cancer, it must be a relatively weak one in epidemiological terms.

These viewpoints clearly do not all require a positive answer to be given in order to make a case, but they are all questions that should be considered in building such a case before, for example, taking legislative action. None alone provides incontestable evidence of causality, especially when taking account of the possibility of confounders, but the best evidence usually comes from the finding of a strong biological gradient (number 6) and of a series of strong associations in separate studies (numbers 1 and 2). Care should be exercised when arguing from number 2 to consider possible **publication bias**, that is the tendency of journals to publish positive results and reject negative ones. Biological plausibility is also a criterion on which not too much weight should be placed, because what is implausible today may become quite plausible with a little lateral scientific thinking; for example, it was argued that the epidemiological associations between air pollution and *cardiac* deaths were implausible and therefore spurious until it was suggested by one of the authors that lung inflammation could have downstream effects on blood coagulability.

It is important that epidemiological results be taken in their biological context, as a means of shedding light on the complex interrelationships between man and his environment. The occupational physician, with feet firmly on the workplace floor and a good understanding of human physiology and toxicology, is in an ideal position to put the findings of this science into its proper context, to the ultimate benefit of industry and those who work in it.

CONCLUSION

Three complementary methods are of use in investigating possible occupational disease – clinical, workplace and epidemiological. The occupational physician needs to have a good understanding of the strengths, weaknesses and value of all three, and to be aware that in combination they are capable of answering most questions about the causation of occupational disease.

4

The management of occupational disease

SUMMARY

- The occupational physician has an important role in managing work-related disease. However, in the modern practice of occupational medicine there is rarely a place in the workplace for prescription of drugs or other therapeutic intervention, except in special cases such as some workplace emergencies.

- In addition to the immediate management of occupational disease, doctors have wider responsibilities in preventing recurrence in the affected individual and in reducing the risks to others. Thus the diagnosis of occupational disease should often lead to modification of the job and/or the workplace.

- While the doctor in industry is usually well placed to assess and to contribute to the management of work-related disease, doctors in hospital or in general practice may often need to seek help from specialist occupational physicians.

- An important responsibility of the doctor diagnosing occupational disease is to ensure that legal reporting requirements are met, although the manner of achieving this varies.

- Finally doctors should be able to advise their patients on matters concerning statutory compensation and, depending on their expertise, issues of causality where a civil action is being pursued.

INTRODUCTION

Occupational disease constitutes an often underestimated proportion of the workload of general practitioners or hospital doctors. When workers are ill, their occupation is not commonly the cause and when work is the cause of injury or disease the occupational physician's contribution to treatment in the narrow therapeutic sense is often limited. Nevertheless, there are important specific aspects of the management of occupational disease, whether it is an emergency or not, that are sometimes neglected, perhaps through ignorance. The purpose of this chapter is to fill these gaps for the benefit of any physician who may come across occupational disease. Some points are covered in other chapters but bear reinforcing.

- The primary contribution of the physician should be to advise on, and hence assist in, the prevention of occupational disease (Chapters 5 and 6).
- Detection of occupational disease should be achieved as early as possible (Chapter 3) because this will usually improve the clinical outcome for the afflicted individual, as well as encourage early steps to be taken to protect other workers.
- Both the individual with occupational disease and the work environment need to be thoroughly assessed. Occupational physicians should be adequately trained in these skills but at the same time must recognize their individual limitations and know when and how to seek further help.
- A few aspects of treatment may be relatively specific to occupational disease.
- Physicians also have some responsibilities in the statutory processes for reporting occupational disease, and in advising workers or their agents in connection with compensation.

It should be clear from this, and from the examples that follow, that the description of the problem in occupational medicine is often more complex than in other clinical specialties where, in simple terms, the physician may merely ask, 'What is the diagnosis? How do I treat it?'. In occupational medicine, the doctor has a wider responsibility, having not only to assess the clinical problem but also to investigate the environmental factors that contributed to it, to take action to prevent further harm to the patient and to others in the same environment and, sometimes, to make a formal report.

The important steps in the diagnosis and investigation of occupational diseases have been dealt with in the preceding chapters. However, in many situations it is necessary not only to determine the nature and severity of a condition and its cause but also to assess the risk of its occurrence or recurrence following workplace exposure to the hazard. This assessment will help to decide the best form of management and will serve as a baseline for subsequent review of the response to its management, or in the event of later relapse. Moreover, proper assessment is important for legal purposes especially when compensation may be sought. In some cases, the clinical presentation might not initially point to an occupational cause as for example with back pain or an anxiety state, and the patient might at the time believe there to be no occupational contribution to the symptoms. Important factors in the failure to recognize occupational disease are long latency and multifactorial aetiology. Nevertheless, the physician should still assess any potential occupational exposure that might be a contributing factor, as the question of such a component to the illness with implications for its management might arise later. Detailed accounts of how to assess disease that may have similar manifestations, whether work related or not, can be found in textbooks of general medicine. However some relevant points will be illustrated, because occasionally physicians in industry do not place enough emphasis on these issues.

The management of occupational disease may present a range of special, interesting and challenging problems in relation to assessing and influencing both the workplace and the patient/worker. Consider the following case history.

Case history 4.1

A 37-year-old female worked in a clothing manufacturing plant. Part of the process entailed making permanent creases to clothing such as trousers. A preparation releasing formaldehyde was needed for this purpose. On one major occasion, and a few more minor instances, she and her workmates had been overexposed to formaldehyde. She complained of symptoms of cough and irritation of the eyes and nose, nausea and general malaise as a result. When seen by the occupational physician, she related that she continued to experience symptoms frequently in the workplace when she had tasks involving the same textile. This occurred in spite of belated steps taken by the company to learn from previous mistakes and to avoid overexposure, and even in circumstances when no formaldehyde was measurable in the atmosphere. These recurrent symptoms consisted of a feeling of anxiety, shortness of breath, numbness around the face and in the fingertips, and nausea.

What possibilities would you consider?

The physician considered various options, including those of continuing exposure to formaldehyde or to other harmful agents, perhaps not yet identified. The possibilities of the exposure concentrations being too small to be readily detected by testing the environment, or increased sensitivity of the employee to the chemicals, were considered. On clinical examination of the respiratory tract the patient was encouraged to hyperventilate by the physician. She then said that she was experiencing symptoms practically identical to the recent ones – i.e. tingling around her lips and fingertips (acroparaesthesia), together with anxiety and generally feeling unwell. Further enquiries revealed that the employee was somewhat resentful of the original apparent lack of either serious intervention or concern shown by her employer, and this was probably justifiable. She felt that she lacked control and information about the exposure and its consequences. Moreover, on one occasion in a department store display she had seen identical garments to the ones she worked on and began to experience exactly the same symptoms as she felt whenever she saw them at work.

The above scenario is consistent with the following interpretation. Exposure to the toxic chemical agent (in this case formaldehyde) had produced symptoms as a consequence of its direct harmful effects on the respiratory tract and elsewhere in the human body. Essential steps to prevent this had not been taken, although subsequently appropriate measures to control exposure at source were implemented. Another harmful consequence of the exposure was a Pavlovian or behavioural conditioning in which stimuli, such as the appearance of the fabric used in the garment, perhaps even the natural smell of the fabric itself, were associated in the worker's mind with the original symptoms, and thus provoked feelings of being unwell, with anxiety, headache, and features of hyperventilation. A two-pronged approach of workplace control and intervention, coupled with detailed individual explanation and reassurance is needed (and was employed in this case) to manage satisfactorily and thus resolve problems such as these. Further psychological intervention might even be necessary to ensure eradication of the conditioning.

The diagnosis of an occupational disease, whether in general, hospital or in occupational practice, should lead to the following steps being taken:

- clinical management of the individual: therapeutic; by exclusion from the cause of the condition; and rehabilitative
- investigation of the workplace by a competent person to reduce risks of recurrence if the patient returns
- consideration of the possibility that others might be affected in the same way

- consideration of the need to report the condition
- advice to the individual on future employment, benefits and compensation issues.

The remainder of this chapter discusses these issues with respect to specific types of occupational ill-health.

MANAGEMENT OF CONDITIONS RESULTING FROM ERGONOMIC FACTORS OR PHYSICAL AGENTS

Ergonomic factors and trauma

Sometimes clinical management can be simple and self-evident as in the following example.

Case history 4.2

A 45-year-old man was referred by a physician to a specialist in occupational medicine with a provisional diagnosis of 'vibration white finger' (nowadays usually called hand–arm vibration syndrome or HAVS), on account of his history of finger numbness and of his use of powered hand tools. However, when assessed by the specialist his symptoms of numbness and paraesthesiae were localized to the distribution of the right ulnar nerve in the hand. Further history taking revealed that he used his hypothenar eminence as a mallet to hit spanners when rusty nuts would not rotate easily, and this had resulted in a localized ulnar neuropathy ('hypothenar hammer' syndrome). He was given advice about his work practice and advised to use a rubber mallet in future, and his symptoms recovered spontaneously.

However, often the clinical problems are more complex and further lessons have to be learnt and additional principles applied, as in the next case.

Case history 4.3

A 28-year-old apprentice joiner had gone off sick with back pain. When seen by the physician he said that the pain had resulted from lifting a narrow wooden architrave (about 5 cm wide and 2.3 m long). On examination the doctor noted that he had some difficulty in touching his toes and on that basis concluded that he was not yet fit to return to work. He remained off work, took analgesics until he was completely pain free and then returned to exactly the same job.

The above assessment and action, although commonplace, are far from ideal. What further information should have been obtained in order to assess the severity of his illness, the prognosis and the action necessary to reduce risk of recurrence on returning to his job?

Five important matters should have been considered:

- the history of the task
- the clinical examination
- the assessment of the workplace
- statutory matters (reporting, benefits, etc.)
- rehabilitation and secondary prevention.

A more detailed history was revealing. It transpired that the wooden architrave was mixed in with a variety of other timbers that were stored at ground level. The sliding out of the desired one, with a bent and stooped back, against the resistance of the other pieces was clearly a risky task. The workplace merited detailed assessment to ensure that the wood was, in future, stored, properly sorted, at a higher and more accessible level.

The objective assessment was not adequate as described. Thus for example, in assessing a worker who is complaining of lower-back pain, one important measurement that may be important in prognosis and subsequent management is that of lumbar spinal flexion. One of the ways of determining this is by the skin marking method. Briefly, with the patient erect a line is drawn in the midline at the level of the dimples of Venus (posterior superior iliac spines), a further mark is made in the midline 10 cm above this and another 5 cm below. The patient is asked to flex as far as comfortably possible while the origin of the measuring tape is held against the top line. The more the lumbar spine can flex, the greater the skin distraction. Most normal people will easily yield to a distance beyond 20 cm between the uppermost and lowermost mark (i.e. 5 cm more than the 15 cm baseline). Additionally, clinical assessment to exclude acute lumbar intervertebral disc prolapse, including nerve stretch tests, tendon reflexes and tests of sensation should have been carried out.

Consideration should have been given to the need to plan for rehabilitation if or when appropriate (see also Chapter 9). In some countries the case would have been reportable; for example, in Britain once at least 3 days of sickness absence had elapsed, the physician should have notified the manager that the incident was reportable as an 'injury' under the Reporting of Injuries, Diseases and Dangerous Occurrences Regulations (RIDDOR). In more prolonged absences, issues of statutory or other benefits (see also Chapter 9) would need to be considered.

Radiation

There are various aspects of the management of certain specifically occupational physical exposures that deserve attention. Exposure to ionizing radiation without adequate safeguards can be a serious medical emergency. An occupational physician facing such a prospect should either have been adequately trained beforehand or at least be aware of the need to seek expert advice as a matter of urgency. In Britain, the radiation protection adviser (RPA) has an important function in assessing the risk of exposure to radiation and in giving advice on its control. The RPA is responsible for monitoring radiation at source and for organizing personal dosimetry through film badges worn on clothing, thermoluminescent dosimeters attached to extremities or direct reading electrometers. The RPA gives advice about segregation, containment, handling and disposal of radioactive materials. The RPA, however, can also help in a retrospective estimate of radiation exposure from a review of the circumstances that have led to it. The physician has a role to play in biological dosimetry in the case of substantial whole body radiation. An appropriate blood sample must be taken early for a white cell count and lymphocyte culture for chromosome analysis, as these indices correlate well with exposure to ionizing radiation at relatively high doses of overexposure.

The acute hazards of non-ionizing radiation to the skin have been exemplified in Case history 2.4 (page 22). The eye is very sensitive to light injury, to varying degrees dependent on wavelength and intensity, but 'arc eye' is a classical example of corneal injury caused by ultraviolet light from arc welding. There may be a latent period of up to a day before symptoms of keratitis develop. It is treated symptomatically but cessation of further uncontrolled exposure is essential.

Thermal hazards

Case history 4.4

An occupational physician was summoned urgently to the kitchen of the canteen of a large workplace when an employee was said to have 'lost consciousness'. The clinical problem was fortunately not a serious one – an 18-year-old female assistant had fainted in a hot part of the kitchen. Luckily she had not been carrying a hot or dangerous load at the time and had not injured herself or any of her workmates. After drinking some fluids and resting, she recovered fully. It transpired that she had recently started this job. She was of very slight build. The physician encouraged her to ensure that she had an adequate intake of fluid and salt. It was agreed that she would initially spend most of her time preparing cold food such as salads, and progressively and slowly increase her exposure to the hotter aspects of her job. Thus she satisfactorily got used to her work environment. In parallel the physician also made recommendations for better cooling, ventilation and rest breaks for all the staff in the kitchen.

In most of today's occupations, the risks of thermal hazards are generally small. Thus in hot, humid kitchens, particularly among workers of small physique, there is a risk of faints. This is especially so among new employees, who may be overzealous and not yet acclimatized. Usually simple environmental steps, such as improvement in ventilation, task rotation, wearing appropriate clothing and acclimatization, are enough to prevent recurrence. Fluid and salt replenishment should be encouraged.

More prolonged exposure to heat, indoors or outdoors, can result in heat stress or heat exhaustion. The patient is unwell and may feel faint or nauseated, or experience cramps, while thermoregulation and hence sweating is maintained. Simple commonsense measures, as outlined above, are usually adequate, but if the condition is not recognized and managed appropriately it may lead to heat stroke.

Heat stroke (hyperpyrexia) is a medical emergency with a very high mortality if not recognized early and treated vigorously. It is characterized by a rise in core body temperature above 40°C, owing to the failure of the thermoregulatory mechanism; in the absence of sweating there is tissue damage, notably to the liver, kidneys and brain. Thus the patient may be comatose or delirious, and may even have seizures. The afflicted worker must be removed urgently from the hot environment, vigorously cooled by wetting and by measures to increase evaporation, together with general supportive measures; an intravenous infusion should be instituted pending transfer to an intensive care unit. Fortunately, this is a rare condition in industry in temperate climates, although it still occurs from time to time, especially in the armed forces on training exercises. In any particular case the occupational physician must assess the circumstances giving rise to these health effects and give advice on measures to prevent recurrence. This should include improvements in the general environment, provision of appropriate clothing, information and instruction about the risks, changes in work practices and removal of particularly susceptible individuals.

Hypothermia may arise occupationally when the worker is immersed in water or exposed to cold air; for a given environmental temperature the former is more rapid in onset than the latter. However, in windy conditions, the chilling effect of the wind, especially on a wet, exhausted and inadequately protected subject, is often underestimated. It is very important for the physician to be aware of the risks and not to miss the diagnosis. The core temperature should be measured, hypothermia being diagnosed usually if it is less than 35°C. The absence of shivering can be a feature of the seriousness of the condition and may be followed by delirium, coma and death. First aid management should start with the application of thermal blankets, but may proceed to intravenous infusion and warming with water not exceeding 40°C until the core temperature reaches 35°C. As with hyperpyrexia, hypothermia is a medical emergency, warranting specialist management of such complications as acid base imbalance. In severe cases, when vital signs are absent, resuscitation attempts should be prolonged, as the low body temperature may protect the brain and other organs from irreversible hypoxic damage for much longer than in the case of normothermic cardiac arrest.

Pressure hazards

Workers exposed to raised ambient air pressures, as in diving, caisson work, or compressed air tunnelling, or reduced pressures, as in flying, are usually protected by specialist medical advice and the support of a hyperbaric chamber. Nevertheless, the generalist should be aware of the risks that may be associated with an abnormal environmental pressure so that specialist advice can be sought in a preventive context, and so that the clinical manifestations after a pressure-related event can be recognized early. Complaints of any symptoms such as headache, nausea, visual disturbance, vertigo, limb pain, paraesthesiae or pareses after work in abnormal pressure environments must therefore be treated seriously and referred immediately to the nearest hyperbaric facility.

MANAGEMENT OF CONDITIONS RESULTING FROM HARMFUL CHEMICAL SUBSTANCES

This part of the chapter contains a number of sections dealing with specific disease categories and their particular management. However, by way of introduction, consider the following non-specific case presentation.

Case history 4.5

A 55-year-old woman had worked for several years in high street dry cleaning shops. In her last employment in particular she had been significantly exposed to perchlorethylene both as vapour and percutaneously. Not only did she have to clear out blocked button traps, and top up the machine with this solvent but also she was in the close vicinity of frequent leaks. She developed multiple symptoms including headaches, nausea, anxiety and Raynaud's syndrome affecting her hands. She eventually gave up the work as her symptoms worsened while exposure remained uncontrolled. Her employers did not have an occupational physician but her complaints, directly and through her general practitioner resulted in the Health and Safety Executive investigating her workplace shortly before she left. Airborne levels of perchlorethylene were monitored and found to be in concentrations consistent with her symptoms, and the employer was obliged to take appropriate action.

Perhaps if this lady's case had been investigated earlier and appropriate steps taken to control her exposure at that time some of her symptoms could have been improved and she could have continued working for longer. However, the fact that at least some investigations were carried out while she was still in employment permitted a better informed clinical management of her case as well as enabling useful data to be collected in the service of justice when she subsequently commenced litigation proceedings against her ex-employers.

Sadly, all too often employees give up their jobs spontaneously or on medical advice when there is circumstantial evidence of an association between their work and their symptoms. Investigations of occupational exposure or of specific biological markers (such as organic solvents in blood or breath, or their metabolises in urine) should be undertaken at the earliest suspicion when the symptoms may still be mild and while the worker is still in employment. Even if the circumstantial evidence is strong or the employee is considering leaving the job anyway, a good case can still be made for these investigations, which may permit identification of the specific agent, and its source, and measurement of the exposure levels responsible for the adverse health effect. They will facilitate appropriate measures to safeguard the worker's health and job and are important in stimulating action to protect other workers. This concern usually springs to mind early in the deliberations of an occupational physician, but is perhaps not so obvious to general practitioners or hospital doctors who naturally address primarily the problems of the individual in their consulting room. Finally, such investigations may provide data that will result in the courts of law being better informed should the matter eventually lead to civil or criminal action.

Assistance with these techniques should, ideally, be sought in the first instance from the occupational physician employed by the firm, because properly trained occupational physicians are well versed in environmental and biological monitoring. However, this ideal route is only available in the minority of circumstances where the firm employs such a person, and in many cases, therefore, the assistance of other occupational health specialists will need to be sought. In the UK, this would usually mean contacting an inspector or doctor employed by the Health and Safety Executive. Although European legislation and Parliaments or National Assemblies in the member states have granted workers the support of government organizations, the concerned physician should not merely point this facility out to the patient and leave it at that. Many workers are lacking in confidence and sometimes do not easily articulate their problem. Therefore a better approach might be for the physician, after obtaining and recording the patient's consent and armed with all the information that can be reasonably gathered (see Chapter 3), to telephone the nearest enforcement authority and ask to speak to one of their doctors or another professional member of the inspectorate. After the two have conferred, a letter should set the seal on the conversation. The enforcing inspectorate can then take further steps to investigate and to manage the suspected occupational disease. These could include seeing the worker clinically and visiting the workplace alone or with a factory inspector, and in due course advising both the worker and the referring physician. Alternatively, occupational physicians employed in the health service or in university academic departments will often be willing to advise a medical colleague informally, although it should be stressed that this may not necessarily be their official responsibility.

Some physicians, both within and outside the workplace, might feel that, because the occupational physician is not responsible for the primary care of the employees, medical treatment, in the strict sense, is never part of this role. However, the occupational physician may have an important treatment function in emergencies, and in other occupational illness where specific training and experience can be a valuable addition to the advice of the other medical attendants. In all such cases, it is imperative to remember the ethical issues governing relationships between patients and their medical advisers.

This being said, one should avoid the fallacy of believing that most occupational illnesses, even the acute ones, have specific remedies – circumstances in which this is the case are the exceptions and not the rule. The following accounts deal with the management of some occupational conditions where the occupational physician should be able to make a useful contribution. It also includes some relatively rare circumstances in which specific therapies in particular antidotes can be used to manage occupational disease, such as poisoning by anticholinesterases, cyanides and certain metals, methaemoglobinaemia, and hydrofluoric acid burns.

Occupational asthma and rhinitis

The mainstay of management of these conditions rests on the correct identification of the causative factors and on the appropriate preventive steps that are discussed in Chapters 3, 5 and 6. Nevertheless, there are certain circumstances when specific therapy is indicated. These are in the treatment of severe symptoms, temporary steps to treat milder symptoms while preventive steps are actively pursued, and the treatment of residual illness once all preventive steps have been implemented.

Occupational asthma, like asthma from other causes, may have a fatal outcome, although this has been reported very rarely. The low molecular weight chemical sensitizers, isocyanates and reactive dyes have been responsible for preventable deaths in the workplace. Continuing exposure, the lack of appreciation of clinical features of deterioration and ignorance of the potential for worsening of symptoms in the hours after exposure has stopped are potential contributory factors. Medical and nursing staff at industrial sites where an asthma hazard exists must therefore be trained and equipped to deal with an asthmatic crisis by the administration of nebulized bronchodilators, such as salbutamol or terbutaline, delivered ultrasonically or by oxygen from a cylinder. This may need to be accompanied by high concentration oxygen therapy. After the immediate emergency is over, two other important steps must be taken. An informed handover of clinical care to the general practitioner or to hospital medical staff supported by an explanation to the employee of the risk of deterioration is essential. Furthermore, the employee (and the manager) must be unequivocally advised against return to the particular job or to another with similar exposures until there has been clinical recovery and the physician and manager have taken all necessary steps to prevent a recurrence.

Case history 4.6

A 40-year-old process worker in the pharmaceutical industry presented to the occupational health centre complaining of shortness of breath. He was a non-smoker and had worked in that industry for 22 years. A few days previously he had developed a cold that he could not shake off and which had gone to his chest. On examination he was clearly distressed and wheezy. His FEV_1/FVC was 1.8/3.9 L.

This improved to 2.6/5.4 L after he was treated in the workplace with nebulized salbutamol. These values contrasted sharply with the results on routine health surveillance a year previously of 4.3/6.1 L. Further enquiry revealed that for the previous week or two he had been working in a different part of the factory from his usual place because of the absence of a colleague. About 12 years previously he recollected having suffered from wheezy bronchitis when he had worked in that part of the plant. A provisional diagnosis of occupational asthma was made and, after his symptoms settled in the occupational health centre, he was given a bronchodilator inhaler, a detailed letter for his general practitioner and was driven home.

The occupational physician's awareness of the diagnosis, and the availability of adequate treatment options had permitted the man's symptoms to be rapidly and effectively relieved. It is not possible to predict the outcome had the treatment not been given on site. He almost certainly would have survived a journey to hospital without treatment, but may have become more distressed in the meantime. Not all cases of acute occupational asthma have made it to the hospital alive.

On return to work, arrangements had been made by the occupational physician for the employee to be recommenced in his usual location, where he had been asymptomatic for at least 10 years. Serial peak expiratory flow (PEF) measurements were commenced. A few days later he returned with the following note from his general practitioner, 'This patient who did have some bronchospasm when he had a chest infection … is clinically well and his PEF today is 610 L/min, which is well above the 95th centile for his height'. The worker refused to continue with the self-recorded PEF tests and further history-taking revealed that he was concerned that a diagnosis of occupational asthma might have implications for his continuing employment.

Fear of the consequences that the diagnosis of an occupational disease may have upon employment, or ignorance of its manifestations, can be serious impediments to both correct diagnosis and management. These points have been well illustrated by the above case. In spite of these difficulties the initial clinical management of this particular case was correct.

Further medical management assumed that this was a sentinel case and a survey of the rest of the workforce was undertaken. This showed that there was a previously unrecognized asthma hazard and steps were taken to reduce the risk of this by containment, local exhaust ventilation and personal protective equipment.

The occupational physician is not uncommonly faced with an awkward situation when an employee, for career advancement or for financial reasons, is willing to tolerate work in an environment where exposure is such as to provoke symptoms of occupational asthma and/or rhinitis. This is unsurprising because loss of employment after the diagnosis of occupational asthma has been shown to result in long-term financial disadvantage. In general, if the sensitization is to protein allergens such as flour, enzymes or animal secretions, it often proves possible to manage such patients by enhanced personal protection (both physical and pharmacological), together with careful control of airborne allergen. With sensitization to low molecular weight chemicals, return to work is rarely possible. A level of control adequate to abolish the occupational asthma must be insisted on, or failing that (and more usually), relocation of the employee. Prolonged exposure in any circumstances almost always results in worsening of the asthma, so the aim should always be to exclude the subject from exposure if at all possible. Short-term compromises between social factors and treatment of symptoms, so long as they are mild, may apply, for example in a postgraduate student who develops laboratory animal allergy but who wishes to complete the project, or in an industrial employee while control measures are implemented. Standard therapy for rhinitis and/or asthma, namely the use of antihistamines, beta adrenoceptor agonists, corticosteroids, leukotriene inhibitors or other therapy as appropriate, would be prescribed by the employee's general practitioner in liaison with the occupational physician, who would closely monitor the situation.

Once exposure to an agent causing occupational asthma has ceased, some employees with this condition may experience persistence of their symptoms. In simple terms, exposure to the hazardous agent may have resulted in a syndrome clinically indistinguishable from 'intrinsic' or 'idiopathic' asthma. The likelihood of this outcome is proportional to the duration of symptoms before exposure is prevented – a powerful incentive for early diagnosis. In these cases management of the asthma should be undertaken and continued in the same way as for asthma of other causes.

Angio-oedema

In the following case history a young worker developed a life-threatening occupational disease.

Case history 4.7

A 20-year-old woman started a job as an animal house technician, dealing mainly with rodents. Workplace exposure had not been properly assessed nor adequately controlled as is required by health and safety law (see Chapter 5). About 5 months later she developed symptoms of conjunctivitis, rhinitis and asthma that improved on spells away from work. Her general practitioner prescribed treatment with bronchodilators but her symptoms persisted. Eventually, after about 1 year in employment she had a severe episode of angio-oedema, with considerable facial swelling and difficulty in breathing, for which she was seen as an emergency in a hospital casualty department, and administered intramuscular adrenaline followed by treatment with antihistamines and corticosteroids. However, no specific action in relation to her job was considered. After this episode she did not return to that work, and eventually resigned her employment.

Arguably, from a medical standpoint the problem was solved. The occupational nature of her symptoms was shown, at least circumstantially; she would no longer work in the animal house and her symptoms would be expected to resolve. However, was the management of this occupational disease really adequate? What problems can you see in the way in which the case was handled, and how might these have been resolved?

The assessment was incomplete. In all cases of asthma, questions should be asked about possible provoking causes, including occupational factors. If such factors are suspected, frequent measurements of peak flow, as discussed in Chapter 3, should be made.

The management of the patient was unsatisfactory. As the symptoms persisted in spite of treatment, further investigation should have taken place. Usually in such an example, referral for a second opinion is advisable; this might have been to a specialist occupational physician. Thus in some parts of Europe, such as Scandinavia or Italy, this might consist of referral to a specialist academic unit, while in Britain the official referral route would be to an occupational physician in the Health and Safety Executive.

In addition, increasingly many occupational physicians in the Health Service or in medical schools can provide such a facility.

There was no attempt to manage the overall problem. Although the patient's problem was reduced (albeit by loss of her job), the workplace problem remained, and other people in the animal house remained at risk. This important aspect of the case can only be addressed by a visit to the workplace, and it is here that the advice of a specialist is particularly important.

The patient lost her job, without financial compensation. In Britain and many other countries, there are systems for industrial injury benefits to be paid to people suffering from certain occupational diseases. The patient in this case should have been advised that her condition was one that would be recognized for benefits. Thus, as discussed later, in Britain, benefits would have been available were she to apply to the Department for Work and Pensions. The disease was not initially reported to the statutory authorities. Again, regulations differ in different countries, but in Britain RIDDOR put the responsibility on employers to report any of a long list of occupational diseases (see Appendix 1). The doctor who makes the diagnosis should inform the employer with the patient's consent or, if this is not freely given, consult with an Inspector in the appropriate authority such as the Health and Safety Executive directly. The regulatory authority is then in a position to take appropriate action. If this step is taken, it is often possible for the workplace risk to be reduced and for the patient to return to work.

In summary, this case contrasts what usually happens with the many issues that often need to be considered in the management of occupational disease. Both the general practitioner and the casualty officer could have obtained enough evidence to take appropriate action, to the benefit of both the patient and her workmates.

An important lesson is that although angio-oedema is a very rare emergency in an industrial context, severe anaphylactic reactions leading to angio-oedema may occur. It is false to assume that this rare but severe event is completely unpredictable. Affected workers often give a history of earlier, milder episodes with urticaria and palpebral oedema. These heralds should be heeded. Moreover, a very small risk may be associated with vaccination. In those workplaces where such risks apply, the appropriate therapeutic agents should be available for use by an occupational health professional. Essentially, these include ampoules containing 1 mL of 1:1000 adrenaline to be administered intramuscularly, usually in a 0.5 mL bolus, as the first line treatment. This should be followed by parenteral antihistamines (such as chlorpheniramine 10 mg), administered intramuscularly or slowly intravenously.

Occupational skin disease

Eczema/dermatitis is the commonest occupational skin disease that any physician will come across. As with asthma and rhinitis, the principal element in the management of occupational dermatitis is avoidance of exposure to the causative agent and to any aggravating factors. Avoidance of exposure does not simply entail advice to wear gloves. The gloves or gauntlets should be adequate in their coverage and resistant to relevant physical damage and to the chemicals in use in the workplace. Thus, for example, ordinary rubber gloves do not provide adequate protection from many organic solvents. Care should also be taken that the gloves do not cause or aggravate the dermatitis. The possibility of allergy to gloves should be considered when dermatitis does not resolve and tends to correspond initially to the area of the glove in its distribution. Moreover, any gloves may cause or aggravate dermatitis by irritation if the skin is weepy or sweaty when they are worn. In severe cases of dermatitis one may have to await substantial improvement before returning to work and then only wearing appropriate gloves. In some cases the wearing inside the glove of cotton inserts that are replaced at least daily can reduce the risk of maceration from sweat and friction. The patient needs to be advised about possible irritants to avoid, whether occupational or otherwise, which, while not necessarily causative, could aggravate dermatitis. These could include washing-up liquids, shampoos and even soap. This can be a time-consuming task with limited retention of the advice by the patient. However, the involvement of an occupational health nurse and the provision of written advice such as an information sheet can help resolve both of these difficulties.

Emollients such as emulsifying ointments and aqueous cream can be a useful adjunct to the treatment of irritant dermatitis associated with a dry skin especially if caused by defatting organic solvents or detergents. They should be applied liberally at least twice daily (just before and after a night's sleep) if it is not convenient to apply topical treatment during the working day. Creams and ointments, however, may make a wet, weepy dermatitis worse. Barrier creams should be considered barriers only in name, because in most instances they provide no protective function at all and sometimes may even act as vehicles to promote the transport of harmful substances into the skin. However, some may have an emollient function or may assist hand cleaning. Topical corticosteroids may be necessary to assist in the resolution of occupational dermatitis as a supplement to, and not a substitute for, cessation of exposure. They should be recommended in close liaison with the general practitioner.

It is best if the physician is familiar with one or two preparations and uses these. The rare but not extinct practice in some workplace medical centres of handing out topical corticosteroids without adequate assessment, protection from exposure or professional advice can only warrant serious criticism. It bears repeating that the management of occupational diseases should include assessment of the workplace and advice to prevent recurrence.

Case history 4.8

A pharmaceutical worker developed itching, redness and subsequently blistering of the fingers and back of the hand. At presentation in the occupational health department she had tense bullae, surrounded by inflamed skin (Fig. 4.1). She was referred to hospital where de-roofing of the bullae was carried out aseptically. After several weeks she made a full functional and cosmetic recovery. History taking and review of the process and the workplace showed that she had been handling a potent alkylating agent (mechlorethamine), while wearing black, natural rubber gloves. The occupational physician found information that such gloves are permeable to this and similar agents and advised that, as well as a review of the workplaces, appropriate alternative gloves should be used.

In this case the managing chemist and the safety officer had made a detailed hazard assessment and taken preventive steps, including the use of rubber gloves. In spite of this, protection was not adequate and the occupational physician was able to make a useful contribution to the management of the problem.

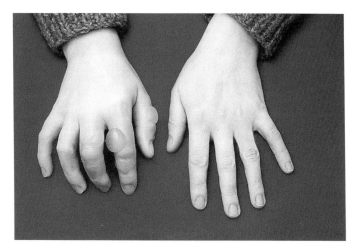

Fig. 4.1 *Patient with tense bullae surrounded by inflamed skin.
See also colour plate 4.1.*

Chemical burns

Emergency management of chemical burns starts essentially with prolonged (more than 15 minutes) irrigation with tap water. Any of the worker's clothes that could have been contaminated should be gently stripped.

Some exposures demand specific steps, as illustrated by the following case history.

Case history 4.9

A 29-year-old worker was etching glass with a preparation containing hydrofluoric acid. As he stretched over the glass surface, some of the agent contaminated his forearm just above his gauntlet. He was instantly aware of the pain and immediately rinsed his skin with water. The first-aider carried on flushing water over his forearm for several minutes, coupled with liberal irrigation with the antidote calcium gluconate in solution, and finally as a gel. He was sent to hospital but luckily the small degree of contamination and the prompt action resulted in only very minor scarring as a result.

Hydrofluoric acid is a hazardous agent that should be singled out as a special example. It is rapidly corrosive to the skin, other soft tissues and bone. If exposure is substantial it may cause systemic upset through hypocalcaemia produced by the binding of calcium to the fluoride ions. Treatment locally should include an antidote (as in the case described), and in hospital intravenous calcium gluconate may be needed to combat the hypocalcaemia. Many chemical burns may need the early involvement of plastic surgeons in case skin grafting should prove necessary.

The eye is of course particularly sensitive to chemical burns and substances such as alkalis – which are present in domestic dishwasher powders and oven-cleaning agents and not only in heavy industry – as well as acids, can inflict terrible damage. All such injuries should be thoroughly irrigated in the workplace and, if there is any doubt at all about residual harm to the eye, the employee should be referred for specialist examination, including fluorescein instillation, using a slit lamp.

Asphyxiation, toxic and irritant gases

Incidents of asphyxiation, whether by chemical poisoning or by displacement of oxygen, are fortunately very rare. They are, however, so serious and eminently preventable that they warrant special mention.

Case history 4.10

In a chemical manufacturing firm, on the first occasion that recommissioned plant was in use after alteration, a process worker donned an air hood as personal protection before commencing a task that could have involved solvent exposure. He was seen to lose consciousness by a workmate who was a trained first-aider. The first-aider immediately pulled off the victim's air hood and carried him away from the immediate vicinity of the reactor vessel. Oxygen was administered by face mask within minutes, and by the time the occupational physician arrived, the worker was regaining consciousness; he eventually made a full recovery. It was discovered that during the alterations the fitting for the air-line had inadvertently and negligently been welded onto a nitrogen blanket line (used to cover certain chemical reactions with nitrogen rather than air to prevent unwanted oxidation).

It is clear that had it not been for the prompt, appropriate and effective action of the first-aider the casualty would have died or suffered brain damage. The investment made by the company and its nurse and physician in training these first-aiders that, in the event of non-traumatic unconsciousness, the casualty was to be urgently but safely removed from his immediate environment, given oxygen and kept in the coma position had clearly paid dividends.

A doctor working in industry has a duty not only to prevent occupational disease (as extensively discussed elsewhere in this book), but also to mitigate the consequences of injuries. This obligation is addressed by considering what disease, poisoning or injury could arise even after implementing preventive action. Adequate material facilities and trained personnel should be made available to deal with adverse consequences at least to a standard that complies with the relevant health and safety (first aid) regulations. These require appropriately labelled first-aid boxes with a specified content to be available. The occupational physician should be familiar with the correct assessment and management skills and should then be able to supervise the training of first-aiders. Many formal training courses in first aid run by outside agencies are excellent, but are often too general and tend towards the management of trauma and non-occupational medical emergencies rather than special occupational problems such as chemical intoxications. In contrast, the trained occupational physician should have both relevant professional knowledge and an understanding of the specific workplace hazards, and is therefore ideally placed to train the first-aid team that he or she is likely to have to work with in an emergency. Moreover, the physician should liaise with the nearest casualty department to ensure that the knowledge and facilities exist to deal with any medical emergencies peculiar to that workplace, such as anticholinesterase poisoning, methaemoglobinaemia, etc.

Many large and responsible firms, usually with an occupational health service, try hard to establish a good working relationship with their local hospital and general practitioners. This liaison can be life-saving in the emergency management of occupational diseases as well as in dealing with less severe cases. Hospital doctors and general practitioners should respond positively to invitations to open days, joint meetings and such like. It is a paradox that some small firms with serious occupational hazards and no occupational health service, and whose workers would therefore rely exclusively on medical skills outside the workplace in an emergency, do not try hard enough to forge such links. General practitioners and hospital doctors who become aware of such workplaces, perhaps through 'herald' patients presenting with minor illness or in other ways, should contact the workplace directly. They should ask to speak to any occupational health or safety professional if there is one or, failing this, to the manager. If this proves difficult, it is better to seek the advice and help of the appropriate enforcing authority, such as the Health and Safety Executive, early rather than wait until a serious and perhaps life-threatening incident results.

Contrary to popular belief, very few poisons can be treated by the use of specific antidotes. Indeed, even time-hallowed dogma on the use of various antidotes is now being called into question. The single most important step in the management of asphyxiation from whatever cause is removal of the victim to a place of safety and administration of oxygen in high concentration (as in Case history 4.10). Some special intoxications are worthy of further mention. In poisoning by cyanide (hydrogen cyanide or its salts) the mainstay of specific treatment used to be the binding of the cyanide to methaemoglobin produced by the administration of inhaled amyl nitrite. Cobalt ethylene diamine tetracetate followed this treatment but this antidote is highly toxic and can kill the worker, especially if the diagnosis is mistaken. It should only be administered to an unconscious patient in whom cyanide poisoning has been proven, at least circumstantially, by environmental measurement. Intravenous administration must be slow and cautious and may result in angio-oedema. Another advocated treatment that is safer and may be equally effective is the intravenous administration of hydroxycobalamin, which combines with cyanide to form cyanocobalamin. Poisoning with other chemical asphyxiants such as carbon monoxide (e.g. from incomplete combustion) or hydrogen sulphide (e.g. from decomposition of sewage) should likewise be treated with high concentration oxygen. When unconsciousness has occurred, urgent transfer to a hyperbaric centre should be considered.

Methaemoglobinaemia can result from exposure by inhalation or by splash to agents such as aniline or nitrobenzene. For reasons that are poorly understood, the electronic configuration of the iron in haem changes and the haemoglobin is converted to methaemoglobin, which is incapable of carrying oxygen. This substance is bluer in colour than normal haemoglobin and this contributes to the clinical cyanosis. Oxygen and rest are very important in the treatment, besides rigorous decontamination. The specific antidote for symptomatic cases consists of methylene blue administered slowly intravenously, although ascorbic acid (vitamin C) has also been employed. One of the authors recalls, as an intern, the dramatic effect his administration of blue liquid intravenously to a blue patient in a casualty department had on watching nurses as the patient turned pink!

Irritant chemicals, such as chlorine and ammonia, and even the less irritant nitrogen dioxide, may cause acute pulmonary oedema, within hours of exposure, and a delayed obliterative bronchiolitis, which may present with breathlessness some weeks after the exposure. The most common industrial gassings are the result of chlorine in the chemical industry and many other workplaces where it is used as a bleach or disinfectant. It even causes problems occasionally in swimming pools and in domestic cleaning where hypochlorites may inadvertently be mixed with acids. Nitrogen dioxide may be generated in silos, by welding and by combustion of cellulose. Many other toxic and irritant gases may be encountered in industry, and occupational physicians should always keep an eye open for places where they could be liberated or accumulated.

Case history 4.11

A 48-year-old man was employed by a local authority as a chargehand at a sewage pumping station. His duties included climbing down into an open sewage channel in the building to scrub down its walls with a brush. There was usually only a small stream of soiled water running at the bottom of this channel. On one occasion, whilst doing this job he noticed that the smell was even more unpleasant than usual. The workers doing this sort of work learn to tolerate awful smells so he continued scrubbing until he started to cough and became short of breath. He also felt faint, but managed to climb out of the channel before losing consciousness. His workmate, who had been out, fortunately came back at this moment, dragged him out of the building and administered oxygen. He was taken to hospital with an acute toxic pneumonitis from which he eventually made a full recovery. Analysis of this gas in the pumping station and subsequent investigation showed that there had been an illegal disposal of chemicals by a large factory into the sewage system the previous night, probably resulting in the release of hydrogen sulphide. This had made its way through the pipes to the station by the time the patient had started work.

This patient was fortunate. Many people gassed in tanks or culverts never make it out, and sometimes their workmates also die trying to rescue them. He nearly died from acute asphyxiation (as in the previous case history), and having recovered from this his lungs had to contend with a toxic pneumonitis. Fortunately his pulmonary oedema settled in hospital with oxygen and corticosteroids.

In the first-aid treatment of exposure to these substances, the rescuers, having first ascertained their own safety, using breathing apparatus if necessary, must then remove the victim and administer oxygen in high concentration. Some advocate the use of inhaled corticosteroids in the workplace when exposure to irritant gases has occurred. This policy runs the risk of being unnecessary in a number of cases and inadequate in the rest. If there has been a non-trivial exposure to an irritant gas that could lead to pulmonary oedema, the best counsel is for the worker to be hospitalized for full assessment. In most serious cases it is wise to give systemic corticosteroids at this stage as there is anecdotal evidence of their effectiveness.

Pesticide intoxications

Many pesticides contain organophosphates or carbamates, potent cholinesterase inhibitors. Occupational exposure may take place through inhalation of mists generated by spraying or through eye or skin absorption. Warm weather makes it less likely that the worker will wear adequate protection, as well as aggravating the physiological consequences of exposure. The symptoms and signs are those of uninhibited acetylcholine-mediated neurotransmission. They range from headaches, nausea, lassitude and visual disturbance, through lacrimation, salivation, abdominal cramp, vomiting, bradycardia and tremors, to pulmonary oedema, convulsions, coma and death. When this type of poisoning is suspected, a blood sample should be taken for cholinesterase assay even if treatment has to be instituted rapidly. The worker, as with many other intoxications where skin contamination is likely, must be stripped and washed thoroughly with soap and water. The attendants must have due regard for their own safety during this procedure. Secretions should be cleared and oxygen administered if necessary. Intravenous atropine in doses substantially higher than the ordinary therapeutic range may need to be administered repeatedly. This drug blocks the cholinergic muscarinic receptors but does not deal with the underlying problem. Tachycardia and pupillary dilatation indicate adequate atropinization. Further management of severe organophosphate (but not carbamate) poisoning includes early administration of intravenous pralidoxime to reactivate the cholinesterase.

Other poisonings

Special forms of treatment may occasionally be needed, usually administered in hospital, as in the following case study.

Case history 4.12

A worker involved in furniture restoration was suffering severe abdominal pain – bad enough to be misdiagnosed as an 'acute appendicitis' (see Case history 1.7, page 6, for his historical and diagnostic details). Because of the elevated blood lead level which accompanied and accounted for his distressing symptoms, he was treated with chelation therapy and his blood lead levels monitored as they fell. His asymptomatic father had a blood lead level of 5.2 μmol/L. Despite repeated attempts to persuade them to follow appropriate precautions of local exhaust, personal protection, and health surveillance, the family unfortunately lapsed from follow-up, and did not follow the advice of the enforcement authorities and are presumably still at risk. In fact his 13-year-old brother was kept from school and recruited to help out while the index case was in hospital.

What are the lessons from the above case study? It does show that chelation may have a limited role in management of some symptomatic cases of heavy metal poisoning. However, one can argue that this is the last lesson to be learnt from this case. It is much more important to bear in mind the points made earlier in this book and in the chapters that follow – namely to prevent disease and to manage it by control of exposure to reduce it to acceptable levels.

National and regional poisons centres have a very important role to play in the management of occupational intoxications. Although they deal most commonly with poisonings by therapeutic substances and household agents, they can contribute in an advisory capacity or by clinical management of cases of industrial poisoning. They are usually accessed by telephone and some can be interrogated electronically.

Management of conditions resulting from infectious agents

In industry there is rarely a need for clinical management of occupational diseases as such. Thus occupationally caused leptospirosis, tetanus, tuberculosis, hepatitis, etc., are treated in exactly the same way in hospital, or convalescing at home, regardless of the source of infection. However, the prophylactic management of exposures to infectious agents warranting specific intervention is discussed in Chapter 6.

In managing infections such as these it may be important to carry out tests to determine the exact strain of the infecting organism as far as is technically feasible. This would help to trace the original source, but equally may be of value in linking any further spread from the index case to others. The management of infectious disease such as tuberculosis may require further effort to trace contacts. Such diseases may also have implications in terms of future fitness for work and work practice. Thus a surgeon who becomes a carrier of hepatitis B might not be permitted to engage in future exposure-prone procedures.

REPORTING OF OCCUPATIONAL DISEASE AND INJURY

Legislation regarding occupational disease has three main aims, dealing with prevention, compensation for sufferers and reporting of cases. The third of these is little known to many doctors, and is often neglected. Reporting is not a mere vexation imposed by the legislators, but fulfils certain functions.

- It provides an opportunity for the episode in question and for issues of compliance with the law to be investigated.
- It should lead to risk management steps for the prevention of similar episodes locally.
- It contributes to national data for assessing the size of the problem and the effectiveness of preventive legislation.
- It thus permits the establishment of better priorities and targets for national preventive strategies.

Although steps are being made towards harmonizing the categorization and classification of occupational disease worldwide, and in Europe in particular, there are still big national variations in the detail; for example, in the UK the mainstay of the legal requirement for reporting occupational ill-health or injury consists of RIDDOR (see Appendix 1). These place the responsibility for reporting squarely on the employer's shoulders. However, in the case of occupational diseases, the employer has to act on a diagnosis provided by a doctor (and not necessarily an occupational physician). It has to be recognized that even for the categories of disease and injury that are reportable, there is evidence of considerable underreporting. The occupational physician should take steps to bridge this gap. Thus employers should be explicitly advised in writing when the physician diagnoses a reportable injury or disease. If the employee does not consent to this, it is recommended that the physician should make a direct confidential approach to the appropriate enforcement authority, explaining the employee's concerns as well as the facts of the case.

Beside the legal responsibilities for reporting, there are various voluntary schemes, participation in which is to be encouraged. The purposes of such schemes may differ from those of statutory ones; for example, to provide information that may be used for research into causes, management and prevention of disease. In the UK the best known is Surveillance of Work-Related and Occupational Respiratory Disease (SWORD) which is part of The Health and Occupation Reporting Network (THOR) which in 2005 expanded to include general practitioners besides the occupational physicians and hospital specialists who previously participated. This involves regular reporting by occupational physicians and chest physicians of a wide range of cases of respiratory disease that could be work related. The list is by no means limited to those conditions that are reportable or prescribed by law, and has confirmed the impression of underreporting of many of these diseases. Occupational and other relevant physicians are strongly encouraged to participate in this and similar schemes such as those addressing urothelial tumours, skin diseases and blood diseases.

COMPENSATION FOR OCCUPATIONAL DISEASE AND INJURY

Money is generally a poor substitute for the suffering and shortening of life caused by disease to the patient, or for bereavement by relatives. Nevertheless, compensation is a mechanism to help provide for lost earnings and other damages. It is important that the physician is aware of the mechanism for awarding compensation for occupational disease. In most countries compensation, broadly speaking, falls into two categories – benefits obtained from the state or some other national fund (such as through the Department for Work and Pensions in the UK) and compensation obtained through civil litigation in the law courts usually from the employer or insurer.

Compensation without recourse to litigation

The following case history illustrates the application of compensation through a national legal provision.

Case history 4.13

A baker aged 60 years working in a hospital suffered from progressively worsening bronchial asthma, needing treatment with beta adrenergic and anticholinergic bronchodilators as well as corticosteroids. He gave no history of asthma in childhood or adolescence, the asthmatic symptoms having started after he began work as a baker. They remitted when he had a spell away from baking but returned when he resumed this trade latterly with the Health Service. He also had a history of rhinitis with polyps and had undergone about five nasal polypectomies. His symptoms became so severe that he could no longer cope with his work. He had never been made aware that his work could cause such symptoms but the history was strongly suggestive of occupational asthma and a visit to his workplace showed substantial exposure to airborne flour. Apparently, previous doctors had not considered the possibility that his symptoms could be occupational. He was given a peak flow meter with instructions for self-monitoring, but the readings did not conclusively show a work-related pattern; after several years of symptoms and with multiple therapy, this was not surprising. He proved to have a very poor exercise tolerance which did not improve after sickness absence, but even if there had been an improvement, there was no early prospect of the hospital bakery reducing his exposure to flour dust substantially.

What was the occupational physician to do? Sadly, premature retirement on grounds of ill-health was the only option as no prospects of relocation to another sedentary job for which he might be fit were found. He might in fact have been short changed by the Health Service twice – as an employee he had not had adequate information and protection, and as a patient the possible relation between his symptoms and his work had gone unrecognized until late in his condition.

What compensation could be available? While some doctors and lay people erroneously believe that the role of social security departments is to guard the national treasury and avoid paying out compensation if at all possible, the reality is rather different. The process is simple.

- The doctor making the diagnosis checks that the patient has been employed in a prescribed occupation (see Appendix 1), and that there is therefore a likelihood that he or she will be eligible for benefits.
- The patient is advised to complete a form making a claim (at the Department for Work and Pensions) for industrial injury benefits, in this case for occupational asthma.
- The patient is told that the process involves an insurance official at the Department for Work and Pensions checking that he or she was employed in a prescribed occupation and then referring him or her to a doctor for diagnosis and assessment of disablement.
- The doctors employed by the Department for Work and Pensions will generally see the patient and, often after consultation with the specialist involved or after obtaining lung function tests, determine the diagnosis and assess disability in terms of 'loss of faculty'. This clinical assessment, based on history, examination and special tests, compares the individual to another of the same age and sex, taking account of his job.

If the diagnosis is agreed, the doctors from the Department for Work and Pensions may review the patient from time to time.

The conclusion of the Department for Work and Pensions may not always be that of the patient or the patient's doctor; for example, in the UK diffuse pleural fibrosis or lung cancer in the presence of asbestosis attract benefits, while pleural plaques alone or lung cancer in an ex-asbestos worker with no fibrosis do not. Where the patient's claim is turned down, there is an appeals procedure through an independent panel (a medical appeals tribunal).

The list of prescribed diseases and occupations is under regular review. There is now a European list and in the UK the independent Industrial Injuries Advisory Council advises the government on which conditions should be eligible for compensation. Any doctor who believes that an occupational disease should be on the list is able to write with the evidence and ask for the matter to be considered. In general the rule is that the disease must be a specific risk of the occupation and not a general risk of other people, thus allowing the connection between cause and effect to be made clinically in an individual.

Compensation through the law courts

There are some very important differences between compensation obtained through Social Security legislation and that obtained in a court of law by a civil action against an employer or ex-employer. In both instances there has to be good evidence of occupational disease and relevant exposure, and a physician with appropriate training may be able to give a good opinion about these points. However, additionally, for a civil case to succeed, the court must be satisfied that the employer ought to have known about the risks and could and should have done more to prevent them in the light of knowledge at the time; that is, the employer was negligent. The employer, in turn, may seek to prove that the injured worker contributed by his own negligence in not taking steps to prevent the disease, that the disease occurred as a consequence of unforeseeable individual susceptibility, or indeed that the worker does not have the disease in question or is suffering little or no real disability. Some of these matters are beyond the area of expertise of many doctors, who should therefore usually confine themselves to matters of diagnosis, level of disability and prognosis. Because the case is heard by a judge and argued by lawyers, the process is both costly and lengthy, and the outcome is never certain. Many cases are settled out of court by a bargaining process, but the possibility that the doctor will be cross-examined should give pause to the wary – only experts should write expert reports! Because of the complexities of the legal process, doctors should be cautious before suggesting that the patient embarks on a time-consuming, expensive and sometimes distressing legal action. If the diagnosis is reasonably secure (in court it is decided on the basis of the balance of probabilities – more likely than not) and negligence is possible, the worker should be referred to his trade union or a lawyer.

Practically anything written by a physician may be the subject of 'discovery', that is, it may be sought by a legal process, reviewed by solicitors and scrutinized publicly in a court of law. An important exception is a report written by a physician specifically for the purpose of advising a lawyer in a case of litigation. However, because such a report is often, by its very nature, intended to help pursue or defend a claim it is often challenged in a court of law. It therefore follows that a physician must at all times exercise the highest standard of care and keep adequate and accurate written records. Thus all consultations should explicitly state the reason, relevant symptomatic and objective findings, the diagnostic and occupational implications, relevant advice imparted and to whom. A medicolegal report should be more detailed, with certain added elements. Thus it should contain a short statement of the credentials, that is the qualifications, relevant experience and employment status of the physician making the report. It should state why the report was commissioned and by whom. The written informed consent of the worker for this purpose must be obtained and appended. After basic personal and social details a detailed occupational, symptomatic and, if appropriate, past and family history is recorded. If the information comes from sources other than the patient, its respective origins should be defined. In many cases it is desirable to review general practice and hospital records and investigations before coming to a firm opinion. Physical examination is important, not merely to the extent that in ordinary medical practice it may establish a diagnosis but also to corroborate (to the limited extent to which this may be possible) the historical assessment. The results of relevant investigations of the patient or of the workplace, together with information regarding their source, should follow. Care must be taken to explain all of this in 'lay' terms so that lawyers and the court can understand it easily. An opinion on the diagnosis should follow, together with an interpretation of the likely causative or contributory factors. The estimated amount of dysfunction, disablement and handicap should be stated. The prognosis, expressed principally in terms of health risk, occupational and social handicaps should follow. Any factors that could have influenced the outcome or could do so at a later date should be stated. An indication of the level of certainty with which the respective conclusions are reached (again remembering that the legal test is the balance of probabilities), if necessary backed up by reasoned argument, is important.

In writing an expert's report the doctor should endeavour to answer all the questions posed by the respective lawyer in an adversarial system such as operates in civil cases in the UK or posed by the court itself as in an inquisitorial system which characterizes many legal proceedings elsewhere in mainland Europe. The doctor should not draw conclusions that cannot be justified. However, the report should address all points that appear to be relevant to the issue, even if they have not all been raised in the referring lawyer's or judge's questions. A useful attitude is to attempt to overlook the source of request for the report and to respond to it in a thoroughly professional and impartial manner, in the knowledge that what the court wants is an expert view of the truth rather than poorly justified support for the case of any of the parties. In England and Wales, reforms to the system require the parties to many disputes now to agree an independent expert whose report is to the court directly and who is required to make clear his or her impartiality.

CONCLUSION

In conclusion, although occupational medicine does not usually engage in therapeutic management of disease in the traditional manner of prescribing pharmaceutical remedies (nor of carrying out surgery), it has a great deal to offer by way of 'management'. This ranges from secondary prevention to rehabilitation and finally to assisting in the provision of compensation for the afflicted workers.

5

Assessment of the risk of work-related ill-health

SUMMARY

- In terms of prevention, it is probably more valuable for a physician to be involved in assessing workplaces prospectively than in carrying out regular health surveillance of workers. This chapter describes the principles of the disciplines that make the largest contribution to ensuring workplace health and safety, by first assessing the relevant risks. These include ergonomics and occupational hygiene, which overlap in some respects.

- Ergonomics is concerned primarily with interactions between man and the physical and psychological environment at work. Some knowledge of ergonomics is helpful to doctors working in industry, both as an aid to diagnosis and also to help in the planning of measures to prevent injury and psychological ill-health.

- Occupational hygiene is concerned mainly with measurement and control of harmful substances and certain physical hazards in the workplace. Thus, an understanding of occupational hygiene allows doctors to give sensible advice on the assessment of risk, and hence of measures to protect workers from harmful exposures.

- Biological monitoring and medical surveillance have an additional important role in the assessment of risks to health from work, after other feasible steps to assess and reduce risk to health have been implemented.

INTRODUCTION

While, in principle, all occupational injury and disease is preventable, in practice this means assessing the risks of injury and ill-health and taking balanced steps to reduce those risks so far as is reasonable and feasible. It is a responsibility of the occupational physician to urge management as far as possible in this direction. While many managers are sympathetic, and only a minority are careless of the welfare of their workers, their primary role is to make a profit or, at the least, to achieve a set financial target. It is a part of managerial decision-making to balance the cost of a particular decision against the likely benefits to the company. When it comes to deciding on measures to prevent ill-health, the equation becomes one of balancing the perceived costs of prevention against the cost of the perceived risk of occurrence. Prevention will usually only be implemented if it has a price tag that is reasonable when compared to the perceived benefits.

How then is the doctor's role fulfilled? An important aspect involves the diagnosis and management of occupational disease, as outlined in Chapters 3 and 4. Because many workplaces in the EU do not have access to an occupational health service (most in the UK do not), the general practitioner or the hospital specialist is often the first person to suspect occupational disease. That doctor is therefore able, by taking appropriate action, to prevent similar injury or ill-health occurring in other workers. Where the company or organization does have access to an occupational health service, preventive measures may be taken at an earlier stage, before ill-health has occurred, if the occupational health professional is aware of the possibility of risk and able to persuade managers to take appropriate action. Management of risk first involves its assessment, followed by planning of action to reduce it, implementation of the plan, and evaluation of the plan's success, just as management of disease first requires clinical assessment, followed by planning and administering treatment and follow-up. This simple logical approach is the basis of all preventive action in the workplace. The identification and assessment processes frequently require experience with a particular industry and with appropriate instruments for monitoring chemical and physical hazards. Some problems may be simple to resolve; others may require extensive and costly changes in plant structure and manufacturing/production process. Selection of appropriate working methods and good design of the workplace and working practices are the best solutions to any problem of workplace ill-health, but they often pose the greatest technical challenges to engineer and plant manager alike.

Most doctors learn something in medical school of the important roles played in disease prevention by improvements in social factors such as housing, sanitation and employment opportunities. Occupational ill-health is prevented in an analogous manner, namely by the improvement of relevant factors in the workplace. Proper design of jobs and of the place where work is undertaken will do much to prevent injury and accident – this is the business of the disciplines of ergonomics and safety management. Careful control of exposure to physical factors (essentially forms of energy) and to substances (usually chemicals but may include microorganisms) that may present a risk to workers is the business of occupational hygiene. These two disciplines operate within a legislative framework, which defines the duties and responsibilities of managers and workers within the workplace. The physician concerned with workplace problems needs to know something of ergonomics, occupational hygiene, and health and safety law, even though these are specialized areas with their own particular professional practitioners. In all cases training and education of workers and managers is crucially important.

It will be noted that the emphasis of this chapter is on prevention initially by assessing the workplace in a proactive manner with a view to making that workplace safer. This should not be a surprise, but many managers erroneously believe that prevention should be based rather on selection of the super-fit or disease-resistant at pre-employment examination. This is, of course, a misconception that flies in the face of efforts of doctors and others to rehabilitate less than fully fit people into the working population. Nevertheless, pre-employment assessment of appropriate people for certain types of work is sometimes necessary, and this is discussed in the next chapter.

Identification of safety hazards and assessment of the risks of adverse incidents such as falls, trips, burns and so on, fall primarily within the remit of the safety officer or the safety engineer. However, this function may fall to occupational health professionals in a number of contexts, either by default when there is no-one else to do it, or else opportunistically when something becomes apparent to the trained eye. Moreover, a doctor or a nurse when seeing a patient in a clinic can often elicit information on the factors contributing to a work-related accident or ill-health. The following cases give relevant examples, but elsewhere in the book this message is often reinforced.

ASSESSING THE RISK OF ACCIDENTS

Accidents at work are a common problem, and their apparent decline in frequency in developed countries such as in the European Union reflects more a change in the emphasis of work to service from manufacture, accompanied by an ever-increasing automation, than a substantial increase in safety consciousness in the workplace. Accident rates in heavy industry remain unacceptably high, the worst offenders being mining, agriculture, metal manufacture, railways and construction. However, no workplace is immune.

Case history 5.1

A physician was contacted by a nurse because an employee in the warehouse of a chemical factory had found a broken glass bottle in a box of miscellaneous chemicals and had contaminated his skin with its contents. The doctor was told that the box was labelled as containing ethyl acetate and the doctor could therefore reassure the nurse and the worker that cleaning of the skin with soap and water and attending to any glass cuts was all that was needed. However, as that bottle had broken, in similar circumstances another bottle might have broken – what could the implications of that have been? The physician asked to see a complete list of all the reagents within that box and other boxes like it, and found that the packing list included nitrogen mustards. These very potent alkylating agents, even in small quantities, can cause serious damage on contact with skin as well as possibly being associated with longer-term genotoxic and carcinogenic hazards. Clearly had one of these bottles been broken the consequences could have been very serious indeed. It was found that a risk assessment in relation to risk category of chemicals had not been undertaken because the company had focussed on the main feedstock products and by-products of its production, rather than the various chemicals used, usually in small quantities, by its research and development department. The physician therefore advised that the single generic assessment of all exposure to the pool of chemicals used by the development department (and the consequent identical packaging and handling policy) was inadequate. Because it was not feasible to carry out a detailed assessment for every chemical that the department might order, it was advised that generic assessments should be conducted by chemical grouping of chemicals. Thus alkylating agents and mustards would have a risk assessment process, and precautions for packaging, handling, etc., that would thenceforth take account of their substantially higher hazard when compared to most simple esters, ethers, ketones and alcohols.

The above case shows how a sentinel 'near miss' led to a systematic revision of the risk assessment process. Subsequent examples will illustrate principles of safety management, ergonomics and occupational hygiene.

Case history 5.2

An occupational physician called on a works manager in a large hospital (to discuss the rehabilitation needs of one of the workers). In the corridor outside he spotted a large yellow-coloured, compressed gas cylinder which unfortunately proved to be full and to contain chlorine. Naturally, immediate steps were taken to move the cylinder outside to the designated safe storage area.

This was an accident waiting to happen. What had gone wrong that could have resulted in catastrophic consequences? The hospital was responsible for chlorinating its own water supply and so received regular deliveries of chlorine. The delivery truck driver simply had a cylinder addressed to the 'Works Manager' and clearly had not been given any special training or clear explicit instructions about his responsibilities and the legal requirements for safe working practice. Therefore he simply took the cylinder to the receptionist in the Works Department, obtained a signature to confirm receipt and deposited it where he was asked to –'there in the corridor outside the Works Manager's office'. The consequences could have been disastrous – if the cylinder had a leaking valve, or had been accidentally knocked over as it stood vertical and unchained in the corridor, its valve could have been damaged to release poison gas through the whole office block!

This event prompted a revision of the risk assessment and safety management systems in that workplace.

Although dictionaries may define accidents as unforeseen events, this should not be taken to mean that they are unforeseeable. Their immediate causes are as varied as are accidents themselves, but ultimately, almost all can be traced back, with the advantage of hindsight, to the coincidence of two factors: an unexpected hazard and an unsuspecting human being. Although the science of risk assessment can produce estimates of the likelihood of events ranging from a worker tripping up and breaking a wrist to that of a jumbo jet crashing onto a nuclear power station, there nevertheless seems no limit to the capacity of man to defeat such predictions. Machines, like people, have an inherent tendency to go wrong, while people may misunderstand or, as in the case of the disastrous events in the USA on September 11th 2001, misuse them. Appropriate action can reduce the risks from both factors, designing safer workplaces and machines, educating managers and workers in safe practices, and reinforcing those messages by safety audits. While the responsibility is primarily managerial, doctors and nurses in industry may play an important role.

Unsuspected hazards

The greatest opportunities for accident prevention arise from the recognition of hazards. Some physical hazards are extremely obvious – scaffolding, holes in the ground, cables strewn across floors, moving machinery and poorly stacked materials, for example. Many become more hazardous as a consequence of a second factor – ice on steps, water on floors, strong winds when working at heights. Poor lighting and noise can mask danger signs and increase risk. All these are relatively easily predictable, and sensible precautions to reduce risk can be taken.

Rather less obvious is the hazard entailed by breakdown of systems. All complex systems, including human beings, have an intrinsic tendency towards disorder, known as entropy. This is demonstrable in people and animals by increased mortality and morbidity in the early stages and towards the end of life. In machines, for example cars and aeroplanes, the same phenomenon is observable with the highest risks of accidental breakdown being early on and after several years of use. It may be kept at bay in machines by regular servicing, a benefit not available to animals (save possibly the humans who receive replacement joints or organ transplants). The natural lives of machines are in general as predictable as those of human beings, as is the likelihood of breakdown of their various components. Thus it is possible to predict risks of accident resulting from such breakdown, although this process becomes extremely complex when systems comprising multiple interreacting structures and machines, such as an oil platform or a nuclear power station, are to be considered.

The keys to avoidance of a hazard are to appreciate its presence and to take appropriate avoiding action. Again this has two components – action by the person responsible for the presence of the hazard, such as the factory manager or the owner of the building, and action to avoid risk by those subjected to the hazard. Thus the risk imposed on individuals by a hazard is critically dependent upon the individual's perception of that risk and action taken to avoid it. Ultimately, when the engineer has completed the processes of designing and building the workplace, the machine or the system, risk depends on factors associated with fallible, often careless, human beings.

The unsuspecting human being

Accidents to people occur, by definition, when the person does not appreciate the risk. Many factors may contribute to this lack of awareness. Among the more important are the following factors.

Gender

In general females are less liable to accidental injury than males. Almost 90 per cent of fatal and 78 per cent of other reportable industrial injuries occur in males, even though the numbers employed are roughly equal. Of course, men tend to select themselves into more hazardous jobs, but even in the same industrial sectors, the gender difference persists. While some of this difference may be related to the fact that, even here, women have the less physical jobs, it seems likely that women take fewer risks than men and generally behave more sensibly.

Age

It might be thought that the young employee is at greater risk of industrial accident than the older worker, as is clearly the case with respect to traffic accidents. Younger people tend to be less experienced, somewhat more impetuous and perhaps have a greater fear of appearing cowardly and a greater tendency to show off. However, although the numbers of reported accidents are greatest in younger employees, when these are corrected for numbers employed in the respective age groups there appears to be little difference.

When age and gender are considered together, there is a tendency for male accidents to peak in the 25- to 34-year age group and for females this is in the 45- to 55-year group.

Industrial sector

Certain industries, as mentioned above, have high accident rates. While part of this is caused by the inherent dangers of the work, there is little doubt that careless behaviour is characteristic of some sectors. This is particularly marked in the construction industry, where neglect of safety precautions such as wearing hard hats or safety harnesses, and failure to shore up the sides of trenches are responsible for many serious injuries and fatalities. Such behaviour is associated with poor training and supervision of a workforce that is often transient and particularly insecure in its prospects of continuing employment.

Psychological problems

Concentration on the job in hand is clearly important at work, and any factors reducing such concentration may contribute to accidents. Episodes like this are probably more common than is realized. Family disputes, financial worries, depression and anxiety can all distract the minds of people at work and contribute to increase in risk from a hazard. Alcohol and drug abuse will have similar effects, and in the workplace the effects of hangover are well recognized as influencing accident liability. Lunchtime drinking will impair the efficiency of a manager; it may prove fatal to a worker exposed to moving machinery. Fatigue is particularly important, and this is reflected in regulations to limit the hours worked by lorry drivers and aeroplane crews. Somewhat belatedly, the importance of this has now been recognized with respect to hours worked by hospital doctors. Shift work has attracted much research with respect to fatigue and causation of accidents, with rather inconclusive results. It should be remembered by senior managers that rotating workers between day and night shifts is analogous to regular aeroplane flights to the Far East and back. If the manager has been heard to complain of jet-lag, then the situation of the workers may be appreciated. It would be expected that effects of shift work on accident rates would be related to fatigue resulting from loss of sleep and disturbed circadian rhythms.

The concept of accident proneness has also attracted research, but it is difficult to see a useful, practical outcome from this. In the unlikely event of such individuals being detectable at pre-employment examination, their exclusion from the workforce at risk would be likely to make no appreciable impact on accident statistics, while at the same time excluding many who would never have had an accident.

Management factors

Managers make the biggest contribution to accident causation. All accidents are, in theory, preventable by appropriate design of the workplace and the tasks within it, and by education and training of the workforce. Even when these steps are taken accidents occur when corners are cut to speed up a job or to facilitate it. When a company is under financial pressure it is likely that this pressure will be transferred down the line, mistakes will be made and accidents will increase.

Case history 5.3

A young man was working at a machine that compressed a mixture of two powdered metallic substances placed in a crucible. All such machines have a guard, which prevents access of hands into the press when it is being operated, and an interlock switch that prevents the machine being operated when the guard is open.

During the summer holiday period, the factory was short-staffed and this coincided with the need to fulfil an order to a tight timetable. The operator found he could keep to his schedule more easily if he overrode the interlock switch, allowing the guard to remain open during the compression. In putting the crucible into the press, he caught his fingers and required amputation of a terminal phalanx.

It may be seen from a case like this what opportunities are presented to lawyers, where a worker may blame a manager and a manager the worker. Both clearly contributed, the most important consequence being the lessons learned with respect to future prevention.

Communication failures

Failure of communication between people themselves, or between them and the machines or control rooms that they operate, is at the heart of many accidents. Avoidance of such failures lies in the realm of ergonomics. Failure may, for example, be a consequence of noise obliterating a warning signal, of incorrect or no messages passed from a manager or colleague to a worker, of a worker failing to understand a badly designed dial, or of a broken or defective signal. Well-known examples include railway train crashes where signals are missed and the *Herald of Free Enterprise* capsize, in which the officers on the bridge were not aware that the bow doors were still open as she set to sea; episodes similar to these but on a minor scale occur in workplaces daily.

Reporting accidents and ill-health

Accidents, which may be defined as unexpected occurrences usually involving injury or damage, are an experience common to us all. The attention of the media is attracted by serious and fatal accidents, especially if they are of a sensational nature. Such episodes, involving loss of life or major damage to property, are of course the tip of a very large iceberg. Fatal accidents attract publicity related more to their unacceptability to society then to their frequency – for example, death from a railway or aeroplane accident (all rare events) are consistently reported in all national papers and on television; deaths from especially gruesome murder are also widely reported; yet deaths in industrial accidents are often only reported in local newspapers.

Measurement of the frequency of accidents, ill-health and other untoward events in the workplace is essential at a national level. Managers of workplaces, aided by their occupational health and safety staff, have a responsibility to contribute to the national and supranational pool of information. For purposes of data collection, it is necessary to define certain types of occupational accident that require to be reported. Every country has its own system, the only consistency being in the reporting of fatal accidents. In the UK, for example, the following accidents are reportable, under the

Reporting of Injuries, Diseases and Dangerous Occurrences Regulations (RIDDOR), to the Health and Safety Executive:

- deaths arising out of a workplace accident
- major accidents, defined as a fracture of skull, spine, pelvis or a long bone, amputation of a hand or foot, loss of sight in an eye, or any accident requiring overnight admission to hospital
- injuries resulting in absence from work for more than 3 days
- episodes, such as leakage of explosive gas, explosions and collapse of structures, that had the potential to cause major injury but did not.

These regulations probably ensure consistent reporting only of the most serious accidents, those requiring a night in hospital or several days off work often going unreported. Behind the official figures lies an unquantified number of unreported and minor accidents. In a survey carried out by one of the authors, it was estimated that almost one in every 10 workers employed in the manufacturing industry and the agriculture/forestry/fishing sectors attends a hospital accident department each year for a work-related injury. Among these, some industries have very high rates of specific injuries; for example, in mechanical engineering, as many as 6 per cent of those employed suffer an eye injury requiring hospital attention each year. In the survey it was found that over 16 per cent of new attendees at the major regional accident department and almost 22 per cent of attendees at the corresponding eye casualty department had work-related injuries. However, because of its overall size, the service sector provided the largest total numbers of casualties of all the major industrial sectors.

Other obligations include the keeping of an 'accident book'. Thus, in the UK employees have a duty, under the Health and Safety at Work, etc., Act, to report to their employer accidents resulting in any injury; the employer in return is obliged to keep an accident book in a prescribed format. Details of the individual, the events surrounding the accident and action taken are recorded. If the employee claims industrial injuries benefit, the employer has to make a return to the Department of Social Security.

The reporting of an accident should not be the end of the process. All reports should result in investigation and preventive action. Both should be based on the matters discussed previously under accident causation. The investigation should take place as soon as possible after the event and should involve interviewing the victim (if possible), witnesses and supervisors or managers, and visiting the site of the accident. While it is a management responsibility, it should be made clear that its primary objective is not to apportion blame but to obtain information necessary to prevent recurrence. In the case of serious reported accidents, the Health and Safety Executive may also investigate the circumstances and, if the employer is thought to have been in breach of the provisions of the law, a prosecution may result. In general, however, the objective of all such investigations is prevention of future episodes. Serious accidents should always result in the production of a report detailing the steps to be taken in this direction.

Thus at factory, industry and national levels, statistics on frequency and severity of accidents are valuable indicators of the effectiveness (or lack of it) of preventive measures. The two components of interest, numbers of accidents and their severity, need to be related to the numbers at risk and the length of time over which people are at risk in order to give sensible information to managers when, as is usually the case, the size of the workforce fluctuates over time. The severity of accidents may be recorded by categorizing different types of injury or by recording indices such as hours or days lost from work.

ERGONOMICS

Ergonomics is concerned with the interaction between the worker and the job. The simplest definition of ergonomics is 'the science of making the job fit the worker'; another is 'the application of human sciences to the optimization of people's working environment'. Ergonomics seeks to improve the match between the job and man's physical abilities, information handling and workload capacities. The subject is synonymous with 'human factors engineering', a term used in North America. Its fundamental importance is recognized in the International Labour Organization, which defines ergonomics as 'the application of the human biological sciences in conjunction with the engineering sciences to the worker and his working environment, so as to obtain maximum satisfaction for the worker which at the same time enhances productivity'. This definition emphasizes the important triad of ergonomic elements: comfort, health, and productivity.

Thus ergonomics seeks to adapt work to human physical and psychological capabilities and limitations. In seeking this goal, it draws on many disciplines including anatomy, physiology, psychology, sociology, physics and engineering. Table 5.1 lists a few of the salient ergonomic hazards in the modern office environment – all doctors should be familiar with these hazards as offices are widespread work environments, in which even doctors spend a significant proportion of their time.

The value of ergonomics is easily understood by all of us who have tried to undertake a job using the wrong tools. The increased difficulty causes the job to take longer, leading to frustration and loss of temper. This, in turn, leads to use of excessive force and increases the risk of a slip of the hand and injury. In the wider world of industry and commerce, such problems arising from poor design of jobs, machines or workplaces may lead to large-scale inefficiencies, risk taking, increase in accidents and 'near-misses', and increases in absenteeism related to dissatisfaction with the job. The doctor working in industry, equipped with an understanding of ergonomic principles, is in a position to understand problems arising from interactions between people and

Table 5.1 *Ergonomic problems in the modern office environment*

Physical
Awkward postures of back, neck or upper limbs while at desk or elsewhere
Frequent repetitive movements at keyboard
Reflection from display screen, poor image contrast
Flicker from lights
Background noise
Unsatisfactory temperature and humidity, lack of control over these
Other people's smoke and other odours

Psychological
Demanding workload with competition for available time
Role conflict or ambiguity, especially for middle managers
Rivalries and animosities between workers
Fear of new technology
Lack of career prospects

their work, to plan solutions to such problems, and to help ensure that equipment is used safely and effectively. Knowledge of ergonomics may be of diagnostic value, for example in the investigation of musculoskeletal disease, of aid in management, as in rehabilitating someone with back pain, and helpful as an adjunct to other preventive measures, for example personal protective equipment will not generally be used unless it is acceptable to employees, by fitting comfortably and not interfering unduly with the task for which it is needed.

Case history 5.4

It was noted during a workplace visit that men working on coal silos were not wearing their safety harnesses. Failure to wear such equipment in the past had resulted in fatalities when workers had fallen and drowned or been crushed in the machine. The men said that the equipment was difficult to wear and in any case did not work properly. A study was planned in which workers were presented with the various types of safety harness available, asked to put them on, and were then hoisted up by a rope attached to a pulley. The results (Fig. 5.1) were revealing, most men having great difficulty donning the equipment, and often doing it incorrectly so that they slipped through or were caught in awkward positions.

The lesson of this simple experiment is that protective equipment needs to be carefully designed and re-assessed with the user in mind. In this case, new designs of harness were necessary, and the manufacturer needed to test these on a panel of relatively

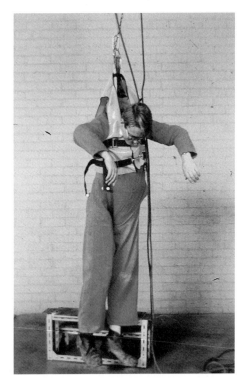

Fig. 5.1 *Consequence of inadequate design of safety harness and training in its use. See also colour plate 5.1.*

unsophisticated workers before releasing them on the market. In any situation when people interact with machines or equipment, the application of ergonomics can prevent later dangerous and perhaps fatal consequences.

Some of the tasks of ergonomics are to achieve optimal working conditions by seeking to reduce excessive workload, to improve working postures, and to facilitate cognitive and psychomotor functions in the handling of working instruments, including avoidance of unnecessary recall of information and the appropriate placement of workers. Ergonomics is best employed *de novo* in designing the job. By designing tasks with human needs clearly in focus much can be done to prevent problems before they arise.

The role of ergonomics in occupational medicine

Ergonomics is almost unique in that it holds hope not only of reducing risk of injury and accident, but also of increasing productivity. By carefully designing a workplace or a job, the worker may be both safer and more effective in the task. The role of ergonomics, therefore, should be relatively easy to sell to managers as a cost-effective means of improving safety.

Case history 5.5

A large and very expensive coalmining machine was designed to extract coal efficiently in difficult conditions underground. The engineering design was complex, but solutions were found and the machine was introduced into the workplace. Once in operation, it was assessed by a professional with expertise in ergonomics. A number of observations were made. The seat for the driver had been positioned in such a way that he was unable to see the drilling head when it was in action, thus requiring the use of an additional man as guide. The driver frequently had to stop the machine in order to stand up to see what he was doing. This failure to consider the sightlines of the operator was a fundamental design fault that cost money – in the need to employ another man and in the inefficiency of a stop-start operation. However, from a medical point of view, it also led to risk of accidents such as injury to the spotter by the machine itself or to the driver from frequent awkward movements. This latter problem was compounded by many other design faults in the layout and spacing of controls. As an example to designers, the ergonomist investigating this machine redesigned a man to fit easily into the machine and operate it (Fig. 5.2)!

In this example the problem was deemed insoluble by managers because of the large investment already made in the machine. However, the lesson could be learnt. Say an injury had occurred to the spotter, what actions might you reasonably urge on management in order to prevent recurrences?

Actions might be divided into immediate and long term. Immediate ones might include clear instructions and education on operation in the presence of a spotter, the use of video equipment instead of a man, and installation of emergency stop buttons. Long-term solutions would involve the provision of ergonomic guidelines for designers, so that future machines could be designed with the needs of the operator in mind. Such guidelines take account of the size, shape and capabilities of workers in relation to the required tasks.

From a medical point of view, the greatest contributions of ergonomics are apparent in the prevention of three very common work-related problems: accidental injury,

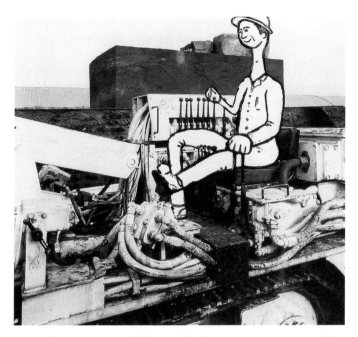

Fig. 5.2 *Man designed specifically by ergonomist to operate complex mining machine. (Courtesy of Mr Steve Mason and Mr Geoff Simpson.)*

musculoskeletal disease, and stress-related illness. When it is realized that these make up the bulk of work-related ill-health, it becomes clear that ergonomics has an important and generally, as yet, underutilized role in preventive workplace medicine. Sometimes a failure to apply ergonomics can have devastating consequences. Indeed, many of the major disasters that occur in industry can be traced back to a problem in the area of interaction between people and their workplaces.

A whole area of ergonomics concerns itself with the design of control systems, be they aeroplane cockpits or the control rooms of diving operations or nuclear power stations. It is not uncommon to find such complex arrays of dials and warning signals in the charge of a relatively unsophisticated worker, who has not been thoroughly trained, particularly with respect to emergency reactions. Proper design of such systems depends on an understanding of the capabilities and reactions of the operator, and training should involve practice in emergency responses, as in the flight simulators used by airlines.

Case history 5.6

Back injuries are the most frequent cause of long-term sickness absence in the mining industry. Contrary to popular conceptions, much of the activity underground relates to transport and the operation of complex machinery. As part of a systematic investigation of the ergonomics of underground transport, ergonomists found that cabs in some locomotives were designed with no thought to the dimensions or capabilities of the operators. Controls were badly sited (Fig. 5.3), access was difficult, and seats in the cab tended to be a pad of plastic material set on a metal ledge. The postures adopted in operating these machines were such as to suggest a high risk of back injury.

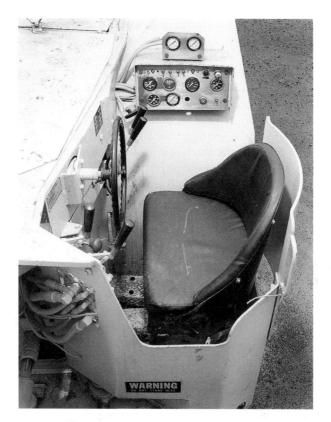

Fig. 5.3 *A badly designed workspace in an underground haulage machine.*

Anthropometric surveys of working miners allowed definition of the appropriate size of the cab, its furniture, controls and doorway. Subsequent redesign of new cabs, using this information, led to a much improved environment for the driver and also gave a potential commercial advantage to the manufacturer.

In carrying out such surveys, it is important to take account of factors such as clothing or protective equipment, which may limit reach and mobility, and the requirements of the task itself, which may require a particular type of person. For example, there is little point in trying to redesign the tasks in a rugby scrum so that the front row can be anything other than 100 kg mesomorphs – sometimes the task dictates the type of person required. However, in most cases in industry this does not apply, as efficient tools and good design of workplaces allow most tasks to be carried out by people of most shapes and sizes.

In some workplaces, problems are remarkably common. It is interesting that as work in the developed world has shifted from heavy physical activity into the office, so the complaints of work-related ill-health come increasingly from the latter source. The design of office work affords a good example of the application of ergonomics, as outlined in Table 5.1.

The office environment is based increasingly on electronic systems. While these have brought great efficiencies and benefits (who would now go back to retyping draft after draft of papers?), they have also brought problems as outlined in Table 5.1. Such problems tend to become focused in particular workplaces on one factor – for example, the visual display unit or the ventilation systems – and sometimes acquire notoriety as 'sick building syndrome'. A simple prospective assessment would be followed by advice on reducing risks (discussed in more detail in the next chapter). There are now well-established guidelines on the introduction and use of office technology based on ergonomic criteria; for example, the layout of screen, separate keyboard, document holder and chair should provide maximum flexibility so that the user can adapt them to personal requirements. The chair should be adjustable, stable but mobile, and usually have arm rests. The screen should be positioned so that it does not reflect light. Work should be arranged so that long continuous periods of keyboard operation are avoided, breaks being agreed during which other tasks (such as filing) are performed.

Psychological problems are less easy to predict, assess and prevent, depending largely on skilled management. One very important factor is consultation between managers and operatives before new systems are introduced, followed by a run-in period during which problems are dealt with and workers are given proper training. Only in these circumstances will the full benefits be realized and antagonism be avoided. It is extraordinary how often the authors have encountered intractable workplace problems stemming from neglect of this simple procedure, which sometimes stems from managers' own unfamiliarity with, and even fear of, new technology.

Ergonomics and illness assessment

While the primary role of ergonomics is in the prevention of work-related illness and accidents, it also has an important role in management of such conditions. Wherever ergonomic factors have played a part in causing symptoms, or run the risk of exacerbating them, alleviation is usually only possible if the job is redesigned or if the patient spends time off work, perhaps permanently. Again, musculoskeletal and psychological illnesses contribute the bulk of problems where job improvement is necessary and there is often overlap between these two categories.

Work may give rise to either acute or chronic musculoskeletal disorders. The acute damage is usually, though not necessarily correctly, attributed to an isolated incident of load handling, such as lifting a heavy load. The more chronic pattern of presentation arises from repetitive work/movements, sometimes known by the American term 'cumulative damage'. The 'acute' disorder may be a stage of a degenerative/cumulative process and so the two types tend to merge in practice.

The main sites of pain resulting from awkward postures or movements are the cervical and lumbar spine, the shoulders, elbows and wrists. Problems with the hips and other lower limb joints are much less common, although long-term degenerative disease of these joints may well be contributed to by physical activity at work. The interrelations between such activity and trauma are complex, as a reasonable level of activity is likely to be protective by ensuring good muscularity and, in early adult life, bone development. In women such activity probably also contributes to lessening risks of postmenopausal osteoporosis. The brunt of repetitive trauma seems to fall on the arms and spine, and is generally related to use of excessive force, often in an inefficient anatomical position. Again, what is excessive and what is inefficient are matters that may be defined by ergonomics.

Orthopaedic surgeons see a range of conditions affecting the musculoskeletal system, often apparently of mysterious aetiology. The workplace is one, though far from the only, cause of many of these syndromes. The general practitioner and the occupational physician tend to see conditions at an earlier stage in their development, when their effects and severity are insufficient to fit them into a clear diagnostic category. At this stage, the application of sensible ergonomic principles may often prevent serious injury or chronic disease.

Case history 5.7

A 55-year-old worker in a citric acid factory was employed in a process drying calcium citrate in a centrifuge. The material was caked to the sides of the tub of the centrifuge, and he had to break it up prior to shovelling it out. He consulted his general practitioner because of a painful right hand, which was impairing his ability to work, and was diagnosed as having trigger finger. The factory nurse suspected this might be related to his job, and asked the occupational physician to investigate. The patient had tenderness and crepitation over the palmar flexor tendons of his right hand, and obvious triggering of his right ring and little fingers. When asked to show the physician his job, he demonstrated how he repeatedly drove a chisel into the concretions of chemical, using the palm of his right hand to drive the chisel down. Study of the task clearly indicated the cause – the tools being used were not suited to the task, and a powered chisel was introduced. The worker was transferred temporarily to non-manual work and over the next 3 months his symptoms and signs gradually and completely disappeared.

Had such a patient been referred to a surgeon, who may have believed from reading the literature that work does not cause trigger finger, the outcome might have been less satisfactory and others might have developed the same condition. Many such syndromes may be seen in the workplace and their solution can be found by an ergonomic assessment. These pains may assume considerable significance to workers as a result of anxiety about possible long-term consequences, particularly when there is media publicity about such syndromes as 'tenosynovitis' and 'repetitive strain syndrome'.

As in the above example, the doctor becomes aware of an ergonomic problem when a patient presents with a complaint of ill-health. If the connection between job and illness is made, cure will depend on appropriate modification of the task. Consider the following case history.

Case history 5.8

Two ladies, one aged 20 years and the other 46 years, consulted their general practitioners. The younger had shoulder and neck pains, the older an acute attack of sciatica provoked by lifting a bicycle out of her car boot. Both were treated symptomatically and returned to their work in the hospital central sterilizing department. Their symptoms continued and they contacted their union representative, believing that their work was contributing to their problems.

The occupational physician was asked to see the two patients. He found no abnormal signs in the younger, while the older had some paraspinal muscle spasm and limited flexion, with a reduced straight leg raising test on the right. Both attributed their current symptoms to the use of a new washing machine in the department.

At this stage, what do you think is the appropriate action? What would you do if you were the doctor?

A detailed history revealed that the machine had been in place for about a month, and the workers were finding some difficulties in using it. One said that it was slower than the previous method, which had involved washing the theatre equipment by hand at a bench.

Clearly, a workplace visit was necessary. The physician asked what was the busiest time, and made the visit then – at 08:00 h the next day. He found that the machine had been introduced without attention to the size and strengths of the workers. Trays had to be lifted from the floor onto the belt of the machine, loaded at a height that was barely possible for the smaller workers, then unloaded at the far end in a mechanically inefficient position. The tray was then lifted off and carried to a trolley. The positions adopted were easily seen to put unnecessary strain on the back and shoulders (Fig. 5.4).

The machine was a big investment and was fixed. What could be done? In fact, the solutions were quite simple.

The physician noted that the heights of the workers, all female, ranged from 142 cm to 168 cm. The job rotation pattern required all to take a 2-week turn on the machine, loading for one week and unloading for another week, every 6 weeks. He suggested that trays were stacked on a table at the loading end, so no bending and twisting was required, the trays simply being carried across at chest height. A platform was recommended at the unloading end for the shorter workers, and the trays were

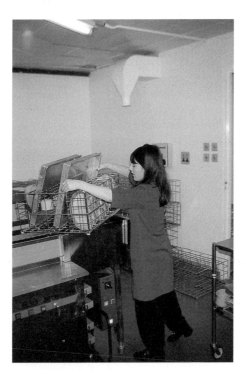

Fig. 5.4 *Bad ergonomics. A short operator in a hospital sterilizing department having to fill and empty trays on a washing machine at the extreme limit of her reach. See also colour plate 5.4.*

orientated so that articles were pulled out towards, rather than away from, the woman on unloading duties. Finally, the trolley was placed adjacent to the belt at the unloading end so that trays could simply be lifted across rather than carried.

Such common sense management hardly justifies the title ergonomics, but the benefits are potentially great. In this situation, one worker was at serious risk of recurrence of her sciatica (incidentally, she was transferred to lighter duties temporarily) and others were likely to develop intractable muscular discomfort, which would eventually lead to sickness absence, resignations and possibly litigation. All could have been prevented by application of ergonomics in the design of the job and the machine. It appeared, rather typically, that the machine had been designed by men for men!

Another point is raised by this story. The older patient went back to her work rather too early, prompted by the need to maximize her income. If you had been her general practitioner, and had some concerns about her ability to cope with a physical task, you would have had three options: to send her back and hope for the best; to advise her not to go back; or to contact her manager about a rehabilitation period. This last important, but rarely considered, option is discussed fully in Chapter 9. If, as in this case, the organization has an occupational physician, the patient could have been referred for an opinion.

OCCUPATIONAL HYGIENE

The discipline of occupational hygiene is concerned with the recognition, evaluation and control of hazard in the working environment. Its practitioners usually come from a background of chemistry, engineering or physics, although biologists and nurses are increasingly being attracted to the discipline. It is usual in large organizations for an occupational hygienist to work closely with physician, nurse and safety officer towards the common goal of ensuring a safe workplace.

The four essential stages to the practice of occupational hygiene are:

- recognition of hazardous work situations or practices
- measurement of the levels of the pollutant substance or physical energy
- design and implementation of control measures
- audit of effectiveness of controls.

Occupational medicine is almost unique amongst the medical specialties inasmuch as there are some areas of practice within it whereby a keen and astute practitioner should be able to identify a number of new causes of disease. Better still, the disease can be prevented. In identifying hazards and assessing risks some degree of lateral thinking and of logic by analogy may be needed. Consider the following example.

Case history 5.9

A practitioner involved with the aerospace industry was confronted by the use of novel chemicals – such as in paints and other applications on surfaces. No human data were available on these, yet it was clearly unsafe to equate 'absence of evidence' with 'evidence of absence'. After consultation with a colleague it was evident that some guidelines could be established as to which agents were likely to be harmful; for example if one looks at Fig. 5.5 a number of documented causes of occupational asthma feature on the right-hand column. They all seem to have two or more reactive nitrogen atoms usually manifest as amines or as other chemical groups. In contrast the chemicals in the left-hand column, although known irritants, do not seem to cause asthma. Therefore a useful guideline would be to consider those chemicals that are di or polyamines or azo-compounds, or similar entities, as posing a significant asthma hazard, even in the absence of evidence one way or the other. This enabled a ranking of the chemicals to be carried out for the purposes of determining which ones warranted specific health surveillance and special protective measures to reduce exposure. Ideally one would seek to substitute these compounds, but often the very chemical properties that make them pose a risk to humans are also the properties that made them attractive to industry because of their capacity to bind to other molecules and therefore result in high performance adhesives or coatings.

It is very important to re-assess the risks to the health of workers whenever there is a change in manufacturing process. Indeed this requirement is explicit in a range of legislation in the European Union. In the experience of one of the authors, a foundry company sold their site and premises, dismantled their equipment and moved to new

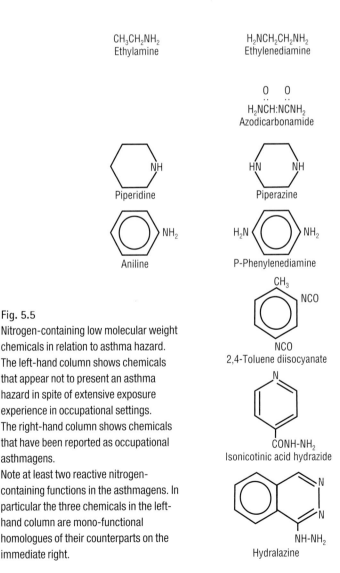

Fig. 5.5
Nitrogen-containing low molecular weight chemicals in relation to asthma hazard. The left-hand column shows chemicals that appear not to present an asthma hazard in spite of extensive exposure experience in occupational settings. The right-hand column shows chemicals that have been reported as occupational asthmagens. Note at least two reactive nitrogen-containing functions in the asthmagens. In particular the three chemicals in the left-hand column are mono-functional homologues of their counterparts on the immediate right.

premises about 5 kilometres away. They felt that they did not need to re-assess the airborne lead concentrations as they had not changed their equipment or methods. It required persistent persuasion from one of the authors to make them realize that they could not possibly guarantee an identical replication of the design or performance of the ventilation system, and therefore a re-assessment was mandatory. The following case shows the health consequences of a subtle change in process that had not been adequately re-assessed.

Case history 5.10

Employees in an establishment handling sterile products began to complain of irritation and rashes of the skin and face after opening and handling sterile packs. When the manufacturer was contacted they responded that the same product had been supplied for years previously without any such symptoms, and the plastic had not been changed. Moreover, they stated that the product was in use worldwide with no similar complaints. However, persistence on the part of the users and of their occupational physician paid off. The manufacturers acknowledged that the sterilization process for the product had changed from a heat (steam) sterilization to ozonization. Although there was no residual ozone in the product, it was possible that exposure to ozone had resulted in irritant epoxides being formed. Re-assessment of exposure and of symptom incidence was prompted. It was discovered that employees in at least two other plants elsewhere in the world had developed similar symptoms associated with this subtle change of product.

Case history 5.11

N-hexane is a neurotoxic solvent. It is metabolized by the body to the diketone 2,5-hexane dione, which can react with the terminal amino group of the amino acid lysine present in nerve sheaths. Within the same week an occupational physician came across instances of workers exposed to the solvent in two different workplaces. In one, the solvent was used in small quantities of up to 1 litre at a time, whereas in another the standard batch used of the order of 1 tonne of the solvent.

In which one of these contexts would one expect the higher exposure to have arisen? Although the answer might appear obvious at first, not enough information has been provided so far to reach the correct conclusion.

Actually, exposure was significantly higher in the first workplace where an impact adhesive dissolved in a mixture of n-hexane and solvent was used to stick laminated veneers into chipboard surfaces. It was applied by hand using a paintbrush. The worker had to bend over to adjust and trim the veneer and clamp it into position. There was no local exhaust ventilation and even general ventilation was poor – the place stank of solvent. In the second workplace solvent extraction was undertaken in a large enclosed vessel that was supplied with solvent automatically through a piped system. The solvent was heated with a steam jacket and returned to the vessel via a large water-cooled condenser. The whole system was closed except for a safety vent from the circuit directly to the outside, distant from the workplace (which was well ventilated in any case).

Recognition

The methods of approaching and examining a workplace have been outlined in Chapter 3. Each stressor or pollutant in the working environment can be classified into one of several classes.

1. **Physical.** These agents include noise and vibration, visible and ultraviolet light, microwaves, ionizing radiation and heat and cold, dependent on incident energy for their effects. In this category of physical hazards one may include the biomechanical stresses, of primary interest to ergonomists, discussed above.
2. **Chemical.** The worker may be exposed to inorganic and organic chemicals in a diversity of physical states as dust, fume, gas, vapour and mist. The toxic agent must gain access to the body, usually by inhalation or percutaneously, in order to have a significant health effect. In each occupational setting, the risk to the individual arises as a function of toxicity and the level of exposure, which determines the dose over time. Not only must the toxic agent be present, but also it must be absorbed in sufficient quantities to create a toxic effect at the critical organ.
3. **Biological.** Biological agents may cause illness in consequence of their infective or toxic nature, or of their capacity to act as antigens and produce a harmful immune response. In recent years biological agents have achieved greater prominence in the workplace, most notably *Legionella* spp. in air-conditioning systems, and the viruses responsible for hepatitis B and HIV, a source of concern for healthcare and some public service workers. The importance of animal and plant antigens, especially the former, as sensitizers has been recognized more widely also.
4. **Psychological.** Stress in the workplace is responsible for much ill-health, as has been discussed in Chapter 2 and in the section on ergonomics.

Evaluation

In Chapter 3 we discussed how to approach a workplace visit. Often the assessment of risk from perceived hazards depends on some form of measurement of the workplace environment. In making such measurements, the hygienist (or ergonomist) will bear in mind the type of hazard and its possible effects on workers. It will also be necessary to know something of the variability of the hazard over time and of any measures taken to protect workers. What ultimately is important is the dose of hazardous agent that the individual takes up, and which is determined by exposure. However, individual susceptibility to a given dose may vary considerably.

Sampling

In order to evaluate risk, the first requirement is to obtain representative measurements in relation to the activities of workers. This is not possible without a detailed knowledge of the whole of the task performed by individuals.

Not infrequently an otherwise apparently safe process becomes unsafe as a consequence of a seemingly trivial procedure.

Case history 5.12

A young man presented to his doctor with a history of nervousness, frequency of micturition and trembling. He had associated this with his work, which involved testing samples of oil for gas content. The process was enclosed and took place under mercury, which he injected from a container. Great care was taken to monitor air levels of mercury in the workplace and blood and urine samples from the workers were also being monitored regularly. His had shown a steady and unexplained rise.

On detailed review of his work, it transpired that at the end of each analytical procedure it was necessary to flush any residual gas out of the enclosed system. This was done in such a way that any residual mercury could have volatilized and been discharged into the air of the workplace. Indeed such transient peaks were apparent on close inspection of the monitoring records. Subsequent control of this part of the process alleviated the problem.

This case history illustrates that a meticulous approach to assessing working practices is essential to good preventive occupational medicine. Even regular monitoring may be insufficient if inadequate attention is paid to its siting, timing or, as in this case, the results.

Measurement of environmental hazards ideally might be made continuously, on-line, from multiple fixed points where the hazard is estimated to be most likely to be present. Such systems were widely introduced for the measurement of vinyl chloride monomer in PVC plants after the risk of hepatic angiosarcoma was recognized. Levels above those allowed would then trigger an alarm and allow prompt action to be taken. Similar systems are in use, for example, for gases in mining and the petrochemical industries. At the other extreme of sampling strategy, one may use a wide array of portable equipment to measure gases, noise, radiation and so on. A number of the commonly used pieces of apparatus are illustrated (Fig. 5.6).

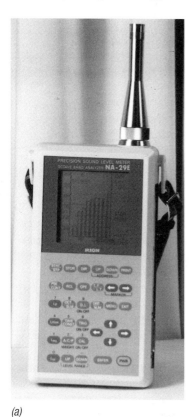

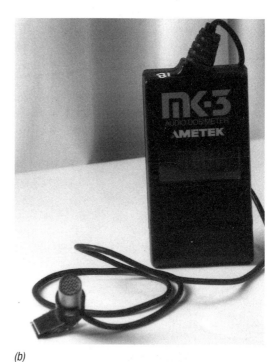

(a)   *(b)*

Fig. 5.6 *(a) Sound level meter with octave band analyser. Used to measure the sound level and frequency spectrum at a fixed location. (b) Personal sound dosimeter, which is used to measure average sound level for an individual worker. The microphone can be clipped close to the ear and the electronic unit attached to the wearer's belt. (continued)*

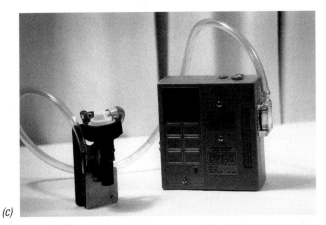

(c)

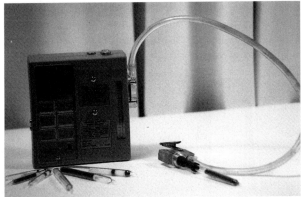

(d)

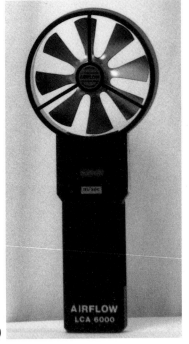

(e)

Fig. 5.6 *(continued) (c) Personal sampling pump and sampling head for respirable dust. The pump can be clipped to the wearer's belt and the sampling head attached to the lapel, close to the nose and mouth. The dust is collected inside the sampling head on a filter paper. (d) Personal sampling pump and sampling head for gases and vapours. The pump unit is the same as for dusts, although operated at a lower flow rate. The sampling head consists of a glass tube containing an adsorbent, specific to the gas or vapour being sampled. A selection of adsorbent tubes is used to measure average air velocity at the entrance to fume cupboards and other ventilation systems. (e) Vane anemometer, used to measure average air velocity at the entrance to fume cupboards or other ventilation systems. (continued)*

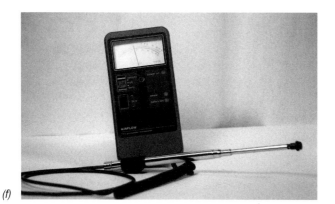

(f)

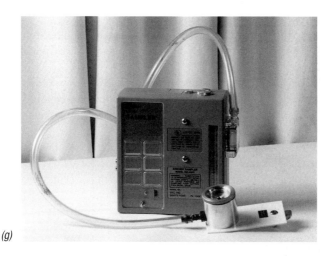

(g)

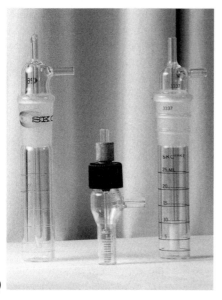

(h)

Fig. 5.6 *(continued) (f) Hot wire anemometer used to measure air velocity in ventilation ducts and other moving air streams.*
(g) Personal sampling pump and sampling head for lead dust. The pump can be clipped to the wearer's belt and the sampling head attached to the lapel, close to the nose and mouth. The dust is collected inside the sampling head on a filter paper. (h) Glass impingers and bubblers, used with a pump to collect gases or vapours and some particles. The glass tubes are filled with an appropriate absorbing solution and air is then passed through the liquid. (Photographs courtesy of Dr John Cherrie.)

Because it is the dose of the hazard that reaches the worker that is important, personal sampling devices are available for a wide range of chemical substances and physical hazards. The most familiar to a doctor is the radiation badge (or personal dosimeter), which measures cumulative exposure to ionizing radiation. Personal noise meters are also available. Gas and dust samplers are usually operated by a pump, attached to the belt, sucking air through a tube of absorbent granules or a filter device on the worker's lapel. Methods for assessing skin exposure to chemicals are currently underdevelopment.

Standards

The act of sampling workplace air of course implies that the measurements obtained mean something in terms of threats to health, in the same way as measurement of blood constituents indicates disease in a patient. There thus needs to be some guidance on the harmfulness of specific levels of toxic substances. While it could be argued that the only safe level of, say, mercury, is no mercury, such guidance lacks practicality in many workplace situations.

A small number of carcinogenic substances are regarded as too toxic to handle, and are therefore banned, but most other harmful substances are believed safe enough to use if levels are kept below a stated maximum. The concept that there is for such substances a threshold, below which harm is unlikely to occur, gave rise to the term **threshold limit value** (**TLV**), which is still used in the USA. Two sorts of TLV are published in that country for a wide range of airborne substances – one that gives a figure averaged over an 8-hour period, and a short-term (or ceiling) value that should not be exceeded over a short period.

In the UK, legislation has moved the focus of adequate control from compliance with an **Occupational Exposure Limit** (**OEL**) standard to applying principles of good practice for the control of exposure to 'substances hazardous to health'. Ostensibly this brings all such substances within the definition of adequate control, regardless of the routes of exposure and whether or not they still have an OEL (about 100 no longer do). Employers have to ensure that these new OELs called **Workplace Exposure Limits** (**WELs**) are not exceeded and that exposure to substances that can cause occupational asthma, cancer, or heritable damage to genes is reduced as low as is reasonably practicable.

Standards of whatever type vary from country to country, and from time to time within a country. They are based upon a combination of epidemiological and experimental evidence as far as possible, but ultimately are often arrived at through discussion, speculation and consideration of safety factors in the absence of any human toxicology or epidemiology. Moreover, economic factors, namely the extent to which industry or society can afford to comply, often influence the setting of an exposure limit. They should therefore be looked upon as guidance for control measures rather than as absolute 'safe levels', and steps should always be taken to keep actual levels as far below such standards as practicable.

Health surveillance

In assessing the risks to health from work there is a whole spectrum of approaches. On the one hand the best way of preventing ill-health is to conduct a prospective assessment of risks even before any workers have been exposed. Clearly, however, this is fraught with difficulties because of lack of information and may be built on some very tenuous assumptions. Further along the line, one may measure exposures to hazardous agents or substances such as noise, dust or radiation in a way that would permit the assessment of risks and therefore lead to steps to reduce further risks before any damage to human health had occurred. If conducted properly and early one should be able to identify an increase in uptake of a harmful substance before it has produced any significant harm; this is the main principle behind biological monitoring.

Health surveillance can be defined in various ways. Classically it has been understood to comprise those strategies and methods to detect and assess systematically the adverse effects of work on the health of workers. It has, however, also been used to include systematic assessments of fitness for work, and/or of health status, that are not directly related to occupation. The following examples relate to the use of the term in the context of the assessment of the uptake of, or adverse health effects from, exposures in the workplace. Within this term one can include:

- biological monitoring, where the agent or a metabolite of it is measured
- biological effect monitoring, where a physiological consequence is measured even if this is not manifest as ill-health
- other forms of surveillance, where ill-health is systematically sought, often through the use of health questionnaires, examination or other clinical methods ('medical surveillance').

Case history 5.13

Workers in a non-ferrous foundry making plumbing fittings were exposed to lead-containing alloys (Fig. 5.7). Although measurements of airborne concentrations of lead were made from time to time, these could not be assumed to reflect uptake accurately, because of factors such as skin contamination, and hence uptake of lead through eating or smoking. Thus as prescribed by law as well as by good occupational health practice, the assessment of the risks to the workers' health included regular measurements of blood lead. The results of the two main categories of workers are shown in Figure 5.8.

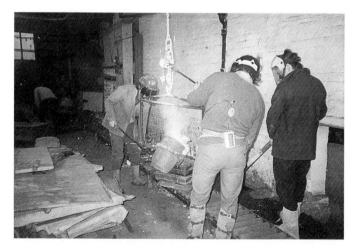

Fig. 5.7 *Foundry workers subject to health surveillance since they are exposed to lead fume from pouring molten metal into casts. See also colour plate 5.7.*

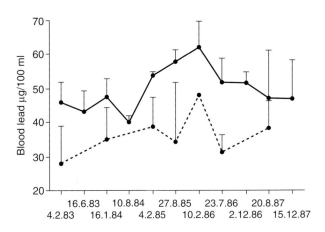

Fig. 5.8 *Blood lead levels of foundry workers. (Solid line refers to workers in melting and casting while the broken line relates mainly to fettlers.)*

As can be seen, one group had appreciably higher blood lead levels, although neither gave cause for complacency. The group with the higher lead levels consisted of workers exposed to lead fume through melting and casting (as distinct from the other group who finished the cooled product). The results of the assessment shown prompted measures for better control of exposure at source, and especially improved local exhaust ventilation. Assessments were still needed at regular intervals until the factory ceased operation.

Case history 5.14

Workers were employed from time to time on a batch process manufacturing a potent anti-cholinesterase. The process was not completely sealed and in parts of it material had to be handled (using an air hood, gloves and other protective equipment) as part of the purification process. From the occupational health standpoint, concern was expressed regarding the potential for serious harm from exposure to the compounds. Management offered the reassurance of the 'full personal protection' and the fact that there had never been any serious instances of poisoning save only people complaining of transient blurring of vision on one or two occasions. However, for good practice this reassurance is not adequate – the need was for direct measurements of exposure to any poison, whether airborne or by skin contact. Unfortunately there were no suitable assays for the substance in question. The physician was concerned there might be biological effects, falling short of overt symptoms, and yet which might be harbingers of more severe consequences later. Therefore he recommended a biological monitoring exercise. This was to consist of blood samples taken from the eight operatives before the commencement of the batch processing, and then at intervals thereafter – with the exercise spread out over a number of weeks. The physician used some of his own blood and also persuaded the chief first aider (who worked elsewhere in the plant) to provide a second control sample on each of the sampling occasions. The identities of the exposed workers and the two controls were obscured and the samples were sent for analysis. Encouragingly, results from the subjects were within normal limits for pseudo-cholinesterase.

There are several lessons to be learned here. There are number of situations in which it is not feasible to monitor exposure concentrations of harmful substances, and therefore one has to rely on some form of biological monitoring or health surveillance. This is especially important where exposure may occur through extraneous routes. Besides the individual variable, exposure, there may be wide individual variation in physiological manifestations as illustrated by this case. The samples therefore need to be taken with appropriate controls (and perhaps sending some blind duplicates to assess laboratory quality). In the above example it was not possible to measure the harmful agent itself nor any of its metabolites in the human body, and therefore it was necessary to measure the biological effect in the hope that this is sensitive enough to identify risks before harm to health results.

There are circumstances in which risk to a working community as a whole is measured, systematically identifying ill-health in individuals – this is called health surveillance. In a sense one could argue that this consists of shutting the stable door after the horse has escaped. However, there are circumstances in which such surveillance is an essential part of the process of protecting workers; for example, exposures to allergens or certain mineral dusts in mining may not be able to be reduced to concentrations at which all individuals are guaranteed protection. In these circumstances, surveillance allows the earliest symptoms to be detected and action to be taken to prevent progression. In the case of occupational asthma, an early indication of rhinitis may be sufficient to alert the doctor or nurse that sensitization has occurred, while in preventing pneumoconiosis, early X-ray changes will allow change of job and prevention of serious disease. This process is known as secondary prevention. The detection of one such case may moreover alert management to a problem and allow steps to be taken to protect other workers.

Before implementing health surveillance the physician should ensure that workers and managers understand the purposes and criteria and the properties of the techniques as listed below:

- **Purposes of health surveillance** are:
  - protection of health of the individual employee
  - detection of any adverse health effects at an early stage
  - detection of hazards and assessment of risk
  - assisting in the evaluation of control measures
  - reassurance of workers potentially exposed to hazards.
- **Criteria for conducting health surveillance** are:
  - there is an identifiable disease or other identifiable adverse health outcome
  - the disease or health effect may be related to exposure
  - there is a possibility that the disease or health effect may occur
  - there are valid techniques for detecting indications of the disease or health effects
  - appropriate measures can be taken to reduce risk if necessary.
- **Health surveillance techniques** should be:
  - sensitive
  - specific
  - easy to perform and interpret
  - safe
  - non-invasive
  - acceptable.

The specific health surveillance techniques to be used depend on the specific exposures and risks but may include the following:

- **Biological monitoring**, e.g. 2.5-hexane dione (a metabolite of *n*-hexane) in urine; COHb in workers exposed to methylene chloride.
- **Biological effect monitoring**, e.g. cholinesterase in blood of workers exposed to certain organophosphorous pesticides.
- **Enquiries, inspection or examination by a suitably qualified person**, e.g. an occupational health nurse administering a questionnaire for symptoms of asthma or rhinitis; or examining the hands for dermatitis.
- **Medical surveillance**, e.g. lung function measurement in workers exposed to substances known to cause occupational asthma; chest X-rays in workers exposed to respirable quartz.
- **Monitoring of sickness absence** – review by the Occupational Health Service for work-related trends in sickness absence.

CONCLUSION

In conclusion, assessment of risks to health from work should best be undertaken prospectively before any worker is exposed. It should start with identifying physical, chemical, biological and psychological hazards ('the possible') and then proceed systematically to identifying the likelihood of harm ('the probable'). Sciences such as safety engineering, ergonomics and occupational hygiene have an important role in this assessment. Re-assessment at regular intervals continues as long as employees are exposed, in a manner appropriate to the risk. Sometimes this entails measuring the uptake of toxic substances, their biological consequences and adverse health effects throughout the working population as an adjunct to other forms of assessment. In any case assessment is never an end in itself but always a means towards reduction in risk. Therefore this chapter and the next are inextricably linked.

6

Reduction of the risks of work-related ill-health

SUMMARY

- All stakeholders, ranging from employers to employees, doctors to politicians, have a role in reducing the risks of work-related ill-health. The first steps to achieve this include debate, a common consensus and attitude resulting in sound policy.

- Elimination of hazards, or at least their substitution by less harmful ones, is an important first step. This applies equally to ergonomics, physical, chemical or biological safety and psychosocial hazards.

- Reduction of exposure and hence of risk can be achieved by segregation, exhaust ventilation or other means depending on the hazards concerned.

- In special circumstances, such as for prevention of the adverse consequences of exposure to biological agents, immunization may play an important role in complementing other measures.

- Although personal protection may have a very important role, its limitations must be understood and it should not ordinarily be relied upon as the first or the main line of defence. This is equally true of psychologically analogous forms of personal protection, such as 'coping strategies', or of post-exposure management such as therapy for 'post-exposure prophylaxis'.

- Although training is very important throughout, it too is of limited benefit if applied to individuals without the appropriate organizational and background risk reduction measures.

- Pre-employment selection has a limited role in reducing the risks of work-related ill-health and, like personal protection, cannot be utilized as a mainstay of risk reduction.

- Legislation is an essential buttress for all of the above – but an improvement in societal attitude must be aspired to.

INTRODUCTION

While the management of cases of occupational disease involves an important element of prevention, the systematic reduction of risks of occupational disease and injury is a novel, or at least nebulous, concept to many clinicians. This chapter provides an insight into risk reduction as a means of preventing occupational ill-health. It starts, following good occupational health practice, by discussing how risks can be reduced in the workplace environment by reducing exposure to harmful substances and physical hazards – thus adding to the concepts of occupational hygiene in the preceding chapter. Then it addresses the reduction of ergonomic risks and of accidents. It goes on to address steps that are specific to certain workers, including immunization, and the role of pre-employment selection. Finally, it illustrates the role of legislation in the prevention of work-related ill-health.

CONTROL OF EXPOSURE TO HARMFUL SUBSTANCES AND PHYSICAL HAZARDS

When asked to discuss methods of preventing occupational disease, most doctors and students instinctively start by mentioning methods of personal protection, such as ear muffs or respirators.

Think for a moment why this is the wrong approach. Say, for example, a farmer had told you to use an arsenic-containing chemical to kill the parasites on his flock of sheep during a summer job as a student, what measures might you sensibly have taken to protect yourself? Personal protection has several disadvantages – it is never 100 per cent efficient (and uncommonly even 50 per cent); it relies on the full cooperation of the wearer; it requires careful maintenance; it may interfere with the task; and it may induce complacency. Better surely, in our example, not to use arsenic. Substitution of safer for less safe substances is the first step to consider. Other steps may include enclosure of processes and exhaust and dilution ventilation.

Case history 6.1

A 53-year-old librarian, who had been in the same job for about 19 years, began to complain that soon after the start of her working day her eyes became watery and her nose started to itch. As the day progressed, her chest felt tight as though she had a 'chesty cold'. She was symptom-free at weekends and her symptoms started to improve within an hour of getting home on workdays. She attributed her symptoms to the turning up of the ventilation in her library about a month previously. She was asked to keep a record of peak expiratory flow at approximately 2-hourly intervals for 4 weeks. This showed an approximately 20 per cent variability between her maximum and minimum peak flow readings and her values were slightly worse during the working week when compared to the weekends. The particulate pollution concentrations in the library were measured using a continuous sampling infrared scattering device. This showed marked rises in dust concentrations from approximately 10 micrograms per cubic metre at baseline up to around six times higher values whenever the ventilation was switched on. Attempts at identifying specific aeroallergens were unsuccessful. The ventilation system was overhauled and found to be heavily soiled, with contaminated filters, evidence of fungal overgrowth and other debris. The system was thoroughly cleaned and a regular service and maintenance schedule instituted. She resumed work and became completely symptom free and has remained well since.

This case shows how simply taking the history of a symptomatic worker, drawing a working conclusion as to the likely cause, and then implementing simple commonsense steps (in this case cleaning out the air conditioning and ventilation system) resulted in an effective improvement in the health and working conditions of the employee. In the above case there were two useful lines of supporting evidence inasmuch as peak flow readings confirmed the temporary relationship of the patient's symptoms with her work, and the dust measurements also showed that the air conditioning and ventilating system, far from improving the environment, was actually polluting it. In spite of attempts at identifying an aeroallergen through the use of Petri dishes with culture media and other approaches not described in detail here, this final link in the chain was never conclusively proven. In practice one often has to accept that not all the pieces of the jigsaw puzzle can be found, yet enough can be identified to permit control methods to be employed to safeguard the health of the employees. In the above case one could argue that even if the peak flow readings were not conclusive, and if no particulate pollution measurements had been carried out, it would still have been the management's responsibility to clean out and service an air-conditioning and ventilation system that was long overdue in terms of maintenance. This is especially so when a worker complained of a clear temporary relationship between her symptoms and the exposure to the air flow.

Case history 6.2

The sister in a gastroenterology unit became unable to enter the endoscopy suite, for which she was responsible, because of rhinitis, lacrimation and wheeze. She reported that she had been obliged to delegate cleaning of the endoscopes to a staff nurse, who developed similar symptoms. Others in the unit complained of sore eyes. The cause was glutaraldehyde (which was considered necessary to prevent possible transmission of hepatitis B and HIV) used in an open container and syringed down the endoscopes. The occupational physician watched the whole procedure, which involved at one stage holding the endoscopes up at arm's length, the glutaraldehyde running down the arm of the nurse. He advised on the provision of an exhaust ventilation cabinet, equipped with appropriate sinks. The doctors on the unit preferred to purchase a special machine for washing the endoscopes – this did the job more efficiently but did not eliminate the source of exposure, and ultimately exhaust ventilation was installed over the machine itself.

This story illustrates the fact that the obvious solution is not always the best one. Prior to the request for advice from the occupational physician, the unit staff had decided that better ventilation was the answer, and had the hospital engineer install an extractor fan. Unfortunately this was put in the ceiling, about 3 metres above the source of vapour, and simply drew air from the door 6 metres away to the ceiling, leaving the vapour to eddy around the nurse's face. Then the consultants thought that if the process were automated, exposure would cease. This did not take account of the facts that the machine had to be filled and emptied and that vapour of glutaraldehyde was able to escape from it. To avoid contact between people and vapour, it was necessary for the vapour to be drawn away from the person, and an extractor cabinet was an effective way of doing this. One final problem occurred in this extraordinary episode – an ergonomic one. In spite of advice on design, the engineers built a cabinet with the sink so far to the rear that the nurses, who were of short stature, had to put their upper body inside to reach it (Fig. 6.1)! Fortunately this was spotted before the unit was used and was able to be corrected.

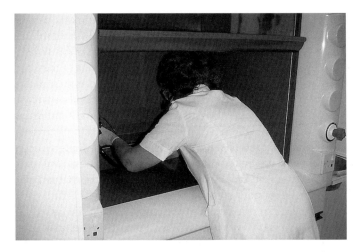

Fig. 6.1 *Fume cupboard in endoscopy unit – designed so that nurses have to put their heads inside in order to wash endoscopes! See also colour plate 6.1.*

Case history 6.3

A small dental surgery employed ten staff in a clinical capacity. The occupational health nurse for that area who was responsible for several healthcare premises saw two employees with possibly work-related respiratory symptoms and alerted the physician. On further systematic enquiry they found that six of the clinical staff (dentist, nurses and hygienists) had respiratory symptoms and most of them had consulted their general practitioners because of these over the previous months. The symptoms had been ascribed to diagnoses such as 'persistent cold', 'sinusitis', and 'wheezy bronchitis'. Assessment of the workplace identified that the staff had been cleaning/sterilizing surfaces using an aerosol spray of unclear composition, and symptoms had dated back to the introduction of this technique. The manufacturers were asked what the preparation contained and, in particular, whether it contained known irritants or sensitizers such as aldehydes. At first they denied this but later admitted that the preparation did contain glutaraldehyde. Substitution of this method of surface cleaning by the use of 'wipes' containing quaternary ammonium detergents and applied with appropriately gloved hands resulted in resolution of the symptoms and prevention of further similar ill-health.

The principles of control of exposure to harmful substances are listed here.

1. **Substitution** of a less harmful for a more harmful substance or operation. Important examples in industry have been the substitution of toluene or cyclohexane for benzene, chalk for talc and mineral wools for asbestos. Where the harm comes from a contaminant or a by-product, for example benzidine in organic dyes, it may be possible to specify a maximum content of the contaminant. Noise injury may also be prevented by specification in the design of new machinery.

2. **Segregation** of workers from the source of harm. This may be by time or distance, as in mining where workers retire to a safe distance at the time of blasting, and when such operations take place on shifts when fewer workers are about. More commonly, however, it involves enclosure of the process so that there is a physical barrier between the source of harm and the workers.

3. **Local exhaust ventilation** is used where the above methods are impracticable. Ideally it is combined with partial enclosure of the process, as in the familiar fume cabinet. Alternatively, the ventilation is applied very close to the point of generation of the dust or vapour. The air velocity required to draw the substance away is called the capture velocity, and this depends on the physical characteristics of the substance and the mechanisms of its release. It is intuitively obvious that lower velocities are needed to clear evaporating chemicals than particles generated by blasting or drilling.

4. Reduction of airborne levels of substances by **dilution ventilation or precipitation**. A familiar example is the use of water and high airflows in mines to reduce dust levels. Electrostatic forces may also be used to reduce levels of dust, commonly in preventing pollution by smoke stacks.

5. **Personal protection.** The law generally requires all reasonable efforts be made to engineer the hazard out or to shield individuals from it. Only then is it permissible to resort to personal protection. Most such devices are not comfortable for long-term use and give only partial protection. Included in this category are respirators, protective clothing and gloves, eye shields and hearing defenders. Clearly in some circumstances they are mandatory – eye protection in welding and metal work, ear muffs in caulking (which today means hammering metal in ships' hulls), and so on. However, they should never be relied upon as the sole, albeit cheap, method of protecting workers. Where they are used, care should be taken in their design, in terms of comfort and wearability, as well as in their efficiency in terms of protection. Some forms of personal respiratory protection are illustrated (Fig. 6.2).

6. **Education and good housekeeping** remain important principles of prevention in all circumstances. Workers should be made aware of dangers by instruction, notices, codes of practice and safety audit. Similarly, managers should be trained in their responsibilities in these respects. Good housekeeping, keeping chemicals in safe places, not leaving dangerous materials (or indeed any materials) lying about, making sure that everything is clearly labelled, vacuuming floors and benches after use, and other such measures will reduce risks of illness and accident and will ensure that everyone is safety conscious.

Problems with control measures

None of these methods is flawless and several should normally be used in combination. Can you think of problems with each of them? After you have considered this – read on: some real-life examples may surprise you.

Substitution

The widespread substitution of solvents such as toluene and white spirit for the leukaemogenic benzene has given rise to the concept of 'safe' solvents. However, these substances are only relatively safe, and their uncontrolled use may lead to neurological or psychological disease, as described in Chapter 2. Similarly, certain fibrous minerals used as substitutes for asbestos may themselves have carcinogenic potential, and require careful handling.

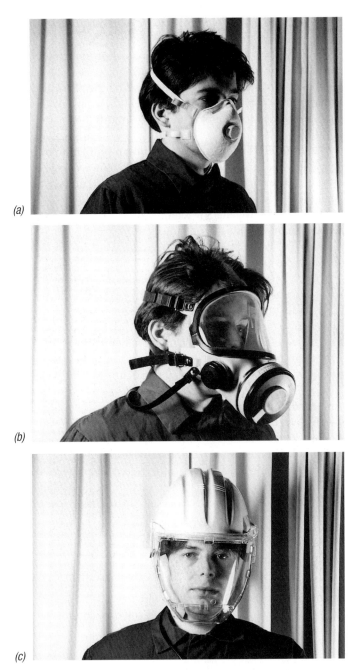

Fig. 6.2 *(a) Filtering facepiece respirator to provide a moderate level of protection against dusts and other aerosols. (b) Full-face powered respirator which will provide a high degree of protection against dusts and other aerosols. (c) Powered helmet respirator. Air is drawn from behind the head, filtered to remove any particles and blown over the face. The unit also provides head protection and a visor to protect the face. (continued)*

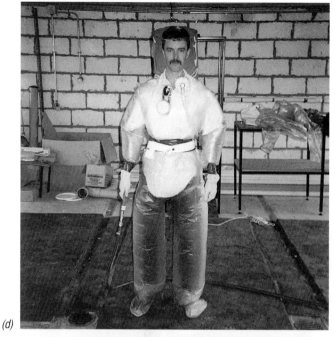

(d)

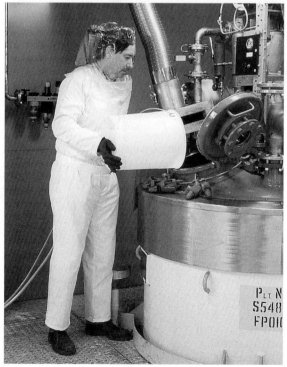

(e)

Fig. 6.2 *(d) Ventilated suit used to provide higher level of respiratory and body protection against radioactive dust. (e) Personal protection including breathing air being delivered through an air hood in the chemical industry. Note also local exhaust ventilation through a flange overlying the reaction vessel next to the potential emission source. (Photographs courtesy of Dr John Cherrie.) See also colour plates 6.2(d) and (e). (continued)*

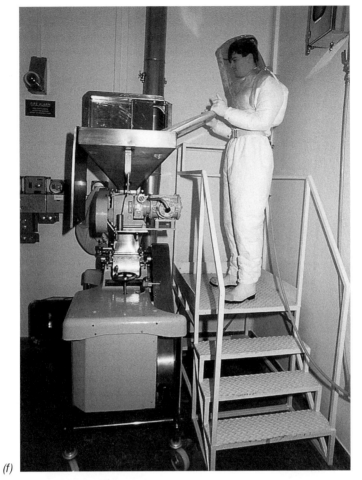

(f)

Fig. 6.2 *(f) Air hood providing personal protection in the pharmaceutical industry during milling. Note also the local exhaust ventilation. Noise is another hazard here. (Photographs courtesy of Dr John Cherrie.) See also colour plate 6.2(f).*

Segregation

A case has already been quoted (Chapter 1, Case history 1.9) in which an organic dye process was properly enclosed, but fitters required access for maintenance and repair. One of these men subsequently developed bladder cancer. Similarly, in a very clean and well-kept bakery the only man who developed asthma as a result of flour allergy was the fitter who had to repair pipes and silos when they burst. Remember, when looking at a well-isolated piece of machinery, to ask how it is maintained or repaired.

Exhaust ventilation

Exhaust ventilation is very effective if properly designed and if the extractor fan is working. A young female technician developed allergic alveolitis and asthma as a result of sensitization to a chemical reagent she was preparing in a fume cupboard in the laboratory of a university medical school. When the problem was investigated, it was found the extractor fan was not working. Three men developed acute mercury poisoning while making repairs in the boiler of a power station. Some other workers in a distant part of the plant had spilt some mercury which had vaporized. The extract fan in the system was running in reverse and the vapour was propelled along pipes to the boiler in which the other men were working.

Dilution

Where dilution is used, the substance remains in the air, but in lower concentration. Unforeseen problems may, however, occur to make matters worse. An operating theatre had a well-designed ventilation system to reduce microbial levels in the area around the patient. Nevertheless, a series of patients undergoing prosthetic heart valve surgery developed infections with *Aspergillus fumigatus*. It was eventually discovered that the fungal spores were being removed efficiently from the air by filters which needed to be changed regularly. The technician changing these was not given any special instructions, and simply took them down into the theatre, substituting the new ones. This process released the captured spores in high concentration. In other cases, the supply of conditioned, humidified air to operating theatres has resulted in humidifier fever among theatre staff.

Personal protection

Sometimes personal protection devices may be even worse than implied by their efficiencies. Face masks are not as universal in their fitting to the human face as manufacturers and wearers would hope, and thus often allow leakage. Filters on respirators need changing regularly or their performance deteriorates. Some disposable respirators become ineffective after use because of being crumpled in a pocket or soaked with water. Respirators are required to be formally tested to various standards – in doing this, testing laboratories have found filters that release respirable fibres, giving higher counts within the masks than outside! Some helmet-type respirators become less efficient if used in moderately windy conditions. Earplugs may contribute to otitis externa, visors may obscure the welding job and thus may not be used properly, gloves may be permeable to chemicals, and so on.

Education and good housekeeping

To be effective, as all doctors know, education has to be a continuing process. After three fatal cases of pneumonia had occurred in a biotechnology factory, all managers were instructed in appropriate preventive measures, and codes of practice were introduced for hazardous operations, of which the most important was water spraying. After an illness-free period of 4 years, another severe case of pneumonia occurred. The victim, who fortunately survived, was a contract worker who had been using a high pressure hose in a cleaning operation. The manager in charge was new, and had not been informed of his responsibilities in supervising contract workers and preventing such hosing procedures.

Problems with physical hazards

Similar principles apply to physical hazards.

Case history 6.4

An occupational physician was inspecting a light engineering department spread over a couple of rooms, as part of an investigation of possible occupational dermatitis. The physician noticed that some of the machinery was very noisy and wearing of personal protective equipment was inconsistent. He made some interim recommendations. These included the replacement of the oldest equipment by quieter and more modern tools, relocation of the less noisy jobs so that they were all together in a relatively quieter area (segregation) and strict enforcement of the wearing of personal protection in the residual noisy area. In the longer term, after consultation with workers and managers, a programme of education, health surveillance for noise-induced hearing loss, professional occupational hygiene assessments of noise, and further steps to reduce exposure was instituted.

THE ROLE OF ERGONOMICS IN HEALTH RISK REDUCTION

In preventing illness and injury induced by work and conditions at the workplace, greatest emphasis must be placed on appropriate design of the job, backed by proper education and training of the workers. Selection of appropriate workers, as discussed below, is also sometimes necessary. However, this is a matter that should only be considered after every attempt has been made to reduce risks in the design of the job.

Job design

Most ergonomic problems in a workplace come to light as a result of sickness absence or complaints by the workers. Almost all are caused by physical or psychological stresses above a threshold acceptable to the workers involved. Many can be traced back to bad, or careless, decisions by managers who had not thought out the implications of these decisions on the workers, and often when the decisions have been implemented it becomes very difficult to resolve the problems. A good example of this has been the office revolution, with widespread moves to computers and visual display units.

Case history 6.5

A 50-year-old female records clerk in a hospital was referred to the occupational physician because of prolonged sickness absence. She had been employed for over 20 years with a very good work record until 2 years previously. Then, after a series of short absences, she had been off work for 6 months with depression. She had seen a psychiatrist who believed problems at work lay behind her illness. In fact, the source of the problem was the sudden introduction of a computer to make her record keeping more efficient. She was given 1 day of training and then had to get on with the new job. Having never used a keyboard before she was slow, and felt the younger clerks in the office were laughing at her. Far from making her job easier, the computer added problems to a job that she had previously done without difficulty, and contributed largely to her psychological breakdown.

This story had a happy ending, thanks to the ability of a sympathetic manager to adjust her job so as to retain her valuable services. The problem in both these cases arose from a sudden requirement to take on tasks for which the worker had not been adequately trained. These problems do not arise because of an intrinsic design fault of the hardware; rather they are a consequence of its careless introduction and use. After all, secretaries have used typewriters for a century without great problems, and a whole generation of adults has now grown up accustomed to staring at television screens. But the widespread introduction of these devices into workplaces means that many, possibly most, people using keyboards do so without the training that secretaries go through, while the very number of visual display units means that ergonomic factors such as lighting and seating may be quite difficult and costly to bring up to appropriate standards.

The design of a job in such a way as to minimize ergonomic difficulties should include consideration of the factors given in Table 6.1, but always in the light of the capabilities, physical and mental, of the employees. The consequences of not doing so may lead, on the physical side, to musculoskeletal injury, on the psychological side, to anxiety and depression, and on both accounts to increased accident rates.

There is clearly no such thing as an ideal job able to be coped with and enjoyed by all employees, no matter how physically or psychologically vulnerable. However, the underlying principles remain; namely constantly re-assessing and striving to reduce risks to health from work, as well as improving general well-being.

In keeping with the principles discussed earlier, you might outline a strategy for prevention of back injury at work. This should consider design of the job, so as to minimize awkward postures or loads, training of the workers in safe handling techniques, supervision or audit to ensure that the lessons learnt in training are applied, and selection of appropriate workers, giving special attention to previous history of back injury. In the UK, for example, Manual Handling Operations Regulations require employers to make an assessment of likely risks involved in operations involving handling loads and to take steps to minimize those risks by redesign of the job, providing appropriate lifting aids and so on.

Table 6.1 *Some important ergonomic factors in job design*

Physical
Loads to be managed: weight, dimensions, frequency, etc.
Rate of work
Hours of work and overtime, shift pattern
Breaks, days off and holidays
Postures and range of movements required
Temperature, lighting, noise and vibration
Ventilation

Psychological
Relations with managers and supervisors
Relations with fellow workers
Demands to produce – piece work, bonuses, etc.
Demands upon intellect
Demands when breakdown or emergencies occur
Lack of demand, or boring repetitive work

Case history 6.6

A 45-year-old man was employed as an operative on a production line in a food factory. In a previous period of employment with the company he had spent some time off sick with back pain. Nevertheless, his job entailed collecting waste in plastic buckets from nine, often inaccessible, points in the line. When the line was faulty, as many as 180 buckets needed to be collected on a shift, whereas on a good day as few as 18 were required. When full the buckets weighed 67 kg and were dragged to a main collection point where they were stacked three high on a pallet for collection.

In the course of this work the man (who was of short stature) sustained a prolapsed intervertebral disc. Back and leg pain were still present 2 years after the episode and had prevented his return to work.

This story, with minor variations, is a very frequent one, although methods of prevention rely largely on the application of common sense.

Case history 6.7

A 30-year-old lady felt an acute pain in her wrist when propping herself up in bed in the morning. The pain subsided and she went to work in the office of a major insurance company. Her job had involved adding figures and keeping books, but she had recently been transferred to other clerical duties and spent much of the day at a computer keyboard. She had never been shown how to use this in any formal way. After a week she found that the pain in her wrist was getting worse and she had to consult her general practitioner. He certified her sickness absence from work, and prescribed anti-inflammatory drugs and a splint. The pain persisted, perhaps partly because of her need to do housework and look after a young child at home. Referral to an orthopaedic surgeon and a rheumatologist followed, and the term 'repetitive strain syndrome', with its implication of prolonged and even permanent disability, was used. The general practitioner referred her to an occupational physician who examined her and found no physical signs, but an awkward typing technique. He was able to reassure her that she was, by then, recovering from a mild ligamentous strain exacerbated by bad typing techniques. He arranged a rehabilitation programme with the company (including keyboard training) and advised that it review its arrangements for training keyboard operators. Followed up, 2 months after return to work, she was symptom free.

This story illustrates several common problems in occupational medicine. A mild condition is often made worse by bad work technique or posture. Lack of training and sudden introduction to work with which people are unfamiliar often lead to injury. Multiple medical opinions, especially if uncertain or negative, lead to anxiety, which, in turn, increases perception of symptoms. Positive action and optimism often lead to improvement.

A whole area of ergonomics concerns itself with the design of control systems, be they aeroplane cockpits or the control rooms of diving operations or nuclear power stations. It is not uncommon to find such complex arrays of dials and warning signals in the charge of a relatively unsophisticated worker who has not been thoroughly trained, particularly with respect to emergency reactions. Proper design of such systems depends on an understanding of the capabilities and reactions of the operator, and training should involve practice in emergency responses, as in the flight simulators used by airlines.

Anthropometry deals with measurement of body size and movement. Its importance in ergonomics relates to its role in ensuring appropriate design of tasks and machines. It is, for example, possible from a survey of a workforce to define the range of height, reach in various directions, and strength of selected muscle groups, and thus to ensure that given tasks or operations within given workplaces are within the capabilities of actual and potential workers. Such surveys are conventionally described in terms of the capabilities or characteristics of the 5th to 95th percentiles, or 90 per cent of the population, and may apply to any aspect of human physique and performance. Static anthropometry leads to the production of limiting values for dimensions, say, of furniture, equipment and buildings. A familiar use is in the design of car seats and controls. Dynamic anthropometry considers functional operation, and includes posture, range of movement, strength, endurance, precision and sight lines, as well as assessment of capabilities in a psychological sense. It is particularly important in the design of tasks, such as keyboard operation, and controls, such as the keyboard itself.

Case history 6.8

A 25-year-old man presented for a pre-employment medical examination prior to enrolling on a nursing degree course. His previous employment had been in the drilling team on an oil rig. He was a fit looking, muscular man but had to be turned down on the basis of recurrent back injury which made him physically unsuitable for nurse training.

The injury had occurred on the oil rig, an environment notable for the machismo of some of its workers. He had been told to haul 70 kg segments of metal piping a height of some 10 metres. This he did with a rope, which his mate tied round the objects while he leant over and pulled them up. While doing this he developed acute lumbar pain and sciatica. After a period off work he returned to the job and again injured his back while undertaking another lifting task. Apparently, no consideration had been given to the use of pulleys to lighten a task which required considerable force in an anatomically inefficient posture.

In such cases, the need for lifting aids is often intuitively obvious. For managers and doctors responsible for workers involved in physical tasks, however, there are published ergonomic guidelines and criteria that can be applied allowing minimization of risk.

However, ergonomic issues in the workplace, probably more than any other category of problems, require what some might term a 'holistic approach'. They often cannot be resolved simply by tackling single hazards (such as controlling noise or vibration, or substituting a sensitizer). Moreover, when workers complain of musculoskeletal symptoms, ergonomic factors such as work practices and workplace design are not the only factors to consider. Psychological factors make an important contribution which cannot be ignored. Consider the case history which follows.

Case history 6.9

An occupational health nurse and physician were consulted by a number of employees of a large company.

A 28-year-old secretary had pain in the dorsal spine and neck. Her workstation was found to be poorly designed for the multiplicity of devices she had to contend with. Besides her computer and its display screen and usual input devices (keyboard and mouse), she had a photocopier, separate printer and telephone and facsimile machine, yet leg room was limited as she tried to rotate her trunk between tasks. Advice was given to her and to her manager to replace the two desks by a single curved work surface, without interfering drawer units underneath. The secretary was also told to vary her tasks and to have regular breaks so that she would not be unduly restricted to her seat at the workstation. Her new furniture was soon delivered and within a fortnight her symptoms had abated.

A 49-year-old office maintenance worker complained of pain in his right wrist. He had to repeatedly hammer cable cleats along skirting boards and in other areas because of the installation of new computer networking. Physical examination did not reveal any abnormality. The advice given to him and his manager was to use a special device similar to a staple gun that was intended for such a task. His symptoms improved significantly, although when followed up they had not disappeared altogether. Moreover, several other employees also presented to the occupational health service with musculoskeletal complaints or with anxiety or complaining of 'stress', although in a number of them, links between their symptoms and the need for ergonomic improvements in the workplace were not always unequivocal.

What factors should the occupational physician consider when faced with symptoms which might be associated with the need to rectify ergonomic shortcomings in the workplace? As previously stated, the occupational history is crucial, and it has to be borne in mind that many musculoskeletal complains causing distress to workers do not have associated physical findings which could be used to monitor progress objectively in response to control measures. An assessment of the workplace accompanied by reasoned advice on design and work practice should follow. However, psychosocial factors arising from work or home contribute to workers' symptoms and need to be taken into account. In conjunction with the worker and other advisers such as the general practitioner, the occupational physician may help with individual factors affecting wellbeing. In the cluster of cases which arose above, the physician became aware of disquiet amongst many staff who presented to the occupational health service. They knew of recent changes in senior management and had heard rumours about 'reorganization' and the need for change. They had been told that new policies were being developed on a wide range of issues from procurement to staff recruitment, and some were uncertain about their future. The occupational physician spoke to the personnel manager and postulated that uncertainty might be affecting morale and hence wellbeing amongst the workers. The personnel manager conceded that communication with staff had perhaps not been adequate during the 'change'. Staff who should have been reassured had not been, while those who needed support in planning for new jobs, or perhaps even retirement, had not been helped thus far. Senior management and the personnel department began briefing staff more openly and provided individual meetings, advice and support for those who needed it. Morale and wellbeing amongst the workforce generally recovered, although slowly and erratically.

Case history 6.10

An occupational physician was asked to advise regarding 'safe weights' for loading industrial washing machines in a laundry. The assessment consisted of two parts: in the first a thorough ergonomic assessment of the workplace was undertaken – including detailed inspection of the process of handling of the laundry and in particular the loading of the machines. It was noted that the load was never completely borne by the employees. Some of the machines were top-loading and for these a canvas cylinder needed to be swung in place and opened. Other machines were front loading and involved tough manhandling of the laundry hanging in the canvas cylinder. The employees were assessed individually both anthropometrically and clinically. Appropriate references were consulted. The recommendation was that for top-loading machines the canvas cylinder was not to be loaded to more than 45 kg, while for front-loading machines a lesser limit of 40 kg should be set – even if the load capacity of the machines was greater. This apparently settled the problem but 8 years later an employee injured his back while handling the canvas cylinder with a load greater than the previously set limit. He successfully sued his employer on the grounds that the employers had not adhered to the limits set by the assessment that they had commissioned.

THE ROLE OF THE DOCTOR IN THE PREVENTION AND MANAGEMENT OF OCCUPATIONAL ACCIDENTS

It should be clear from the foregoing that prevention of industrial accidents depends on an awareness of the fallibility of people, the dangers of machinery and workplaces and the risks inherent when the two interact. Prevention thus depends on ensuring as far as possible that the workplace is safe, that people in it are constantly aware of hazards and take active steps to reduce risk, and that systems are set up for regular safety checks or audit.

The prevention of accidents, or indeed the prevention of disease, is not primarily a medical matter. Doctors, by virtue of special training in the causation of **diseases**, are able to play a leading role in advising government, the general public and individual people on their prevention. In contrast, most doctors do not have a special understanding of **accident** causation (and hence prevention); rather we have confined our attention to the management of accidents once they have occurred, both by emergency treatment of individuals and by coordinated medical management of major disasters. Thus other specialists have developed interests in accident prevention, the study of which has become of academic and practical interest to, *inter alia*, psychologists, engineers and ergonomists. In particular, responsible industries usually employ specifically trained safety managers, and national organizations exist in many countries for training and certification of those concerned with safety in the workplace.

The greatest responsibility lies with management, who should normally include in their number someone with special responsibility for safety. But individual workers must also be made aware of their duties for the safety both of themselves and of their colleagues. In the UK, under the terms of the Health and Safety at Work, etc. Act, workers may nominate their own safety representatives, who should carry out regular safety inspections and report problems in writing to management, usually via the safety committee. Managers also should be responsible for regular audits of safety.

Setting up safety committees and appointing safety representatives is not in itself sufficient. The representatives should receive formal training, as should any managers with safety responsibilities, and all workers should be made aware of the importance of safe working practices and of action necessary to reduce risk. Dangerous areas should be clearly labelled and access restricted as far as possible, and machinery should be equipped with guards and other appropriate safety devices. Ultimately, it is the awareness by individuals of risk and their willingness to avoid actions that might have dangerous consequences that is the area where the greatest impact can be made in preventing accidents. Individual, often apparently quite trivial, acts of carelessness may have disastrous consequences.

Case history 6.11

Paper manufacture involves passing the fibrous pulp between pairs of very large rollers arranged in series. Access to the rollers is necessary in order to service them and to deal with tears or folds in the paper, but such access occurs only when the rollers are stationary. The platform allowing access is guarded by a rail and clearly labelled 'no access when machinery is running'. Nevertheless, on one occasion an experienced operator climbed over the rail to help feed the paper between the rollers while they were working, by kicking at it. He slipped on the wet floor, his foot was caught in the machine and his body was delivered in fragments moments later.

This horrifying story is repeated somewhere, with minor differences, every month in workplaces throughout Britain. It emphasizes the need for safety training to be taken seriously by everyone. Management should have a written safety policy and should set an example themselves by always wearing appropriate safety equipment, such as boots and eye protectors, in designated places.

There is much scope for originality and initiative in devising safety training and promoting safety awareness in an organization. Safety fairs, videos and quizzes with prizes all have more impact than lectures or written information. Incentives, such as safety bonuses for parts of the organization with least accidents, need to be used with care, however, as they may result in a failure to report injuries. In all these activities, the occupational physician or nurse, with their knowledge of the consequences of accidents in terms of human suffering, can play an important role.

In accident prevention, therefore, the doctor usually has only the role of other educated and sensible laymen. However, the doctor working in industry will often assume a more active role, related to knowledge of particular hazards of the specific industry, study of accident statistics and some expertise in the human factors related to accident causation. This may include, for example, examination and exclusion from hazardous work of people with conditions such as epilepsy, diabetes or alcoholism that may put them or others at increased risk. In most industries, accident prevention should be regarded as a team effort, with managers, trade unionists, safety officials and health professionals of various sorts contributing. In general, the leader of the team would be expected to be a manager with special knowledge of the hazards of the workplace. The doctor's advisory role would depend on what particular expertise he or she possessed. The doctor working in industry does, however, have a more significant role in the management of accidents. This includes training and maintaining the standards of first-aiders (although this may be the responsibility of nurses or other appropriately trained people), the planning and implementation of methods for the immediate management of injuries, and ensuring that legal requirements for accident reporting are observed. Some large or particularly dangerous workplaces may have their own medical centre with a fully equipped accident department. Most have a first-aid room. The doctor (or nurse) working in industry would normally be responsible for supervision of any treatment centre other than the most basic first-aid facility.

In dealing with major accidents, the doctor working in industry has a number of responsibilities with respect to accident management. These may include first-aid provision and training, immediate medical care, documentation, reporting and, of course, planning for prevention. The doctor should also be involved in planning a strategy for dealing with major incidents in such workplaces as chemical factories or nuclear reactors, where serious episodes are possibilities. Dealing with the major incident is clearly the responsibility of senior management, with the doctor usually having an advisory role in planning and a facilitatory role in the event of an accident. Plans will be specific to the particular work site, and must foresee the possibility of explosion, fire, release of clouds of toxic gas or radioactivity, and multiple casualties.

Nowadays such planning must also take account of the possibility of terrorist attack. Detailed analysis of possible worst-case scenarios will be necessary, and appropriate action planned in conjunction with the local fire and police services, local hospitals and the ambulance service. Hospitals in the vicinity of hazardous industrial sites should be aware of possible injuries or gassings that might occur and should incorporate these possibilities into their major accident plans. The doctor in industry would be wise to assist local hospitals in running simulations of such accidents in cooperation with local authority services.

First aid provisions vary from country to country. In the UK, regulations govern the provision of first aid in the workplace, and the Health and Safety Executive regulates the training of first-aiders. Over and above these provisions, the doctor working in an industry where there is a risk of particular accidents, such as poisonings or gassings, should make arrangements for immediate treatment on site, including administration of oxygen and antidotes if appropriate. Contact should be made with the local accident departments to inform them of possible emergencies and, in the case of risk of chemical poisonings, there should be ready access to the manufacturers' data sheets, which give the chemical constituents, medical hazards and first-aid measures that may be necessary in the case of poisoning.

Case history 6.12

A chargehand in a petrochemical plant was responsible for injecting dimethyl disulphide from a container into an oil pipeline. This was done simply by turning on a tap that released the liquid chemical under pressure into a hose connected to the pipeline. On one occasion, as he did this, the hose ruptured and he was sprayed all over with the chemical. The chemical has a distinctive, extremely unpleasant smell. He managed to turn the tap off, but had to walk 200 metres to the first aid post where he was stripped and showered. By this time he had become short of breath, and oxygen was administered while the data sheet was being found. This said that dimethyl disulphide was a respiratory irritant and it was therefore concluded that respiratory support for possible pulmonary oedema might be needed. He was transferred, breathing oxygen, with the data sheet to the local hospital, where he was detained overnight and appeared to make a recovery. Subsequently, however, he developed persistent shortness of breath as a result of steroid-resistant airflow obstruction, and was thought to have suffered an obliterative bronchiolitis.

In general, the first-aid management of industrial accidents is straightforward, involving support of vital organs and transfer to hospital, taking care to avoid making matters worse by inappropriate treatment. The management problems in hospitals come not from trauma but from poisonings, and the availability of a data sheet giving the name of the chemical and its adverse effects is a great help. In such cases, one of the national poisons centres may be contacted for advice. Even so, in many cases the best management of such rare episodes (as in the example quoted) is not known. In the case of acute respiratory irritants, there is anecdotal evidence that early administration of corticosteroids may reduce the risk of later obliterative bronchiolitis.

INFORMATION, EDUCATION AND TRAINING AS TOOLS IN RISK REDUCTION

Although this subject has been touched upon earlier, in the section on 'control', it is of such pervading importance that it merits further attention here.

Case history 6.13

While walking through the corridors of a hospital, an occupational physician noticed a painter wearing a surgical mask and latex gloves while painting radiators with an organic solvent-based paint (as evidenced by its odour and the fact that it was clearly dissolving the gloves!). A two-phase educational opportunity was immediately grasped. In the first instance the painter was advised that neither the gloves he was wearing nor the mask were affording him any protection at all. Indeed the gloves were probably increasing his exposure to solvent by allowing its dissolution in a medium applied to his skin. Second, the estates manager was contacted and advised to institute a proper policy of education and training of in-house staff as well as other measures to control exposure.

It is clear that a well-informed, safety-conscious worker is less likely to suffer work-related injury or illness than an ignorant one, just as a driver who reads and complies with the provisions of the Highway Code is less likely to have an accident. Safety and health training should be a part of every organization's strategy, its level and intensity being dictated by the perceived risk in the workplace. If the risk is no greater than tripping over or having a heart attack at work, then first aid provision and training is all that is necessary, but in most workplaces, as the reader will by now realize, risks are usually somewhat greater. Upper limb disorders in offices, back injuries in manual workers, deafness in noisy places – all these are preventable by appropriate modifications in the workplace but are more likely to be prevented if the workers are informed of risk and of protective measures. It is not sufficient to leave this to the trade union, whose representatives at shop floor level have sometimes been known to be more interested in negotiating 'danger money' than in ameliorating conditions.

The range of methods of information and education is large, and each organization should plan its own strategy. Joint management–worker safety committees are a useful forum for planning such activity, which may include posters, leaflets, lectures and seminars, quizzes and videos. The last of these are increasingly popular, but it is important that they are seen to be relevant to the workplace where they are shown. Some organizations make their own, and may run management competitions for the best one made.

The first British Medical Inspector of Factories, Sir Thomas Morison Legge, propounded a number of aphorisms, which are much quoted by occupational physicians. Among these are the following, all of which apply to this day (but to working women as well as men):

- unless and until the employer has done everything, and everything means a good deal, the workman can do next to nothing to protect himself, although he is naturally willing enough to do his share
- if you can bring an influence to bear, external to the workman (that is, one over which he can exercise no control), you will be successful; and if you cannot, or do not, you will never be wholly successful
- all workmen should be told something of the danger of the material with which they come into contact and not be left to find out for themselves, sometimes at the cost of their lives.

Education and training should not of course be confined to the shop floor, but should be provided at all levels in the organization. Uninformed managers and company directors can pose a far greater risk than uninformed workers as their decisions may result in the loss or saving of many lives. In the UK in recent years, management ignorance of workplace hazards has become a serious problem.

THE ROLE OF IMMUNIZATION

Immunization as a means of preventing disease can be an important tool in specific workplaces, most notably health care and the emergency services. The need to consider immunization in an occupational setting arises for various reasons:

- it can protect the employee from ill-health that may be a specific consequence of work, e.g. administering BCG (Bacille Calmette-Guérin) to mortuary workers, or active hepatitis B immunization of healthcare workers or police potentially exposed to blood
- a similar consideration may apply to prophylaxis for overseas travel, although the source of infection is not necessarily directly occupational
- immunization, besides fulfilling the above function, can also protect the health of members of the public as well as employees, e.g. immunization of surgeons against hepatitis B
- immunization may also offer protection unrelated to specific work risks, e.g. immunization against influenza virus.

Immunization policies, like all other issues in health promotion, should not be looked at in isolation but as part of an overall strategy and given correct priority.

Case history 6.14

An occupational physician who was new to a particular workplace received a postal reminder inviting the repeat annual ordering of influenza vaccine. Further enquiry revealed that it was custom for all the workforce to be offered influenza vaccine once a year and approximately one-third accepted. The physician's assessment of the workplace identified various respiratory hazards and indeed that some workers suffered from occupational rhinitis and/or asthma. The physician's advice to the manager and to the safety committee was that steps should be taken to control respiratory hazards in the workplace and that influenza vaccine in that particular workplace should only continue to be offered (in line with the current Department of Health guidelines) to individuals at a particularly high risk, such as those suffering from cardiac or pulmonary disease.

When learning lessons from the above case, it does not necessarily follow that the same conclusion would have been applicable to all workplace circumstances. It is likely that in other contexts, e.g. healthcare workers in the front line or other indispensable staff, a different conclusion might be reached. There is some evidence that vaccination against influenza may reduce the sickness absence rate of employees and therefore make them more available to carry out work for their employer.

Immunization should be put in its proper context, as part of an overall plan appropriately targeted and ranked in priority. Good information systems need to be in place to record which groups of employees have been targeted, have had appropriate information and education, have been offered immunization, and the date of its administration. Arrangements for recall and review need to be similarly effective and efficient.

Patients may also need to be protected from an infection that is relatively harmless to most healthcare workers but which would have serious consequences for some categories of patients. Here a typical example is vaccination of healthcare workers against rubella in order to reduce the risk of transmission of rubella (German measles) to patients who might be in the early stages of pregnancy.

Finally there may be a slightly more controversial purpose of immunization. If immunization was completely free from risk, and from perception of risk, such policies would be most unlikely to present difficulties. It is important to ensure that employees are fully informed of the reasons for the vaccination policy, the evidence for effect as well as for possible lack of effect or side-effects. Where the purpose of the immunization is essentially to maintain high productivity rather than to ensure health and safety, it is even more important that the programme should be a voluntary one without compulsion.

The principles behind immunization in the workplace, largely applying to healthcare workers and the police, can therefore be summarized in the following list.

- Identification of infections for which immunization may be part of a control strategy is the first step.
- A full, detailed evaluation is then needed for each of the possible immunizations based on information such as background frequency of the infection or of the carrier state, job-specific risk assessment (including implications for workers as well as patients), effectiveness of the specific immunization procedure, side-effects, and finally health economics. By addressing these issues in the context of each other and of the whole control strategy, the appropriate immunization priorities are set.
- Identification of the target population for each immunization follows.
- Methods are needed for calling workers for immunization, logging of relevant employee and immunization details, provision of information to workers and to management (in summary form).
- Mechanisms for recording, investigating and reporting apparent unwanted effects need to be in place.
- Subsequently means are needed for recall of workers for completion of immunization and/or for postimmunization serology (where relevant).
- Review of occupational health service immunization activity and outcome, e.g. confirmed side-effects, and postimmunization serology (where relevant) is essential to complete the quality assurance process.

Prophylaxis following exposure to infectious agents

This section considers the management of exposures to infectious agents warranting specific intervention. This occurs most frequently in healthcare or laboratory contexts but may also be encountered in other situations involving the emergency services or local authority employees; for example, a municipal worker or a postman may be bitten by a dog and need appropriate antibiotics; a sewage worker could be exposed to *Leptospira* spp.; while a gardener could sustain an injury needing anti-tetanus prophylaxis. As in other previously described circumstances, a good history with pertinent questions is essential to assess exposure. Having assessed the risk of transmission of infection following exposure and determined that active treatment is warranted this can follow either of two routes: immunization (passive and/or active) or drug treatment. Post-event immunization against such conditions as tetanus and tuberculosis is well covered in non-occupational texts but the management of special infective exposure incidents deserves special mention.

Case history 6.15

A medical registrar was summoned urgently to a patient suffering from systemic lupus erythematosus who was on treatment with high dose steroids and who had been readmitted severely shocked. Very shortly after the doctor's arrival the patient sustained a cardiac arrest. Attempts at resuscitation including mouth-to-mouth respiration were unsuccessful. The next day, blood cultures from samples taken during the failed resuscitation attempt showed a heavy growth of *Neisseria meningitidis*. The registrar sought advice and was administered chemoprophylaxis, and fortunately suffered no adverse effects. (He was prescribed 600 mg of rifampicin orally twice daily for 2 days, although more recent chemoprophylactic alternatives offered to healthcare workers with direct exposure to nasopharyngeal secretions from patients with meningococcal infections are ciprofloxacin or ceftriaxone.)

With the increasing effectiveness of anti-retroviral therapy, it has now become standard practice to offer prophylactic therapy to those exposed to HIV-infected blood. These situations are illustrated by the following case histories.

Case history 6.16

A nurse in a casualty department was undressing a semi-comatose young man. who was suspected of being a drug addict. While removing his jacket, she pricked her finger on a needle in his pocket. This turned out to be attached to a syringe that contained blood from a recent self-injection and the needle had penetrated quite deeply. The wound was encouraged to bleed. A blood sample was taken from the patient for subsequent testing for hepatitis B and HIV antigen (the patient had already said he was HIV positive) and the nurse was immediately given a booster dose of hepatitis B vaccine, having previously had a course with a good antibody response. According to the policy operating at that time, she was seen and counselled within 1 hour by the infectious diseases consultant and given zidovudine (Syn AZT: azidothymidine) intravenously followed by 2 g by mouth daily in divided doses for 4 weeks. On further follow-up, with her informed consent, the HIV status was monitored and fortunately she did not become positive.

This was an unusually clear-cut case, where there was little doubt that a risk of infection existed. It has been estimated that the risk in such circumstances is about 2–5 per cent for hepatitis B and about 10 times less for HIV. The prevention and post-injury management of hepatitis B risk is straightforward because active and passive immunization is readily available, but the management of HIV exposure is much more problematic. In this case, the physician's first step is to assess the problem, by trying to determine the likelihood of infection of the source, although this can present ethical problems, which are discussed below. The worker should be counselled about the risks and consequences of infection, and the implications of testing. Thus insurance firms tend to look adversely at applicants who have had a test for HIV antibody undertaken, regardless of the reason for this or the outcome. A suitable compromise may be merely to take serum on presentation and after an interval of a few months and store it, only to be tested with the worker's consent at a later date if clinically indicated. Finally, the circumstances of the case must be reviewed in consultation with the manager to take action to prevent future episodes by introducing appropriate policies, information and changes in work practices.

As in the above case, antiviral drugs may be administered to exposed employees, after an individual case-by-case risk assessment after needlestick or similar injuries from HIV positive sources. There is evidence in humans that appropriate chemoprophylaxis may reduce the risk of seroconversion and there are case reports where such protocols have manifestly failed to protect individual employees. Moreover the drug in question may have severe side-effects, including bone marrow depression. The reader is advised to keep up with the publications that will continue to appear on this subject for up-to-date advice; for example, current recommendations for HIV post-exposure prophylaxis feature a 4-week course consisting of zidovudine 250 mg (or 300mg) twice daily, lamivudine 150 mg twice daily and nelfanivir 1250 mg twice daily. In any case, careful documentation of the event and follow-up is essential. The exposed employee should be advised to have serum stored in order to keep the option open for testing at a later date if so counselled and agreed. Postviral exposure prophylaxis is a rapidly evolving field and the reader is advised to search the literature rather than rely on textbooks; for example, agents such as hepatitis C may pose special challenges, yet there may be agents such as interferon which might find use in addition to other chemotherapeutic antiviral agents in these circumstances. Once the risk of transmitting infection has been thoroughly assessed on an individual basis by an occupational physician, often in conjunction with another relevant specialist, the employee and the employer should be advised about it and consideration given to appropriate redeployment. If voluntary reporting schemes or research projects are in progress, the physician should be encouraged to participate in the data collection for these activities.

Case history 6.17

A domestic assistant employed by a contract cleaning firm in a hospital injured herself on a hypodermic needle while cleaning behind a radiator pipe in a geriatric ward. She reported the matter to her supervisor, who referred her to the casualty (accident and emergency) department. The doctor took a vaccination history, but unfortunately, and not surprisingly, it was not possible to establish the likely patient on whom the needle could have been used. Her wound was cleaned and she was given hepatitis B hyperimmune gamma globulin intramuscularly in a dose of 500 units, and started on a vaccination course to protect her against hepatitis B.

In general where an immunologically unprotected worker sustains a needlestick or similar injury breaching the skin, or else a splash to a mucous membrane or inflamed skin with blood which is not known nor demonstrated to be free from hepatitis B virus, immunization is appropriate. The conventional treatment consists of the administration of hepatitis B hyperimmune gamma globulin, as in the case above. This should be given as soon as possible after the exposure, and in any event within 2 days, together with the commencement of active immunization with hepatitis B vaccine. Other management such as wound toilet may be necessary. A detailed assessment should include careful inspection of the needle and any syringe or other device that it may have been attached to, as well as the wound it inflicted as these can give a rough estimate of the size of the inoculum. A narrow-bore needle as used for venepuncture to withdraw blood, or for parenteral therapy, or an intravenous cannula obviously carries a higher risk than an apparently clean wide-bore needle (as used for making up drug solutions in phials). If the source was clearly identified, the hepatitis B status of the patient on whom the needle had been used could be determined. In situations of exposure to blood-borne pathogens, risk assessment may be difficult. The age and medical histories of the patients on the ward in this case suggested that infection with HIV would have been most unlikely, although great care should be taken in attempting to determine or guess the lifestyle, past history and therefore potential infectivity of patients. In assessing these cases, if the ward, department or other context of exposure was determined one might find that it consisted of a renal dialysis unit with known hepatitis B-negative patients or, alternatively, if the department dealt with infectious diseases or with gastroenterology the risk would be presumed to be higher. This information should be carefully sought and recorded. The likelihood of hepatitis B infection was deemed more likely, although still not very high. However, the infectivity of hepatitis B from needlestick injury is higher than that for HIV. Moreover, the effectiveness and safety of prophylaxis against hepatitis B is certainly better than that in the case of HIV. Considerations such as these informed and guided risk assessment, hence the management in the above case.

Special ethical dilemmas may arise when attempting to determine the risks of infectious exposure of employees. While many physicians responsible for the care of patients who may have been the source of body fluids to which a healthcare employee has been exposed will disclose risk factors or the results of investigations (such as hepatitis B status) at the request of a physician caring for the employee, this extent of cooperation is not universal. Furthermore, the current ethical consensus in respect of HIV infection is that it is not acceptable for a patient to be tested without full informed consent accompanied by appropriate counselling. This requirement is generally held to be paramount and therefore to take precedence over assessing the risk to employees. Although it appears incongruent with other policies and practices in regard to occupational health risk assessment, it has at present to be respected.

Other serious ethical problems may also arise when employees in certain occupations may be carriers of hepatitis B and HIV. In the vast majority of occupational contexts, such infection in itself has no implications for fitness for work, unless the consequent physical impairment is such as to present a disability in undertaking tasks effectively or safely. However, in occupations such as invasive surgery, dentistry, vascular catheterization, extracorporeal perfusion (in theatres or in renal support units) and obstetric procedures during which bleeding can occur, there is a small, but finite, risk of infection with hepatitis B or HIV being transmitted from employees to the patients they care for. Various bodies have produced guidance on this; for example, in the UK the recommendation of the Expert Advisory Group on AIDS is that 'healthcare workers who have or suspect they are infected with HIV must seek expert advice on whether there is need to limit or alter their work practice'. It must also not be forgotten that employees have wide responsibilities, under Health and Safety at Work legislation, to reduce the risks to others and to cooperate with employers in ensuring health and safety. Employees engaged in jobs such as those mentioned above must seek the advice of the occupational health physician if they know or suspect that they might be infected with hepatitis B or HIV. Full counselling on the social, domestic and occupational implications of possible infection must precede testing. The doctor should, if possible, be in a position to confirm the employer's commitment to safeguard the confidentiality and employment of employees; ideally this matter should have been discussed and a policy agreed with management before the first case occurs. Unless these reassurances are explicit, honoured and believed, employees will be very reluctant to come forward for help and advice, in spite of all the pronouncements of various professional and other bodies. Clinical investigations can help confirm or estimate some aspects of the risk of transmission; thus in employees who have a history of hepatitis B (HBsAg positive) or who have apparently not responded to hepatitis B vaccination, serological measures of the 'e' antigen (HBeAg) are an index of high infectivity if positive.

The role of worker selection in prevention

Screening and discrimination

Some readers may wonder why this section appears so late in the chapter. The reason is that for most employees and most types of employment the reduction of risks to health from work should be brought about by improving the work environment rather than by stopping employees from pursuing their chosen jobs. While, in general, jobs should be designed so as to make them safe to be carried out by any employee, some of them of necessity involve tasks that are beyond the capabilities of some individuals. Such circumstances lead to the requirement for pre-employment selection procedures. When this is necessary, it is appropriate to think first of the precise physical and psychological demands of the job, and then to decide on appropriate requirements.

Of overriding importance in countries with appropriate legislation, as in those of the European Community, is consideration of disability discrimination law. This is discussed in more detail in Chapter 9, but in essence it requires employers and trade/professional associations to treat disabled individuals no less favourably than those without disabilities. Clearly there is plenty of room for debate about what constitutes a disability, and an escape clause, 'without good reason', also allows discussion as to how far a reasonable employer is required to go. Mental impairment, a serious disability, would exclude an individual from employment requiring high intellect, while the physically impaired would not reasonably be expected to gain employment in the police or armed forces. There are, however, many grey areas that are usually resolved locally by application of good sense but that, if this is not the case, may give employment opportunities to lawyers.

Fitting the person to the job or the job to the person

A familiar example might be the selection of medical students. What are the demands placed on a doctor? How far did the selection procedures of your medical school go towards picking out those most capable of doing the job? In retrospect, looking at your experience and that of your fellow students, do you think these procedures could have been more effective?

In many cases in the past, selection into medical school has been on the basis of results in school examinations alone. This provides a test of intelligence and ability to recall facts, two factors that are undoubtedly important in the practice of medicine, and that probably ensured that a majority of those selected would survive the traditional pre-clinical course. But how far does it select those capable of coping with the stressful early years of training and able to deal effectively with the many years ahead in clinical practice? A moment's thought will allow you to see two possible approaches to this problem – more careful selection, by aptitude and psychological testing, or modification of the tasks. Recently in medicine in the UK the emphasis has been,

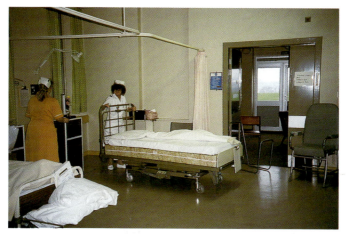

Fig. 2.1 *A familiar environment.*

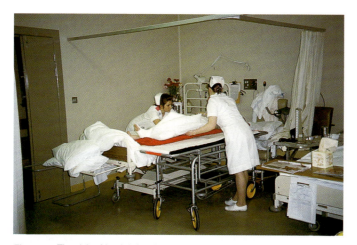

Fig. 2.2 *The risk of back injury in nurses can be measured.*

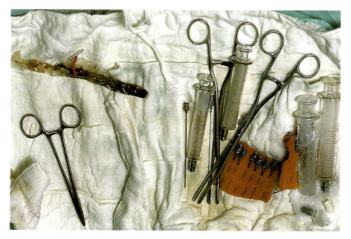

Fig. 2.3 *A day's collection of 'sharps' from the hospital laundry.*

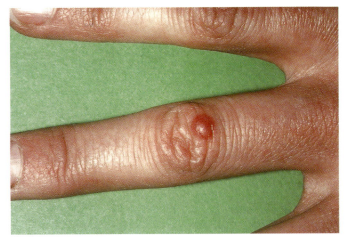

Fig. 2.5 *Early lesion of orf in a hospital registrar.*

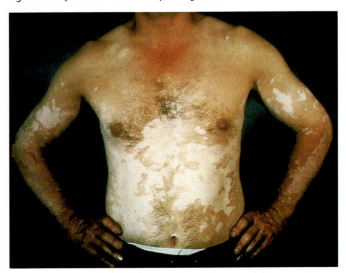

Fig. 2.6 *Vitiligo caused by exposure to phenolic compounds (photo courtesy of Dr C.J. Stevenson).*

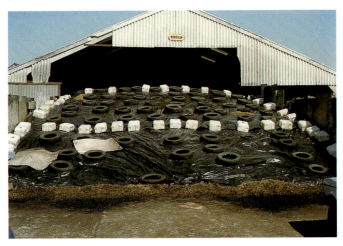

Fig. 2.7 *An open-air silage heap. Any gas given off will be rapidly dispersed.*

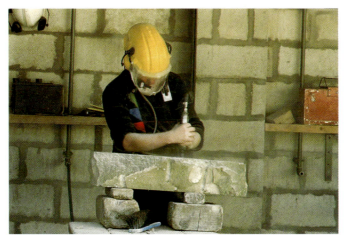

Fig. 2.8 *Buffing sandstone, a cause of HAVS.*

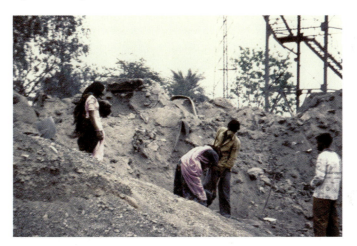

Fig. 2.10 *Unprotected young female workers recycling lead oxide in an Indian lead refinery; a dramatic example of what not to do.*

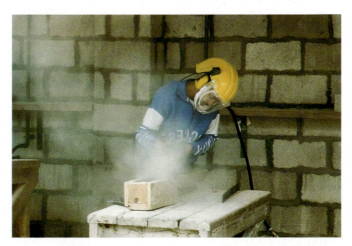

Fig. 3.1 *Stonemason generating cloud of quartz dust in cutting sandstone.*

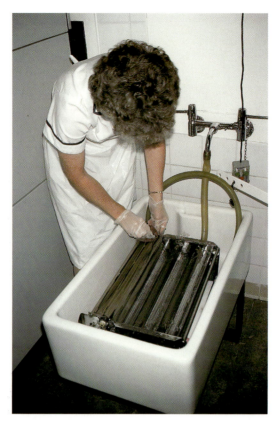

Fig. 3.6 *Washing a unit from the X-ray processor. Normally this is enclosed but has to be removed on a regular basis for cleaning, allowing exposure to chemical vapours.*

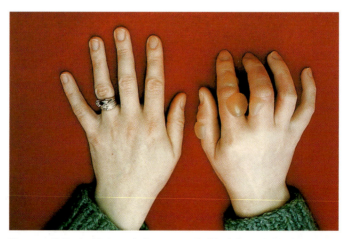

Fig. 4.1 *Patient with tense bullae surrounded by inflamed skin.*

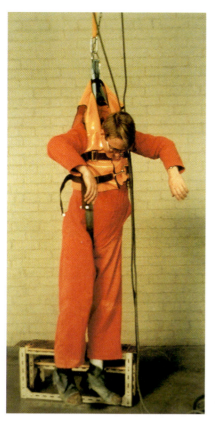

Fig. 5.1 *Consequence of inadequate design of safety harness and training in its use.*

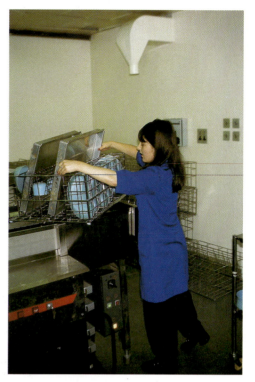

Fig. 5.4 *Bad ergonomics. A short operator in a hospital sterilizing department having to fill and empty trays on a washing machine at the extreme limit of her reach.*

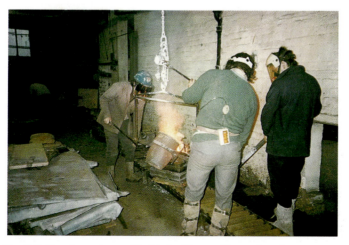

Fig. 5.7 *Foundry workers subject to health surveillance since they are exposed to lead fume from pouring molten metal into casts.*

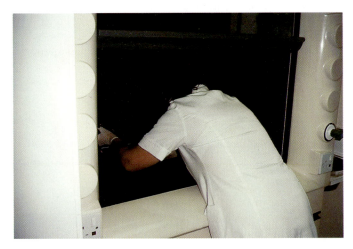

Fig. 6.1 *Fume cupboard in endoscopy unit – designed so that nurses have to put their heads inside in order to wash endoscopes!*

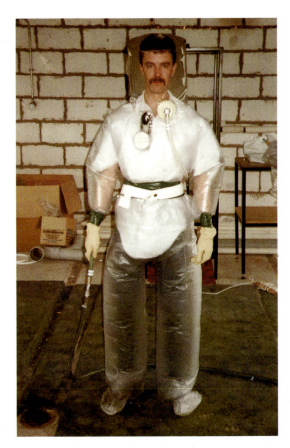

Fig. 6.2 *(d) Ventilated suit used to provide higher level of respiratory and body protection against radioactive dust.*

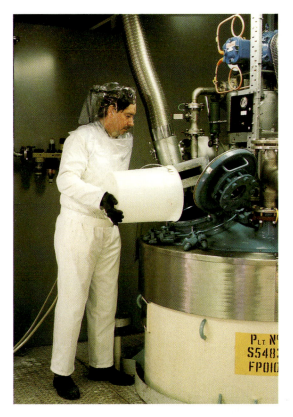

Fig. 6.2 (e) Personal protection including breathing air being delivered through an air hood in the chemical industry. Note also local exhaust ventilation through a flange overlying the reaction vessel next to the potential emission source. (Photographs courtesy of Dr John Cherrie.)

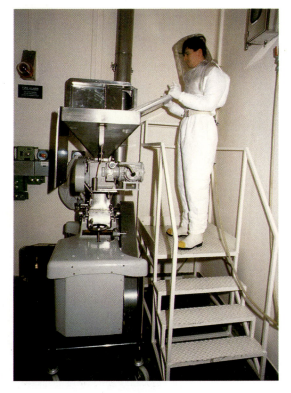

Fig. 6.2 (f) Air hood providing personal protection in the pharmaceutical industry during milling. Note also the local exhaust ventilation. Noise is another hazard here. (Photographs courtesy of Dr John Cherrie.)

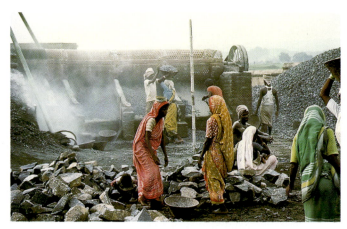

Fig. 7.1 *Women and children working at a roadside stone-crushing plant in rural Bihar, India. High, lifelong dust exposures are inevitable.*

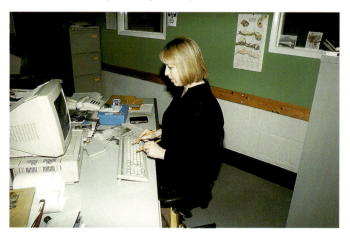

Fig. 7.2 *Office environment: the expansion of microelectronics into everyday life has brought with it unforeseen hazards. In this case, defective technique has led to muscular problems in the operator's forearms.*

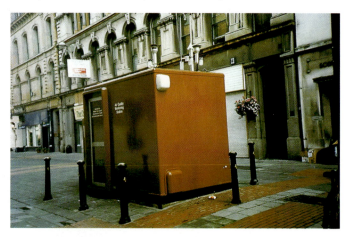

Fig. 7.4 *Air pollution monitor in central Belfast, measuring continuous particle concentrations.*

probably rightly, on the latter, at least with respect to modification of hours of work and length of training, where progress has been substantial. The former approach has not until very recently been seriously considered, and provides interesting research opportunities for the deans of medical schools.

Similar considerations apply in many other jobs, and most include some selection procedures, usually aimed at selecting people who can work most efficiently and effectively. As automation has spread through industry, the emphasis has increasingly turned from physical to mental capabilities, but some jobs still require high standards of physical fitness and it is appropriate to have specific criteria for such work; for example, police and fire fighters, the military and divers all have jobs that may place high physical demands on the individual. It is appropriate that candidates for these jobs should measure up to certain defined criteria because it is unlikely that the jobs can ever be made significantly less stressful; physical breakdown of an individual in such work could put others at risk.

The essential point is to think first of the criteria for performance and safety relevant to the job, and then to consider whether these demands could be modified in order to make the work more accessible to disabled people. It is then appropriate to decide on what selection procedures are necessary. Regrettably, this is often not the way the matter is approached.

Case history 6.18

A Health Board in the National Health Service decided that its occupational health service should generate income. It had recently decided that it could obtain a more cost-effective hospital cleaning service by contracting it out to a privately owned firm. Without consulting the occupational health service, managers decided to write into the contract that all cleaners should have a pre-employment medical examination, for which the company was charged.

The job of hospital cleaner was very poorly paid and often part-time. It therefore attracted people who were only likely to stay until something better turned up. Moreover, the work was arduous, as the company had contracted to do the work with fewer people at lower salaries than was previously considered desirable. The consequence was a very high rate of staff turnover. This initially had the effect of producing income for the occupational health service (even if at a considerable waste of nursing and medical time), but did not have any impact on selecting appropriate people for the job. Moreover, after a short period the company realized that it was wasting money on having people examined who would shortly leave their employ, and adopted a tactic of taking workers on first, subsequently referring them for health screening. This ensured that only those likely to stay a reasonable period were examined, and from the company's point of view was a sensible solution, although it caused problems when people were detected to have disease (usually chronic skin conditions) that made them unsuitable for such work.

What went wrong here? The decision to require health screening was made by a manager simply to obtain income, without real thought as to the medical justifications for it. A moment's thought about the medical requirements for hospital cleaning jobs would have led to the conclusion that if anything was needed it would be a written statement from prospective employees that they did not suffer from any of a short list of illnesses, examination being offered only to those who admitted to having one. As it was, much time was wasted to no obvious effect, and the real costs outweighed the value of the income generated.

If you are asked to carry out pre-employment examinations, you should ask the following questions.

- What are the physical and mental criteria for the job?
- What detectable medical conditions would preclude individuals from that work?
- What is the most cost-effective means of detecting those conditions?
- Could exclusion of such individuals be construed as discrimination?

The third question must take account of the likely frequency of the condition in the population, as well as its detectability on physical examination. Most conditions are best detected by a screening questionnaire rather than by medical examination, saving the latter for those who answer positively.

Indiscriminate use of medical screening, usually to generate income, has contributed largely to the low esteem in which occupational medicine has been held by members of other medical specialties. It is important for those practising occupational medicine to consider critically its value in terms of preventing ill-health, mental and physical, before becoming involved in it.

Screening and genetics

Since the elucidation of the human genome, there has been a hyperbolic tendency to ascribe to this knowledge an ability to predict future illness and likelihood of fatal disease. This is, of course, only true of a very limited number of rather rare conditions; the idea that we shall all be provided with a chip containing our own genome and advice on how to modify our lives in order to postpone the inevitable remains for the moment in the realms of fantasy. Nevertheless, the concept has caught the public's imagination and will no doubt be promoted by the pharmaceutical industry. On the other side of the coin, the application of genetics to epidemiology has given us a powerful tool with which to investigate the relative influences of genes and environment in the determination of disease. It is worth remembering that, fate having given us our genome, the environment is the main determinant of our health and time of death. Thus, dramatic changes in population mortality and morbidity attend changes in political governance, as for example over the period of communist control in eastern Europe or during periods of despotism and sanctions in Zimbabwe or in Iraq. Such environmental determinants largely explain the differences in morbidity within as well as between countries.

Those who promote the idea that selection of workers might be influenced by knowledge of the genomes of individuals do not take account of the principles of occupational medicine discussed above, nor of disability discrimination legislation. Even where a particular constitutional factor has been shown to increase the risk of developing an occupational disease as a result of a given exposure it does not necessarily follow that exclusion from employment on the basis of that factor is justified. Consider the following example of a common, at least partly genetically determined, condition – asthma.

Substance X can cause occupational asthma, and atopic individuals have twice as high a risk of developing occupational asthma from occupational exposure to it under the prevailing conditions than non-atopic individuals. A simple skin-prick test will clearly identify a proportion of the applicants as atopic. Thus we have the following table:

	Applicants	Will develop asthma	Will not develop asthma
Atopic	30	6	24
Non-atopic	70	7	63
Total	**100**	**13**	**87**

As the above table clearly shows, non-atopic individuals have a 10 per cent chance of developing asthma in this workplace, while atopic individuals have a risk of 20 per cent.
If you stopped the atopic individuals from being employed:

- how many cases of asthma would you prevent?
- how many cases of asthma would still occur?
- how many people who would not have developed asthma would have been deprived of the opportunity to do that job (and perhaps been discriminated against)?
- what could you advise management to do instead of barring atopic individuals from employment?

The law generally requires exposure to be controlled so that 'almost all' the population could be employed day in, day out without an adverse effect on health resulting. Is 70/100 'almost all' the population? In these circumstances you would probably wish to persuade management to control exposures, by the measures discussed earlier in this chapter, rather than to exclude atopic individuals.

What applies to a clear-cut case of genetic predisposition will apply with equal or greater force in the many circumstances where genetic polymorphisms may appear to be associated with marginally or theoretically increased risks from exposure, say, to chemicals. In many such cases, it is likely that the genetic influences are very weak compared to easily detectable environmental exposure influences; indeed, they will often depend on the simultaneous presence of two, three or even more polymorphisms in genes responsible for enhancing or reducing the toxic effects of chemicals.

Pre-employment screening and risk reduction

In spite of the above generally sceptical views on the value of pre-employment screening, there are nonetheless a number of important instances where such assessment can be a useful means of reducing risk. The usual method is to require candidates for a post to fill in a short health questionnaire that is screened by an occupational health nurse. The physician could then review any individual whose health record raised questions. This allows the detection of individuals who would benefit from special measures to assist them to adapt to the workplace if required, as well as detecting some of those who would prove unsuitable. This method of screening, like almost all pre-employment assessments, is poor at detecting those who will prove to cause managers problems from repeated short-term sickness absences. Only occasionally is it possible to point to successes.

Case history 6.19

An applicant for the job as a porter in the hospital service was reviewed by the occupational health nurse and, because of suspicions about his alcohol consumption, was referred to the occupational physician. The applicant in his late thirties was a very heavy drinker and had stigmata of alcoholic liver disease. On questioning he admitted to having been offered aversant therapy (disulfiram) but of having refused it. He clearly had no intention of curtailing his alcohol consumption. The physician considered that his attendance, performance and safety at work were likely to be poor and advised the personnel department that the applicant was unfit for the job. The applicant contacted the trade union shop steward, who threatened a strike on the basis of discrimination. He obtained a letter from his family doctor stating that he was fit for work. The personnel officer offered him the job in spite of the physician's advice. Within a month he was acutely admitted in an abusive and bellicose state to the alcohol detoxification unit. His colleagues complained to managers that they could not work with him and would walk out if he returned to work. The personnel officer asked the occupational physician to review the worker and give advice regarding relocation, but the physician stood by his original advice that the risk to other workers or patients was too great. He did not revise his original recommendation that the man was unfit for employment in the healthcare sector. The man never returned to work and the personnel department never questioned the occupational physician's judgement thereafter.

What would have been the consequence if the worker had injured himself or a patient while in his inebriated state?

LEGISLATION AND PREVENTION OF OCCUPATIONAL DISEASE

The preventive measures discussed so far rely for their effectiveness on knowledge of risk and a willingness to take action to reduce it. This alone is insufficient, unless it is covered by legal sanctions in the event of negligence leading to injury or illness. Thus, most countries have a framework of health and safety law, backed by a system of enforcement, and analogous to those parts of the criminal law seeking to protect citizens from other forms of violence. In addition, people injured as a result of their work generally have the right to sue their employers in the civil courts for negligently causing such injury, the onus being on the injured party to prove negligence.

Almost all countries have their own legislation, within often widely differing court systems. In this section we discuss initially the system in the UK, which because of the careful thought that has gone into its more recent framing might be regarded as a model for such legislation and for methods of enforcement. We also refer to systems in the European Community, whose laws take priority over those of the member states, and in the USA.

The Health and Safety at Work, etc., Act, 1974

Prior to 1970, health and safety law in the UK was a mess, with some 500 separate pieces of legislation covering a multitude of dangerous substances and situations at work, and administered by nine separate Government departments. It was gradually realized that rigid enforcement of the law would be impracticable, leading to reduction of industrial competitiveness and overload of the court system. The mass of legislation was therefore reviewed by the Robens Committee, which concluded that, in spite of this law, there had been no significant reduction in the number of people killed and injured at work. A new Act was therefore framed, intended to cover all eventualities by putting a general obligation on employers to ensure, as far as reasonably practicable, the health and safety of their employees. This Act is known as the Health and Safety at Work, etc., Act and the primary responsibility for its enforcement falls on a Cabinet Minister.

Some basic knowledge of the Act is important to all doctors in the UK, because (with the associated Regulations, as discussed later) it embraces all the structures necessary for ensuring the prevention of occupational disease and injury. The essential features of relevance to doctors are as in the following list.

- It requires all employers to provide, as far as is reasonably practicable, a healthy and safe workplace.
- It requires employers to take care not only of their employees but also of other people visiting the worksite. This of course includes contractors as well as visitors and paying customers.
- It requires site operators to prevent, as far as practicable, emission of toxic substances into the general atmosphere.
- It requires manufacturers to ensure that their products are reasonably safe, and to provide information on safety precautions to be taken in their use.
- It requires **employees** to take reasonable precautions for the safety of themselves and of others.
- It makes provision for the appointment of trade union or employee safety representatives and requires employers, if requested by such representatives, to set up safety committees.
- It established the Health and Safety Commission (HSC), with a Chairman appointed by the Secretary of State and members appointed after discussion with representatives of industrial management, employees and local government. The HSC is responsible for administration of the Act, for promoting research, for providing an information and advisory service, and for submitting proposals for regulations to the Secretary of State.
- It established the executive arm of the HSC, the Health and Safety Executive (HSE), managed by a director and two other members, assisted by area directors. This has responsibility for enforcing the law, having taken over the various original Inspectorates. These include the factories, chemicals, agriculture, offshore oil and gas, nuclear and railways inspectorates, and what used to be the medical branch of the Factories Inspectorate, the Employment Medical Advisory Service (EMAS). EMAS, which includes doctors and nurses trained in occupational medicine, has responsibility for advising the inspectorates on medical matters, carrying out medical investigation and surveys of workplaces, giving advice to employers and others on occupational medical matters and carrying out research. These doctors (medical inspectors) are the specialists to whom doctors in the UK should normally turn for advice when confronted with suspected occupational disease.

Regulations under the Act

There remain a number of Regulations specific to certain particularly dangerous substances, including lead and asbestos, situations, such as underground mining, or physical dangers, such as noise and ionizing radiation. Any doctor involved with an organization or industry in which these hazards arise must be familiar with the relevant

Regulations, which give specific guidance on control, monitoring and so on. Otherwise the law has been much simplified by the introduction of the general *Control of Substances Hazardous to Health Regulations*, originally implemented in 1988, but since amended and widely known by the acronym COSHH. These cover all substances (other than those few, notably lead and asbestos, covered by specific Regulations) with the potential to cause harm in the workplace. The workplace is anywhere where a person might work, and substances include microorganisms. The COSHH Regulations may be summarized quite simply.

- They require an audit of the workplace to detect any potentially harmful substances in use.
- The employer or a representative should then review the use of that substance and decide on whether its use may constitute a significant risk to individuals. If not, a note is simply made of the assessment.
- If a risk appears possible, appropriate steps to reduce the risk should be taken, and a note of these should be made. Regular review of compliance with these procedures is necessary.
- In such circumstances, the employer must consider whether environmental monitoring or surveillance of the workforce is necessary. If either of these is the case, again records must be made and kept for up to 40 years.

In general, the emphasis is on control of substances at source, so that workplace monitoring is only required infrequently and worker surveillance very rarely. The latter needs to be considered when there is a reasonable likelihood, in spite of the precautions taken, that workers will develop harmful effects, and that there are valid techniques for detecting the condition when it does occur.

Case history 6.20

As a result presumably of successful promotion by the manufacturers, the use of glutaraldehyde had become widespread in hospitals, and in one such it was found to be used in some 40 different units. It was pointed out to users that they required to make a COSHH assessment in each case, and that this would clearly involve consideration of the use of safer alternatives. Because its only real application is in the sterilization of instruments, such as endoscopes that could have been contaminated with hepatitis B- or HIV-infected blood and that require rapid re-use, it was believed that this would result in a sharp drop in its use. A year later, a repeat survey showed that its use was undiminished and that a COSHH assessment had been undertaken only rarely.

Like all the examples given in this book, this is a true story. If you were the occupational physician in this hospital, what would you have done at this stage? Remember, the inspectors of the HSE could come in at any time, or a person complaining of symptoms could call in a medical inspector or even take an action in court against the hospital.

The second survey also revealed that an appreciable number of nurses were suffering symptoms attributable to glutaraldehyde exposure. The hospital administration was advised, again, of the potential risks they were taking with their employees, and it was suggested that they strictly controlled the use of glutaraldehyde to areas where there was no satisfactory alternative. The hospital infection control committee was asked to advise on appropriate alternatives. Extraction and enclosure procedures were instituted where glutaraldehyde was used and all employees working in such areas were required to attend for 6-monthly medical surveillance. Central control of glutaraldehyde dispensing through the pharmacy, and the inconvenience of medical surveillance, resulted in a sharp drop in its use. Alternative sterilization methods became the norm.

The type of surveillance of individuals may vary. It may involve as little as the employer keeping a health record of exposed employees or as much as regular monitoring of blood (e.g. mercury workers) or examination by a doctor. In many cases, questioning and examination by an occupational health nurse is what is required, reporting any suspected problems to a doctor.

All the Regulations, including the new Manual Handling Operations Regulations, take roughly the same practical form; they:

- assess risk
- implement controls to reduce those risks
- provide personal protection only when all other appropriate measures have been taken
- if necessary, provide environmental monitoring and/or surveillance of exposed workers.

It can be seen, for example with respect to noise in the workplace, that the objectives would be to control the level by using quieter machinery or by soundproofing the process and, if this were not wholly effective, to provide ear protection to exposed workers. In such noisy workplaces, it would be wise to monitor levels regularly (a requirement under the Noise at Work Regulations with levels over 90 dBA) and to provide audiometric screening of the workforce.

Regulations issued by the Health and Safety Commission with the approval of the Secretary of State for Employment are part of the law and their provisions are mandatory, breach being an offence. However, for the purpose of giving practical guidance, the HSC also issues Codes of Practice covering and explaining the Regulations. These are written in relatively simple language, and are obtainable from Her Majesty's Stationery Office bookshops.

Enforcement

Law is of course useless unless it is seen to be enforced – witness the widespread lack of observance of speed limits in Britain. The role of enforcer of safety and health legislation falls to the Inspectorate of the HSE. Inspectors have wide powers to enter workplaces, to inspect them and take samples and to require premises to be sealed off. If necessary, they can obtain the help of the police. They are able to issue enforcement notices of improvement requiring matters to be put right within a specified time, or of prohibition of further activity where circumstances are thought to be particularly dangerous. Employers have the right of appeal against these to Industrial Tribunals.

Much of the work of inspectors involves routine inspection of workplaces and education of employers. They may, however, be contacted by workers, trades unions or others concerned about safety and health hazards at work. In cases of serious breaches of the law, inspectors may take employers or site owners to court, where fines or even imprisonment may be imposed. There has been a welcome tendency in the UK recently for the courts to take such offences, often resulting in loss of life, more seriously and to impose severe punishment. Nevertheless, it remains true that the consequence of killing an employee at work is often less severe than that of killing someone by dangerous driving.

Legislation in other countries

The European Union has issued through its Commission a series of Directives in the field of health and safety. They have proceeded on the basis of individual hazards, setting standards, which are then enforced by the appropriate national agencies. These include Directives on noise, visual display units, the manual handling of loads, carcinogens and biological agents. European Directives are arrived at by consensus between representatives of the national governments and their experts and, once promulgated, give a time limit within which member nations must comply and after which they are legally binding and enforceable.

In the USA the Occupational Safety and Health (OSH) Act was enacted in 1970. Like the later British Act, it puts a general obligation on employers to maintain a safe workplace. The responsibility for enforcement rests on the Department of Labor, through the Occupational Safety and Health Administration (OSHA). OSHA sets workplace standards and has emphasized in particular the regulation of carcinogens. Its powers are similar to those of the British HSE, and it also emphasizes voluntary efforts to improve health and safety, providing education and consultative services to industry. The OSH Act also created a research arm, the National Institute of Occupational Safety and Health (NIOSH), as part of the Public Health Service of the Department of Health and Human Services. This organization also produces Criteria Documents, giving the evidence necessary for standard setting, and provides an information and advice service on occupational health problems. The OSH Act does not cover the self-employed nor, as in Britain, does it cover industries, such as underground coalmining, already covered by separate Acts.

CONCLUSION

In conclusion therefore the prevention of occupational ill-health through steps for risk reduction should follow an appropriate hierarchical strategy where as much as possible is done to reduce risk at source rather than relying unduly on personal protection or behavioural change to achieve these aims. These general principles apply equally to chemical exposures, to physical hazards, to ergonomic issues and to accidents. In any case, education, information and training are essential mainstays – not simply at a tactical level but to ensure that workers and managers have ownership as well as control of the key issues. Immunization and post-exposure prophylaxis have a special role in defined circumstances in relation to biological agents. Pre-employment assessment is, generally speaking, of limited value. Legislation is important to underpin the above provided that it has adequate 'teeth' but the ultimate goal has to be to effect a culture change among both managers and employees.

7

Work, industry and the general environment

SUMMARY

- Health and illness in individuals and populations depend upon the interactions between genetic susceptibility and environmental hazards. The former can be regarded as fixed, and even the explosion of new knowledge of the human genome is unlikely to make a major contribution to changing the worldwide patterns of disease. It is likely, however, to contribute to better treatment of disease and may, in an occupational context, lead to better definition of health-based standards.

- The environment, especially change in it, is the main reason that people fall ill prematurely. Man influences his own environment, as do all living things on the planet, and environmental change may be expected to have profound effects on patterns of health and disease. Realization of this has led to a measure of international agreement on sustainable development, whereby economic development is planned in the light of environmental considerations.

- Profitable industry is essential to development, and pollution can be regarded as an index of inefficiency. Industry can cause adverse health effects by pollution of air, water or the land, as well as by the harmful effects of the processes and products themselves. Such effects may be subtle, unforeseen and sometimes very wide-ranging.

- Local pollution episodes may cause great public anxiety, often out of all proportion to the likely risks to health. Such anxieties arise usually from confusion in the public mind between hazard and risk, a confusion that may be taken advantage of by pressure groups. The management of such episodes requires an impartial assessment of risks to be made and discussed openly with all involved.

- Consideration of people in their environment, their adaptation to it and their failure to adapt, is central to the practice of good medicine.

INTRODUCTION

It is hardly possible to open a newspaper nowadays without reading some medical story. Commonly these take the form of reports of a new cure for some dread disease, characterized as a 'breakthrough', or of a new suspected cause of illness, 'hidden danger in your mobile phone'. Such stories must help to sell newspapers and are read and sometimes believed by our patients. Certainly, the public is better informed about and more interested in medical matters than ever before, and the information available through the internet is now almost limitless. At the same time, this mass of information (and sometimes disinformation) may prove confusing to the less sophisticated or scientifically untrained reader. An important source of concern in the media is environmental causation of disease, often focussed specifically on the activities of industry and on pollution. In fact, in a broad sense the environment, acting on the genetically susceptible, is responsible for all illness. This chapter discusses some of the general environmental issues relevant to doctors whose work takes them into contact with industry.

GENETIC SUSCEPTIBILITY

Since the last edition of this book, the entire genome of a number of individual human beings has been read and published. Many claims have been and will be made about the significance of this exercise with respect to the future health of mankind. Many can be discounted as examples of the tunnel vision or fortune-seeking interests of those involved, being directed at the most expensive and technological end of medicine with the least likely benefits in terms of public health. However, it will undoubtedly focus debate increasingly on the old 'nature versus nurture' argument, and some individuals may call for genetic information to be used in selecting disease-resistant individuals for, or rather excluding susceptible ones from, hazardous work. This is an argument with which occupational physicians are already familiar, with respect, for example, to atopy and occupational asthma, and which can easily be rebutted (see Chapter 5).

Some genes may cause specific diseases, such as those responsible for cystic fibrosis. Some may subtly increase risks of disease, such as those associated with common conditions like asthma and diabetes. Others may modify the way in which the body metabolizes environmental substances with potential toxic effects, such as tobacco and components of the diet. All may be relevant to environmental and occupational medicine. In the first two cases, the gene may only be expressed under certain environmental conditions – an interesting example may be a gene for myopia, which codes for growth factors in the eye that are only expressed under the influence of close visual work. In the last case, it is very likely that many genes will be discovered that influence risks of occupational disease, given adequate exposure, and that future occupational standard-setting and hygiene practice will have to take account of this. This is already making it more difficult for epidemiologists in defining exposure–response relationships on which such standards ideally depend, because these relationships may differ substantially in different genetic groups. As just one example, certain genes determine the presence or absence of glutathione S-transferases, enzymes involved in the phase 2 metabolism of organic chemicals, and some of the null variants appear in up to half of the population in European countries. Indeed, it has been pointed out that such common null polymorphisms make it likely that the human genome project will in fact miss many important disease-predisposing genes. If the absence of one of these enzymes increases risks of lung or skin cancer when the individual is exposed to polycyclic hydrocarbons or of neurotoxicity when exposed to solvents or organophosphates, then clearly standards should be set to protect the vulnerable half of the population. It thus seems likely that future occupational epidemiology will increasingly have to take account of common genetic polymorphisms when there is a reasonable hypothesis that such polymorphisms may influence the relationships between exposure and effect.

The other side of this coin will be a need to accept that occasional rare associations between toxic exposure and disease may be causal. It has always been easy to dismiss such associations as being chance occurrences and published case reports as being mere anecdotes. Many physicians will have wondered, as has the author, if there is any link between a rare disease in a patient and his work with a particular chemical. The response to the usual inquiries is that nothing like it appears to have happened before, and often this is true. Now we are beginning to realize that some chemicals seem to affect only some people – it seems plausible that this will prove to be the case with organophosphates, as used in sheep dips for example. A particular difficulty may arise when the presence in an individual of multiple genetic polymorphisms results in the absence of several enzymes required for detoxification or the presence of variants that increase toxicity. Such problems pose an important challenge to epidemiologists.

Case history 7.1

A 54-year-old man presented with chronic fatigue, shooting muscular pains and paraesthesiae in feet and hands. He had worked on farms all his adult life, and twice annually until 5 years previously has spent several weeks each year dipping sheep with organophosphates. He admitted to episodes of influenza-like symptoms on several occasions in the past after dipping, but there was no history of a viral illness prior to development of his chronic fatigue. On examination he had reduced vibration sensation on his lower legs but no other abnormalities were found. His condition persisted over several years of observation without significant fluctuation and he had to sell his farm. Genetic testing showed him to have the null genotype for both glutathione transferases *mu1* and *theta1* and an intermediate acetylator status for n-acetyl transferase. All these common genetic polymorphisms could result in reduced ability to detoxify chemicals, and may explain why some individuals exposed to chemicals develop disease and others do not. This is not yet established epidemiologically, but it is at least a plausible explanation of this patient's illness.

The process of setting occupational and environmental standards has traditionally taken account of individual susceptibility in what might be regarded as an arbitrary manner, largely based on the assumption of something of the order of a tenfold variation between individuals. Increasing understanding of the genetic basis of such variability in human populations is likely to lead to much greater sophistication in making such calculations. One possible consequence may be a move towards the maximal exposure limit approach for a larger number of substances, pressure being put on those who expose individuals or populations to toxic substances to strive for concentrations as low as practicable under a limit value.

In spite of the above speculations, the human genome project, driven as it is largely by interests related to the cure of disease, is likely to have relatively little impact on the practice of occupational medicine in the short term. In the longer term it is conceivable that individuals seeking employment will have available their own genome and will wish to ensure that it is compatible with exposure to the hazards of that workplace. Discussion of this, and the ethical issues arising, can safely be left to a future edition. In contrast, it is reasonable to predict that future understanding of bacterial and viral genomes will have major influences on design of vaccines and our ability to protect workers from microbiological hazards in the workplace.

THE ENVIRONMENT AND ILL-HEALTH

The principal determinant of health and illness is the environment. Indeed, it has been man's increasing ability to control and bend this environment to his advantage that has allowed geneticists to have a glimpse of the possibility that the genome might also have some role; as environmental hazards are eliminated and risks reduced, so genetic influences become more easily perceived. The major killers of children and young people in the West are accidents, although of course infectious diseases and malnutrition continue to occupy this position in the poorer world where the social conditions of the Western industrial revolution still persist (Fig. 7.1). After accidents come a group of congenital disorders and rare tumours, many of which are likely to have an important genetic component, although environmental factors such as rubella and drugs affecting the developing fetus may still play aetiological roles. Almost all the major diseases of older people have well-demonstrated environmental determinants – tobacco, diet, psychological and physical stress, and infections being the most important.

The predecessors of occupational physicians, the public health doctors of the 19th and early 20th centuries, recognized the dominance of the environment in causing disease, and therefore the potential for prevention by environmental intervention, when they initiated the movement for improved sanitation and working and living conditions of that epoch. This dominance persists today. Think, even, of a few common diseases in which genetic factors are known to be important. Cystic fibrosis, asthma,

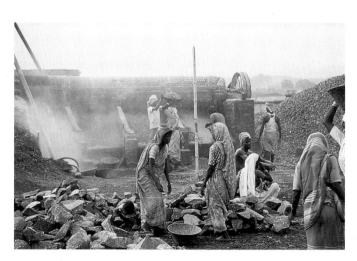

Fig. 7.1 *Women and children working at a roadside stone-crushing plant in rural Bihar, India. High, lifelong dust exposures are inevitable. See also colour plate 7.1.*

and type 1 diabetes might come to mind. The genetics and molecular mechanisms of cystic fibrosis are now well described, but the main determinants of survival (which varies greatly between individuals) seem to be nutrition and infection. It is the balance between the susceptibility of the individual and the stresses imposed by the environment that determines the outcome, and to date manipulation of the environment has paid enormous dividends in the management of the disease. Asthma genes are less convincingly described, although several that modify risks of different phenotypes have been discovered and many others will be. But the disease has doubled in prevalence in many prosperous countries over the last two decades – evidence of a major life-style-related factor. Recent studies suggest that dietary factors and changing patterns of interaction with microorganisms may be important influences on early immune development as well as airway reactivity. Similarly, type 1 diabetes has likely genetic determinants, but studies in twins, differences in prevalence in different countries, and increases in prevalence in some populations again suggest important environmental, perhaps dietary or infective, factors.

Case history 7.2

A 57-year-old woman presented complaining of episodic painful blanching of her fingers, progressively worsening over about 5 years. Her fingers were thin and tapering with taut sclerotic skin. Similar skin changes were apparent around her lips. A diagnosis of scleroderma was made. The occupational history revealed that she had worked all her career in a high street dry cleaning shop, using the solvent 'perc' (perchloroethylene). She reported that there had been frequent leaks and blow-outs and on one occasion the Fire Brigade had been called out.

While this patient's scleroderma may have been simply misfortune, it is at least possible that long-standing uncontrolled exposures to perchloroethylene may have been responsible. In the individual case it is rarely possible to be sure, but a doctor entertaining such suspicions may be in a position to prevent similar consequences in other exposed workers.

As in this example, between the extremes of diseases such as the pneumoconioses, where genetic factors are clearly of trivial importance, and those genetic diseases where the environment plays an important role in determining the expression and deterioration of the condition, lie many diseases of as yet unknown aetiology. Think, for example, of autoimmune diseases such as rheumatoid arthritis and scleroderma, of the neurological conditions motor neurone disease, Parkinsonism and multiple sclerosis, and of sarcoidosis, ulcerative colitis and Crohn's disease. In all these cases there is evidence of the operation of both genetic and environmental factors; in several even, occupational factors have been described: for example, silicosis and autoimmune disease; chemicals and the above three neurological diseases; and beryllium and sarcoidosis. At a day-to-day level, the occupational physician will think immediately of musculoskeletal and psychological stress-related conditions as illustrating the interaction of environment with predisposition.

From Gaia to Rio

The term 'Gaia' was suggested to its originator, the geochemist James Lovelock, by the author William Golding. Literally the ancient Greek for Earth, Gaia embraces the concept of a self-regulating homeostatic chemico-biological planet. Lovelock, taking the view of an observer from outer space, noted the presence of gases in our atmosphere that were too reactive to be in stable equilibrium, and proposed that the earth and its biological population act as a dynamically self-regulating system. Over the 3000 million years of its existence on our planet, life has evolved from simple microorganisms able to build themselves from and reproduce on basic chemicals such as methane, oxides of carbon, cyanide, and hydrogen sulphide, to the huge variety of bacteria, protoctists, fungi, plants and animals of today. All are interdependent, with each other and with the environment in which all live. Growth in the population of any one biological component is limited by the resources available to the whole community of species.

This biological view of life on the planet may lead, depending on one's philosophy, to markedly contrasting attitudes. One is perhaps fatalistic – that whatever we or any other species, such as a new virulent microorganism, do will not matter. The life system on earth has already survived (and taken advantage of) at least three major extinctions of species, the best known of which was that of the dinosaurs and of almost all animals larger than a mouse as a consequence of dramatic climate change which probably followed a meteorite impact. Such extinctions can and will happen again. Seeing mankind as simply one small part of this geo-biological whole in a perspective of billions of years leads to a certain detachment. The other attitude is more centred on our own position, as the first species actually able to comprehend some of the consequences of our remarkable power to reshape and modify our own environment. Increasingly this has given us insight into the importance of biodiversity and of the need to conserve non-renewable resources if the advantages we derive from cohabitation with all the other species on the planet are not to be squandered.

This line of thought leads one in directions that may be alien to many doctors. We have been educated to think of microorganisms as the enemy, to be eliminated wherever possible. One even hears talk of eliminating mites to prevent asthma, as though such an exercise were feasible or likely to be effective (incidentally, asthma is just as prevalent in areas where mites do not live as in those where they do). Pasteur would have been surprised at this attitude, knowing the profound benefits of bacteria to humanity, not least in their ability to produce alcohol. We could not survive without our commensal gut bacteria. Now, of course, in the increase in bacterial resistance to antibiotics, we are seeing the consequences of carelessly waging an unwinnable war against fellow organisms with an in-built evolutionary advantage – the ability to mutate within hours rather than millennia. The future lies in cooperation, and in cohabitation, but with increased immunity to the adverse effects of interactions between organisms.

Mankind has been equally cavalier in his relationships with the inorganic environment. The powerful capitalist and communist economies of the developed world were built with little consideration until recently of adverse environmental effects. The industrial revolution started in the West in the late 18th century and continues today in the developing world as the West has moved into the era of microelectronics (Fig. 7.2). For all of this period we have treated the earth's resources as effectively unlimited and the earth itself as an adequate means of recycling waste products without detriment to ourselves as a species. But, as was pointed out at the end of the 18th century by the Rev. Thomas Malthus, the consequences of a population outgrowing its food supply are war, pestilence and famine. On a global scale we are now witnessing the adverse consequences for some populations of concentration of wealth and resources in other richer ones. But, perhaps even more importantly, we are also beginning to realize that such uncontrolled

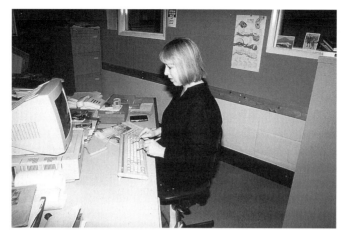

Fig. 7.2 *Office environment: the expansion of microelectronics into everyday life has brought with it unforeseen hazards. In this case, defective technique has led to muscular problems in the operator's forearms. See also colour plate 7.2.*

behaviour in the quest for greater wealth may have previously unforeseen consequences for the chemical and biological equilibrium of the planet. It is worth a thought that when we, or our politicians, speak of securing the planet for our grandchildren, we are failing to acknowledge that our self-interested behaviour has for generations been at the expense of the welfare of children in less advantaged societies.

Recognition of the interrelationships between the environment and public health has developed gradually. European states introduced Public Health Acts from the mid-19th century to control epidemics of cholera and typhoid fever; engineers achieved the separation of sewage from drinking water, while town planners improved housing conditions. The prosperity derived from industry, trade and the development of intensive agriculture allowed a general improvement in nutrition and an increase in life expectancy through the developed world, leading to population growth. In contrast to our neighbours in the poor world, we have become accustomed to safe water, nourishing food and secure housing. A century after these matters were first tackled in the West, action was taken to control air quality, following recognition of the association of episodes of air pollution with excess death rates in urban areas.

Case history 7.3

The winter of 1952 was a particularly cold one and during December a week of cold, still weather led to increased burning of coal in domestic fireplaces across Britain. In the large cities the smoke from tens of thousands of chimneys climbed a few feet into the air where it hit a body of dense cold air, a temperature inversion. The smoke, containing particles of soot and gaseous sulphur dioxide, formed a dense layer over the cities, shutting out sunlight and turning day into night. Many people, especially men, had taken up the habit of smoking during the Great War, and these individuals, now in their fifties and sixties, were beginning to suffer the early cardiorespiratory consequences of the habit. Within 24 hours of the start of the smog episode, the emergency rooms of hospitals began to fill up with men dying of acute exacerbations of chronic lung disease and of heart attacks. By the end of the week, some 4000 excess deaths had occurred in London, constituting one of Britain's greatest environmental disasters.

Such episodes on a smaller scale were repeated in cities each winter throughout the industrialized world. In Britain, the proximity of the 1952 episode in London to the seat of the Government had a similar educative effect on parliamentarians as had the stink from the polluted, cholera- and typhoid-ridden Thames in an earlier generation, leading in this case to effective smoke control regulation.

The public health and legislative actions resulting from these advances in understanding were all aimed at improving health at a local level. It was perhaps the recognition in the 1970s that acidification of lakes and rivers in Northern Europe was related to long-distance transport of pollution across national boundaries and its precipitation as acid rain, that injected an international dimension into the debate. Not long after, the toxic effects of chlorofluorocarbons on ozone were discovered, followed by the demonstration over the Antarctic in 1985 of a hole in the stratospheric ozone layer, a layer that protects the earth from harmful ultraviolet rays. Finally, a link was suggested between the demonstrable century-long atmospheric rise in carbon dioxide concentrations and the increase in the temperature of the troposphere – the global warming debate had begun.

Of course, global temperature change with dramatic consequences for contemporary life on earth had occurred before without mankind's contribution. But in the present case it is at least possible that we as a species may be responsible for causing such change and also, by appropriate action, may be in a position to prevent the worst of its consequences. There is now general agreement that global warming is occurring, but less agreement on its causes and likely consequences. Among the possible consequences of wrapping ourselves in a warm blanket of carbon dioxide, through over-reliance on combustion of wood and fossil fuels and degradation of the earth's photosynthetic capacity, may be:

- increasing desertification in the hot countries, with further problems for subsistence agriculture
- spread of vector-borne disease to more temperate regions
- rises in sea level with flooding of low-lying lands
- even melting of the Arctic ice cap, decreasing salinity of the northern Atlantic and reversal of the Gulf Stream, leading to dramatic changes in the climate of northern Europe.

It may be that the possible effects of global temperature rise have been exaggerated, as some argue; we cannot know for sure as only time will allow verification of such predictions. Nevertheless, the toll in life and human misery exerted on both sides of the ocean by the reversal of Pacific currents known as el Niño is sufficient warning that changes in weather patterns can be disastrous for societies. The ability of scientists to measure such changes and to model possible consequences has awoken governments to what is, after all, the rather common sense view, that we cannot continue indefinitely to use up resources that cannot be renewed.

It was against this background that representatives of most of the world's nations met in 1992, in Rio de Janeiro, at the first United Nations Conference on Environment and Development. This 'Earth Summit' was a unique event, and resulted for the first time in international agreement on sustainable development. One of the central objectives of the Rio accord is to 'minimize hazards and maintain the environment to a degree that human health and safety is not impaired or endangered and yet encourage development to proceed', that is, to promote sustainable development. This was the first time that economic development had been linked to environmental protection, encouraging governments to break down the barriers in policy making between these areas and to think about managing change in the long term. This now forms the basis of policy in the countries of the European Union. In essence the guiding principles are:

- sustainability, over the long term
- consideration of environmental effects, including not only those on human health
- risk assessment based on relationships between exposures and effects
- use of sound scientific evidence
- proportionality between costs and benefits
- that costs should fall upon the polluter – the 'polluter pays principle'
- to err on the side of safety, the 'precautionary principle'.

THE WORKPLACE AND THE ENVIRONMENT

Although starting from opposite points of view, capitalism and communism can both be seen as systems for organizing society in order to achieve, in the words of Joseph Priestley that were adopted by Jeremy Bentham as the main tenet of his Utilitarian philosophy, 'the greatest happiness of the greatest number'. Among those who influenced Bentham around the end of the 18th century were doctors who reacted to the entrepreneurial ideal that characterized the Industrial Revolution by espousing the professional ideal, the concept that those of good fortune might devote themselves disinterestedly to improving the lot of those less fortunate than themselves. Such concepts led to the public health movement and also had in them the seeds of democratic socialism, leading to the forms of government that now characterize the countries of the European Community. The essential feature is a society based on capitalism constrained by government regulation. Karl Marx took a different view, and communism has provided (at what proved to be an unacceptable cost in the former USSR and Eastern Europe) a form of stable government for many people in poorer parts of the world. Now, in its Chinese manifestation, it is also evolving towards the centre ground.

To move from such important global issues to what most people, understandably, think of as 'the real world', the environment in which they and their families hope to survive and prosper, how may the obvious conflicts between a desire for personal prosperity and the need for sustainability be resolved? The ideological battle between capitalism and communism is re-enacted in microcosm in industry on a daily basis. The manager wants profits for self and/or shareholder while the employee wants a share of those profits and does not wish to be exploited. The government, by regulation and inspection, attempts to see fair play, and in doing so often manages to attract the hostility of both parties. The doctor, working in industry, is often in a difficult position in trying not only to ensure the best outcome for a particular individual but also to protect the interests of the employer so as to ensure the greatest happiness of the greatest number.

The occupational physician spends most of his or her time considering the relationships between environment and disease, be they obvious causative links such as psychological and physical stress or the ability of a worker to return to the work environment given a certain level of disability. But there is also a rather wider issue that the physician needs to consider, namely the contribution of a workplace to degradation or enhancement of its local environment. This is an issue that, for the reasons discussed above, is of increasing concern to the general public, including shareholders, to insurers and to governments, and is one on which the views of medically qualified people are often sought. Environmental policy now features frequently in the annual reports of companies to their shareholders.

INDUSTRY AS A CAUSE OF ILL-HEALTH IN POPULATIONS

It goes without saying (although it is sometimes ignored by pressure groups) that productive and profitable industry is essential to society as a generator of the materials and wealth necessary to provide the means for survival of the population. But just as all life forms produce waste gases and materials, so does industry. In an earlier, but not for everyone golden, age human waste was recycled – carbon dioxide by plants and excreta as fertilizer on the fields – allowing sustainable development over millennia. Clearly, the less waste produced, the more efficient the organism or the industrial process; much recent change in industrial processes has been aimed at just this. A good example has been the enormous improvement in the efficiency of the internal combustion engine, and therefore its cost-effectiveness, in response to society's desire for cleaner air. Reduction of waste makes good economic sense.

The three ways in which an industry can produce harm to health of the population are by pollution of air, pollution of water and soil, and by the intrinsic hazards posed by the process or products themselves. The rest of this book is concerned with these effects within the workplace itself, but this chapter considers the effects on the general environment, effects that go further than one might at first think.

Pollution of the air

Air pollution is the most obvious potentially harmful effect of industry on the environment. The smogs, so familiar to those who lived in the great industrial cities of Britain during the 1940s and 1950s, have now largely been replaced in the West by a more hazy and noisome type of pollution generated by vehicles. However, visitors to the great cities of the East, such as Cairo, Bombay, Calcutta or Bangkok, can see and smell pollution derived from both older industrial and domestic and newer vehicular sources. There is a complex relationship between pollution and national prosperity, the former first increasing with the latter and then, as the country becomes prosperous, decreasing again. In some parts of the world, natural sources such as volcanoes and forest or bush fires make important contributions, but deliberate burning of forests for clearance in the tropics has recently been responsible for widespread pollution in Southeast Asia.

Two types of air pollution are of interest to the public. The first is general ambient air pollution, mainly a concern of those who live or work in large conurbations but also occurring in a rural or suburban form. The second is pollution from a local source, such as a power station, an opencast mine, or a chemical factory. Both types attract the attention of pressure groups (on both sides) and may lead to situations where medical expertise is required for their resolution. A third type of air pollution, inside buildings, has come to the public's attention more recently.

General air pollution

The constituents of air pollution reflect their sources, and in the Wes
derived from the internal combustion engine and industrial
domestic/workplace heating making a contribution in the colder montns. ..
terms, the most important pollutants are probably particles, nitrogen dioxide, sulphur
dioxide, ozone, carbon monoxide, lead and polycyclic aromatic hydrocarbons. Other
pollutants that may contribute to ill-health include benzene and aldehydes.

Particles

Particulate matter in the air is responsible for haze, impairing long-distance visibility. It
is often not appreciable when at street level, but is obvious from a tall building or when
landing in an aircraft. Nanometre-sized particles (ultrafines), mainly of carbon, are
generated by all combustion processes, while other ultrafine particles are formed by
photochemical combination of ammonia (derived from animal urine) with sulphate
and nitrate derived mainly from combustion gases. These very small particles are
inherently unstable and clump together in grape-like bunches with diameters below
about 1 μm (Fig. 7.3). Larger particles are generated by wind and wave activity on
surfaces and by abrasive processes on roads, fields and in industrial processes.
Submicron particles remain suspended in air for prolonged periods and can therefore
be carried great distances. They carry on their surfaces a range of chemicals reflecting
their sources and the molecules in the air around them. They are thought to be the

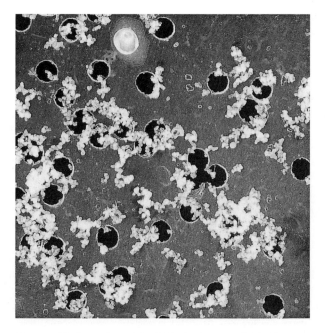

Fig. 7.3 *Electron micrograph of diesel exhaust particles. The
pores in the filter are 200 nm in diameter.*

 articles with which adverse effects on health have been associated, being inhalable and having a good chance of being retained in the peripheral lung.

Conventionally, particles are measured as PM_{10} or $PM_{2.5}$, that is particulate matter less than 10 or 2.5 μm in aerodynamic diameter. As such, they have been associated epidemiologically with increasing risks of death from and exacerbations of cardiopulmonary disease in the elderly, of hospitalizations from and doctor consultations for asthma and chronic airways disease, and of deteriorations in lung function. In the longer term, there is evidence of an association with living in areas of high particulate pollution and death from cardiorespiratory disease and lung cancer. To date no clear evidence of thresholds has been found for these effects. It seems likely that increases in particles in the ambient air are responsible for acting as the final insult that delivers the *coup de grâce* to someone already close to death, or for tipping someone on the edge of illness into the arms of a doctor – the so-called 'harvesting effect'. There is no evidence that particles in the concentrations prevalent in the air of Western cities have any adverse effects on healthy people or that they are able to initiate, as opposed to exacerbate, asthma. We are nevertheless all exposed to them throughout the day (Fig. 7.4).

There has been much debate about how such effects could occur at concentrations so low; they have been demonstrated at well below 100 μg/m³, for example. This argument has not been resolved, but the answer may lie in the number of particles rather than their mass, large numbers of ultrafines having a very large surface area and being able to generate toxic free radicals on their surfaces. It is possible that the lung views such particles, with their toxic surfaces, as potentially invasive microorganisms, capable of penetrating into the blood and causing systemic infection. Thus a defensive strategy, mediated by macrophages, might be designed to attack them in the alveoli and also to provoke a systemic defensive reaction, the so-called acute phase reaction. In this way even the adverse effects of particulate pollution on the circulatory system might be explained.

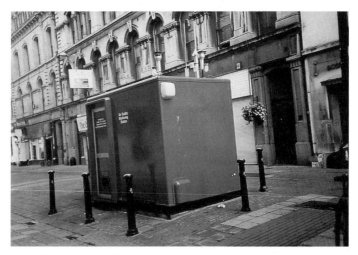

Fig. 7.4 *Air pollution monitor in central Belfast, measuring continuous particle concentrations. See also colour plate 7.4.*

Nitrogen dioxide

Nitrogen dioxide is produced by reaction of ozone in the air with nitric oxide produced in combustion processes; gas cookers in the home, vehicles, and industrial combustion are the main sources. Levels rise in the ambient air in winter when heavy traffic and a temperature inversion coincide. It is a mildly irritant gas that may cause exacerbations in individuals with airflow obstruction such as asthma and chronic bronchitis. In high concentrations in industrial accidents it may cause fatal bronchiolitis or pneumonitis. Some recent evidence suggests that it may be responsible for some of the cardiac effects attributed to air pollution. However, in the author's view it is more likely that in such studies it is acting as a confounder for particle numbers, with which it is closely associated, as both have a common source.

Sulphur dioxide

The chief source of sulphur dioxide is the burning of sulphur-containing fuels such as many coals and oil. Worldwide, volcanic activity is also an important source, while in Western cities diesel combustion is now the primary source. Levels have fallen rapidly in the West following smoke control legislation and removal of coal-burning power stations to rural areas (Fig. 7.5). It is also an irritant gas with similar effects on health to nitrogen dioxide.

Ozone

Ozone is formed as a result of the action of sunlight on precursor chemicals, oxygen, nitrogen dioxide (which it converts back to nitric oxide) and volatile organic compounds generated both by combustion and by plant metabolism. As mentioned above, in the stratosphere it absorbs harmful ultraviolet rays and acts to protect life on

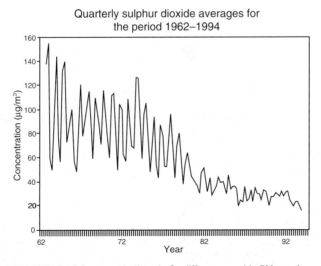

Fig. 7.5 *Particle concentrations in Cardiff, measured in PM$_{10}$ and showing a steady downward trend over the years. Similar falls in PM$_{10}$ and sulphur dioxide have been recorded in all major cities in Britain.*

earth. However, in the troposphere it is an irritant gas, acting through release of free radicals, which may cause increased upper respiratory symptoms and exacerbations of respiratory disease. Because of its mode of generation, it is unusual as a pollutant in occurring at higher concentrations in the summer, in sunnier climates, and in rural rather than urban areas. The latter fact relates to its reacting with nitric oxide derived from vehicles to form nitrogen dioxide and oxygen.

Carbon monoxide

Carbon monoxide is produced by incomplete combustion. Being odourless, it is an important cause of fatal poisoning in houses with defective flues on gas appliances. It also causes occasional unexpected fatalities in industry close to retorts, ovens and in coalmines. The introduction of North Sea gas and catalytic converters on cars has made it a much less common cause of suicide in many European countries than it once was. However, as a direct cause of domestic deaths of young people, usually in house fires, it is the most important pollutant gas. It acts both by inhibiting oxygen transport by red blood cells and also as a poison of cellular enzymes. An important source is cigarette smoke, and smokers characteristically have higher levels of carboxyhaemoglobin in their blood than can be acquired by breathing urban air. Smokers will therefore often contribute the gas to the air around them rather than build up higher concentrations in the blood.

Case history 7.4

While advising an Asian zinc-refining company on its health and safety policy, the author inspected the accident records. While many serious episodes had occurred, fortunately few had been fatal. One, however, caught his eye; a 23-year-old man on night shift had been responsible for stoking a retort. He was found in the morning by his replacement, lying dead at his place of work. His death was certified as having been due to heart attack, but inspection later found a defective flue leaking carbon monoxide.

Epidemiological studies have shown associations between ambient urban carbon monoxide concentrations and mortality, but it is likely that these are the result of confounding, the gas acting as a marker of vehicle exhaust. Ambient concentrations are falling in cities where newer vehicles are fitted with catalytic converters, and in Britain would generally be regarded as within safe limits. Physicians usually become involved where individuals suffer adverse effects as a consequence of faulty gas devices. The symptoms of headache, nausea, dizziness and loss of consciousness, especially when occurring among several members of a family in their home, should always be treated seriously and an urgent inspection by the gas company should be arranged. Chronic exposure to toxic concentrations or acute non-fatal exposures may lead to long-term irreversible neurological damage. Concentrations of carboxyhaemoglobin in non-smokers range up to 1%, smokers may have levels around 2–3%, and the earliest evidence of impaired exercise tolerance or anginal symptoms in people with cardiac disease appears around this level. Headaches usually indicate concentrations around 20% and collapse and death occur at levels from 30 to 50%. Individuals with impaired coronary or cerebral circulations are likely to be susceptible to the serious effects at lower concentrations.

Lead

Lead is of course an important industrial poison, subject to strict regulation in the workplace. As an ambient pollutant, the most important source is water, delivered through lead pipes. As an air pollutant, most lead is derived either generally from the exhausts of cars using petrol to which lead has been added or, locally, to fugitive emissions from refineries. Once in the air, lead is deposited onto crops and into dust, and thus may find its way into the mouths of people. Most concern about ambient pollution by lead has related to the possibility of its influencing the mental development of babies and young children, and there is evidence of an inverse association between blood lead and intelligence quotient in children. While the relationship could be a result of residual confounding in the reported studies, it is a sufficiently consistent finding to have resulted in action in most Western countries to reduce the use of lead in petrol. This has already been associated with reductions in average blood lead concentrations in populations.

Polycyclic aromatic hydrocarbons

Polycyclic aromatic hydrocarbons are produced in all processes involving incomplete combustion of carbon-containing material. They are well-known industrial carcinogens, having been the likely explanation of the scrotal cancer of sweeping boys described by Percivall Pott in 1766, of the shale oil cancers in the late 19th century and, more recently, of the lung cancers in coke oven and aluminium smelter workers. They also occur in high concentration in tobacco smoke. The three best known, classified as probable human carcinogens (IARC group 2A), are benzo[a]pyrene, benzo[a]anthracene and dibenz[ah]anthracene. Vehicle exhausts are the major sources in most cities and may be part of the explanation of higher lung cancer rates in urban compared with rural dwellers.

Local air pollution

Local sources of air pollution often attract a great deal of attention from the public, pressure groups and the media. Curiously, this occurs almost exclusively in rural areas that usually enjoy very good air quality, rather than in urban areas where people have become used to generally more polluted air. It is possible for matters to get out of hand and lead to a great deal of expensive investigation and, often, needless anxiety. Sometimes there are genuine health risks but often the prime motivators are unjustified anxiety or concerns about potential loss of value of local property, so it is desirable that a logical and cost-effective method of investigation of such episodes should be used. A couple of examples will illustrate the types of problem.

Case history 7.5

A coal company sought permission to open a surface coalmine close to a village. The usual precautions were to be taken, including separation of the mine from residences by a hill and the building of a special road for removal of the coal. During the planning process, a local doctor led the action group opposing the development, informing the inhabitants that it could lead, among other things, to increased risks of asthma, cancer and birth defects. The local people required no evidence in support of these statements, as they trusted their doctor. Understandably, great anxiety was generated, inquiries were held and a great deal of public money was spent before the authorities decided that the mine could go ahead. The people of the village nevertheless remained anxious and convinced that harm would come to them.

This sort of story is a common one, repeated whenever a local pressure group decides to oppose an industrial development. Behind it lies an understandable mistrust by the public of big business, based on the long experience of exploitation of those living in deprived areas. A local 'wise man', usually a doctor or a scientist, is persuaded to lead the opposition and he uses his understanding of the uncertainties of epidemiology and toxicology to stress possible adverse effects. The industrial concern, in contrast, stresses the precautions to be taken and the likely benefits, usually in terms of employment opportunities, to the community. Where there is ignorance of possible consequences, or if the parties are badly advised, investigations can get seriously out of hand and become very costly. Usually, however, the likely consequences can be estimated quite easily; for example, the hazards to a population from an open-cast mine will include noise pollution, dangers from increased traffic flows, dust from excavation and fumes from vehicles and excavators. These are all predictable, have known effects, and can be covered by an appropriate risk management strategy. The developer should be required to show that these steps will be taken and how that action will protect the community.

Case history 7.6

A chemical works was intermittently emitting coloured smoke from a chimney and a number of residents claimed that it was causing their children to suffer with asthma. A local retired scientist took the issue up and claimed that the smoke contained dioxin and was carcinogenic. Headlines in the local newspaper increased public anxiety and the local authority and the pollution inspectorate were called in. A major study of the chemicals in the smoke was carried out and inevitably several were of known toxicity; many others were of unknown toxicity. Fears were increased and it was decided to carry out a survey of the health of the local population. Failure to include a control group meant that the results were equivocal, but ensured further increase in anxiety as abnormal findings were attributed to the factory. Eventually, appropriate control of the emissions was brought about, but anxiety remained in the community, with the potential for later legal action.

This story indicates the way in which matters can get out of hand, in this case when there is an air of confrontation between the factory and the local people. This usually prevents a successful conclusion, because of mistrust and anxieties, even if the pollution is controlled. The extreme is reached when legal action is taken, because this inevitably stresses the dangers and prolongs the conflict.

Part of the public anxiety in relation to local air pollution stems from knowledge of the really serious episodes that occur from time to time as a consequence of major industrial accidents. Anyone who lives close to a large industrial complex may be forgiven for some anxiety after the series of accidents over the past two decades. At Seveso, Italy, an explosion in a chlorophenol plant released dioxins and caused an outbreak of chloracne in the local population. At Chernobyl in Russia, meltdown in a nuclear generator released ionizing radiation across an enormous area and caused many radiation deaths and an epidemic of thyroid cancer locally. In Bhopal, central India, thousands were killed or poisoned by an explosion causing a leak of methyl isocyanate. In all of these episodes, a cloud of toxic material generated by an explosion and fire contaminated the surrounding area, or in the case of Chernobyl a large part of the continent. In the case of Bhopal it was responsible for many thousands of deaths from asphyxiation and lung damage. Smaller episodes and near-misses occur regularly and require careful coordinated planning by local agencies and the hazardous industries to control. Occupational physicians should always be aware of the possible local consequences of an explosion and fire in their workplace, and play their part in the emergency planning procedures with health authorities, fire services and police.

Indoor air pollution

Interest in the indoor environment as a source of air pollution has increased in recent years as a result of the description of 'sick building syndrome' and of possible associations with asthma. The former, better referred to as building-related illness, described the occurrence of multiple non-specific symptoms among groups of individuals working in air-conditioned buildings. In a few cases, genuine allergic alveolitis has been described in association with contaminated humidifiers, but usually the symptoms are minor but annoying – a feeling of tiredness, headaches, stuffy nose, etc. No single cause is responsible, but these symptoms have been shown to be more common in people in artificially rather than naturally ventilated buildings.

A more serious problem associated with air-conditioning is its colonization with *Legionella* spp., leading to outbreaks of pneumonia among occupants and visitors. Any system involving recirculation of water used to humidify the air entails this hazard, and the risks need to be reduced by appropriate design and maintenance methods. Episodes of pneumonia have occurred in people visiting buildings and in the communities close to them when the water droplets escape into the local environment.

Case history 7.7

An airport fire fighter was admitted to hospital after suffering for 3 days from a febrile illness. He was tachypnoeic and ill; chest radiography showed bilateral consolidation. He had a stormy course requiring assisted ventilation, but eventually recovered. Immunofluorescent stains of his sputum showed *Legionella pneumophila*. Investigation of his workplace discovered the same serotype in the showerheads at his base. His work involved frequent practices in heavy kit, and he was in the habit of showering at least once and often several times daily.

The most deadly domestic pollutant is carbon monoxide, escaping from defective flues and combustion sources, usually gas or wood burners. This is a regular cause of death and neurological injury in the home, and is also the main cause of death in house fires.

Case history 7.8

During a routine out-patient clinic, the author reviewed a 65-year-old man whom he had looked after for some years for asthma. He seemed uncharacteristically vague and forgetful. Two months previously, he and his wife had been on holiday in Spain and had rented a chalet. The maid had found the two of them unconscious in bed one morning. He survived after oxygen treatment in hospital but recalled little of the event and was left with significant cognitive impairment. His wife died. Investigation revealed a defective gas water heater leaking carbon monoxide.

Several other pollutants are worth mentioning. Second-hand tobacco smoke is now well established as a cause of lung cancer and as an irritant increasing risks of asthma.

Radon gas seeping into poorly ventilated houses from rock formations is also a cause of lung cancer. Risks from this can be reduced substantially by keeping bedroom windows open. Very high concentrations of nitrogen oxides occur as a result of gas cooking, and may be responsible for increases in risks of asthma and chest illnesses in women and children. Again, good extraction in the kitchen can control these risks. Formaldehyde, an irritant gas, can seep out of walls that have been insulated with foam, and this may cause sore throats and upper respiratory symptoms in individuals living in new houses. As time passes, the concentrations fall, especially if ventilation is increased.

Mites and fungi should not normally be regarded as pollutants, but as natural fellow inhabitants of buildings. Viewed biologically, people may be a nuisance to them by attacking them with chemicals, so sometimes they may annoy us by provoking allergies. The same is true of cats and dogs, mice and gerbils.

Pollution of the water and land

Pollution of water by sewage was the cause of the epidemics of cholera and typhoid fever that led to the public health engineering triumphs of the 19th century. Since then most inhabitants of developed countries have had the benefit of bacteriologically clean water. Nevertheless, problems may still occur, as when excessive amounts of aluminium sulphate, a purifying agent, were inadvertently dumped into the public water supply rather than into a storage tank at Camelford in England, or where drinking water passes through lead pipes in older buildings. Occasionally major disasters occur; the most notorious of these was the Minamata episode, when methyl mercury from a chemical factory was discharged into Minamata Bay in Japan. This has led to severe neurological disease, including congenital cases, in over 2000 people who ate fish from the bay.

Heavy metals are a particular problem because of their persistence in the food chain, and may remain a hazard long after the initial discharge. Pesticides and fertilizers may gain access to water from agricultural land and the latter may lead to overgrowth of poisonous algae. The main potential sources of water pollution are agriculture, mining, chemical and oil industries, urban storm run-off and domestic and industrial waste. In developed countries strict regulations control the treatment and disposal of effluent from workplaces, and accidental or deliberate toxic discharges are relatively uncommon. Occasionally, unforeseen episodes come to light, however.

Case history 7.9

A team of sewer workers was investigating a blockage in a small tributary and found it to be clogged with blood. In their job they were well aware of infective hazards, particularly hepatitis A, and suspected a possible risk of infection from HIV and hepatitis B. Investigation showed that the sewer drained the premises of an undertaker, whose practice was to embalm the bodies and flush the blood down the drain. This method of disposal of blood is commonplace, for example in hospital operating theatres and post-mortem rooms, and is probably safer than attempting to treat all such spillages as human waste. Appropriate advice and personal protection were provided for the workers.

It is easy to regard disposal down a drain as a satisfactory means of disposing of toxic material, but it should not be forgotten that people may have to work down sewers, and others work at disposal and treatment plants. Hazardous waste regulations cover what may and may not be disposed of in this way, but these regulations may be overlooked, particularly by small companies seeking to save money. The author has seen a number of sewer workers poisoned as a consequence of such disposal, for example of volatile hydrocarbons. In one case, the worker fell unconscious and was only rescued by the prompt action of a workmate wearing breathing apparatus. A recent film based on fact, *Erin Brokovich*, tells of a lawsuit by residents of a community whose drinking water had been polluted by hexavalent chromium from a nearby utilities plant. Such episodes of careless disposal of waste or seepage of toxic substances do occur, and may lead to ill-advised cover-up operations by industry, heightened fears of adverse effects among populations and very expensive lawsuits.

A particular problem is that of contaminated industrial land that has come into the public domain, as for example when houses have been built on it. Perhaps the most obvious and alarming consequence may be leakage of methane, with its attendant explosive hazard. Alarms may be raised, however, about more subtle effects, such as fetal damage, miscarriages, brain damage to children, and later cancer in people living in the vicinity.

Fears arise from a lack of public understanding of the difference between hazard and risk. That a material, for example asbestos, is known to be hazardous is often sufficient to persuade people that its presence alone is sufficient to cause disease; this is plainly not the case if people do not inhale it. Whether such fears are justified may be assessed only from an understanding of what chemicals are present and whether (and to what degree) they can access people, either by surface contact, ingestion or inhalation. It is always unwise to attempt a bland reassurance without making an appropriate risk assessment. Such an assessment may be complex, involving issues such as uptake of toxic elements into vegetables that are then fed to children. In many circumstances, however, consideration of the likely pathways of chemicals to people leads to reassuring conclusions. It is useful to remember that many elements (e.g. zinc, selenium, copper, manganese, iron) are normal and indeed essential components of human enzymes and other molecules, and harm only arises if the cumulative dose exceeds the body's capacity to deal with it. Other elements, such as lead, and molecules such as polycyclic aromatic hydrocarbons, have no role in human metabolism and can be regarded as wholly toxic. The likelihood of their uptake by individuals will differ in different circumstances, but it is usually possible to estimate from knowledge of activities and local conditions. In some cases, biological monitoring of selected individuals may be possible to test any theoretical estimates.

An approach to management of a suspected pollution episode

The most difficult problems to solve are those involving proving a negative. This is known to environmental pressure groups, who may use it to their advantage. Once a rumour has been started it can easily gain some credibility if supported by a 'scientist' and may be very difficult to counter. However, the problem is not insoluble if one remembers the difference between risk and hazard. Pressure groups almost always talk in terms of hazard, the potential to cause harm, rather than risk, the likelihood of such harm occurring. The management of a suspected hazard is of course to estimate real or likely risks to the people involved and then to take steps to reduce those risks.

Case history 7.10

In the course of renovations to a 1950s office building, asbestos was found to be present in ceiling spaces. The area was sealed off, and contractors were called in to remove it. The workforce, seeing men in white protective clothing, gloves and respirators going to work where they themselves had recently been sitting, not surprisingly became concerned. They quickly became informed about asbestos and discovered that it could cause cancer, even sometimes in people who were not directly working with it. The management embarked on an extensive asbestos monitoring programme and found fibres to be present in low concentrations in various parts of the building where employees had previously worked. Some of these fibres were asbestos. Anxiety was increased and many questions were raised, including not only about cancer risks but also about the possibility of harmful effects on spouses at home or on unborn children.

In discussion with management, it was suggested that outside medical advice was needed and that this should be obtained from someone acceptable both to management and workforce. Managers agreed that full information would be provided and that a report would be made available to all interested parties. Discussions were held with unions and managers together, who cooperated fully. A walk-round survey was carried out and all asbestos measurements were reviewed. Estimates of any likely individual exposures were made, and found to be very small, in terms of both duration and concentration. A list of questions was obtained from the workforce, and an open discussion meeting was held at which anyone with anxieties was encouraged to ask questions.

In this case it proved possible to put people's fears into perspective by illustrating how unlikely any adverse effects were from the acknowledged but trivial exposures some people may have received. A report was written detailing the facts and risks and was made available to all in the building. The consultant made himself available to discuss any further individual's worries, and one such was dealt with by telephone.

This story illustrates two important points in dealing with such an episode. First, someone who clearly demonstrates independence of either side in a dispute is usually going to be more readily trusted than someone who is perceived as having been called in on behalf of either party. This does not exclude an occupational physician employed by the industry concerned, so long as that individual demonstrates clearly his or her impartiality and is trusted by both sides. Objectivity rather than advocacy is what is needed.

A somewhat more difficult problem occurs when risks are not known. Sometimes it is possible to make sensible judgements based on analogy and understanding of toxicological mechanisms, but sometimes epidemiology may prove necessary. A unique opportunity presented itself when the oil tanker *Braer* was wrecked on the Shetland coast.

Case history 7.11

During a winter storm, with hurricane-force winds, a large tanker carrying a full cargo of light crude oil lost its steering and was wrecked on the shore of Shetland, a group of islands to the north of Scotland. As the ship broke up, the oil flooded out and was blown by the gales, as an aerosol, over a wide area of the southern part of the main island, including a local village and several farms. Many problems were foreseen, and the local island council set up a committee to deal with the emergency. As part of the management, it was expected that worries about possible health risks would need to be dealt with. Steps were taken to reduce foreseeable risks by giving appropriate advice and by relocation of some individuals.

Within the first days of the episode a list of likely effects of being exposed to an oil aerosol was compiled. This included sore throats, rashes, exacerbation of asthma in those who already had the disease, and eye irritation. It was also anticipated that the hard labour and long hours involved in protecting livestock in the appalling conditions would lead to non-specific complaints of fatigue among farmers. It was also predicted that within days the media would find a 'scientist', who would be prepared to increase public anxiety by stating that the oil was likely to contain benzene, that benzene caused leukaemia and that therefore the villagers were at risk of this disease. This proved to be the case, although the newspapers had to go as far as the south of England before they found him!

In this episode it proved possible to carry out a questionnaire survey of the exposed population and of an unexposed population living in the northern part of Shetland very shortly after the episode. Concentrations of benzene were also measured during the storm. The survey showed only the expected symptoms and with the objective measurements it proved possible at a public meeting to explain the health consequences of the episode. A follow-up survey was carried out to assess the persistence of any symptoms, and again a public meeting was held to discuss the results. The outcome of the investigation was to conclude that short-term irritant effects had occurred but that long-term effects were unlikely, because overall doses of toxic substances had been very small.

The result of this was that the majority of those involved got on with their lives without further anxiety. A few remained sceptical and a couple pursued litigation against the owners of the tanker on the grounds of respiratory illness. It is at least reasonable to suppose that their asthma may have been made worse by working for long hours outside at the height of the storm.

This episode illustrates the value of dealing in facts rather than speculation. It was fortunate that the episode happened in an area that might have been designed for an epidemiological study and that the authorities were able to address the problem so sensibly and to raise the funds quickly. It is very likely that this prompt action saved both public anxiety and money in the long term, as ignorance of facts allows rumours to flourish.

Many episodes confronting occupational physicians involve relatively unsophisticated populations. Occasionally however, the population perceiving itself at risk is highly sophisticated, and this brings its own problems.

Case history 7.12

A senior lecturer in an ancient university was sitting in his office when metallic mercury dripped from the ceiling onto his desk. It did not escape his notice that mercury is neurotoxic and that all those occupying the building worked with their brains. The building in a previous era and over many decades had been a physics laboratory, and it was discovered that mercury had been used and spilled to such an extent that it had saturated many floors and wall spaces. A very extensive and expensive clean-up operation was completed, but a problem remained in that not all mercury could be detected or removed. The staff involved, mostly social scientists and many female, were concerned about residual risks to themselves and to any unborn children. Recent discussion in the press of possible hazards from mercury dental amalgam had served to heighten anxieties.

In this case the discussion of risk involved such matters as thresholds and the shape of the exposure–effect curve at low concentrations. A management strategy was agreed upon to ensure that the place was made safe enough to occupy. Rooms in the building were characterized by mercury concentrations following detailed surveys, and procedures to decontaminate those with detectable concentrations were set in place. Blood and urine mercury levels were measured in those who had occupied contaminated rooms. Monitoring of rooms allowed them progressively to be declared safe and reoccupied. A concentration at which health risks were thought negligible was determined, based on application of large safety factors to concentrations at which effects were known to occur. Open meetings were held with staff at which questions were answered as honestly as possible, acknowledging uncertainties and concentrating on known and plausible risks.

As with the Braer episode, this approach served to provide what was considered to be justified reassurance to the majority in the building, who saw the major efforts being made to decontaminate the building and appreciated the precautions that were being taken to protect them. However, as is usually the case, a small number sensed a conspiracy to conceal the truth from them and remained dissatisfied.

In dealing with such episodes, it is probably unrealistic to expect to convince everybody. The important point is to convince oneself that the measures being taken are appropriate to ensure the health of those affected and then to put this honestly to them. If this is done and plenty of opportunity is given to ask questions, the large majority will understand. Those who do not, who use the opportunity to seek reparation or to cause industrial unrest, will usually not find themselves supported by their fellow workers. On the other hand, if this open approach is not taken from the beginning, an invitation is given to such people to gain credibility, with foreseeable consequences.

Every such episode is different, but a logical common approach can be used in their management. The key features of this might be to:

- discuss the issues with representatives of those involved, obtaining a list of anxieties, symptoms, etc.
- consider the various ways in which individuals in the population concerned could come into contact with the toxic substances concerned
- visit the site to refine the above assessment
- measure the relevant toxic substances in the medium (air, water, food) in which it might access humans
- assess the likely concentrations to which individuals might be exposed and make a judgement as to whether these entail risk
- discuss the results with those involved; if a risk is predicted, explain what actions are being taken to reduce it and by how much
- consider a health survey of the population, if a risk is predicted, remembering to include an unexposed control group; dummy questions can be introduced to assess bias
- keep representatives of those involved informed at all times about the progress of the investigation.

There is of course an element of judgement in what constitutes a risk, and individuals' views will differ on this. Open discussion, including comparison with other well-known and accepted risks, will often lead to a resolution satisfactory to the large majority, particularly if it is coupled with a commitment to risk reduction.

HAZARDS OF THE PRODUCT

The best known example of a product causing risks to the health of the population is the manufacture of cigarettes and other tobacco products. In the first half of the 20th century there was a general belief that cigarettes were beneficial to health, at least by having a soothing effect on the smoker. This all changed with the reports of Doll and Hill in the 1950s, and subsequent studies have shown the extraordinarily harmful effects that the industry has on public health worldwide. Nowadays few doctors would regard cigarettes as having any real use, although one still comes across nurses who regard them as a therapeutic tool in mental hospitals. An example of a useful product contributing to environmental health risks is asbestos. A material with many uses in industry, several of which are potentially life-saving (fire proofing, brake linings, transport of clean water, for example), was found to cause a number of fatal diseases in workers. Its ubiquity then led to the realization that many people not actually working with it might be exposed para-occupationally and thus to the anxiety that its very presence in the environment may lead to disease in the general population. This anxiety has turned out to be ill-founded, but there is no doubt that risks of mesothelioma are increased in a wide range of jobs where only incidental exposure occurs.

Examples of industrial products leading to widespread illness include those where deliberate contamination has occurred in order to maximize profit, as in the Spanish cooking oil episode in which olive oil was contaminated with cheap non-edible oils and sold from door to door. This led to an outbreak of severe and sometimes fatal neurological and pulmonary vascular disease in hundreds of people. On an even larger scale, pesticides, for example, are responsible for thousands of deaths among the poor in the tropics as well as probably causing illness among sheep dippers in the West. However, the greatest interest in harmful effects of industrial products recently has been in food.

It is a paradox that those of us who live in the rich world are better fed and have access to a greater variety of food than ever before, yet food poisoning is on an almost exponential rise and more and more anxiety surrounds the possible harmful effects of food production. The reasons for both aspects of this paradox are the same – poorly regulated capitalism. Worldwide competition has allowed the food industry in the rich countries to flourish and indeed to provide such relatively cheap food as to lead to population over-nourishment. Rapid international transport makes available, to those who can afford it, food from anywhere in the world. Wealth has led to an abundance of choice and, increasingly, to ability to buy ready-prepared foods. Competition in the agriculture and food production businesses has led to short cuts being taken, abuse of antibiotics as growth promoters, and unnatural animal feeding practices. A culture of haste in food preparation in the home has led to ignorance of the traditional and bacteriologically safe methods of cooking. Microorganisms and prions find their niche, and we now have not only classical *Salmonella* spp. infections but also *Escherichia coli* O157, bovine spongiform encephalopathy and, hence, new variant Creutzfeldt–Jakob disease.

Even more subtly, apparently beneficial changes in the composition of the food we eat may have unexpected side-effects. The use of industrially produced fats as margarines and cooking oils, for example, has reduced the ratio of N-3 to N-6 fatty acids in our diet and also introduced the unnatural *trans* fatty acids. The increasing amount of processed as opposed to fresh food has reduced the amount of antioxidant vitamins in many Western diets. The author of this chapter has speculated that these subtle changes in diet may lie behind the increase in population susceptibility to allergic diseases, asthma and diabetes that has occurred in wealthier countries.

One final example of an industry with great potential both for benefit and for harm is the pharmaceutical industry. The public perception of this industry is that it is wholly beneficial, engaged in a mission to improve public health and cure disease. An alternative view is that it occupies a highly competitive area of capitalism, with the potential for big profits for shareholders and therefore a huge incentive to produce successful drugs and to promote them in order to recover costs and pay dividends. There is clearly a huge opportunity for unethical behaviour, which is why this is one of the most regulated industries of all. In terms of environmental health, it is interesting to note how the pharmaceutical industry has responded to recent challenges. The HIV pandemic has perhaps brought out the best, with highly innovative research leading to a dramatic improvement in the prognosis for many sufferers among the educated and articulate in the West. Unfortunately, the cost of the drugs is such that they will not make any impact on the worldwide problem, again emphasizing the differences between the rich and the poor worlds. The problem of cancer provides another story. Here the public could be forgiven for thinking that we are in the midst of a major epidemic, and that only further massive investment in the industry will provide an answer. In fact, only a few cancers are increasing in age-adjusted incidence, and chemotherapy has so far only produced a very costly cure in relatively few types. In contrast, understanding of causation (e.g. cigarettes, sunlight, diet) holds reasonable hope of progressive reduction in incidence at low cost.

An effect of the successes of the industry in curing some diseases is to distort public and professional priorities in research towards finding a magic bullet rather than finding a manageable cause; for example, we now know that cervical cancer is often a sexually transmissible disease, and therefore largely preventable by appropriate public health measures. The prospect of a cure for cancer envisages rich rewards for the pharmaceutical industry, but to find a microbiological or other environmental cause which could form the basis of a public health strategy tends to be left to a few lateral thinkers, who may find it difficult to obtain grants.

Another consequence of the success of the pharmaceutical industry has been an increase in public reliance on drugs. In the West, up to one-third of the adult population takes vitamin pills or other dietary supplements on a regular basis. Rather than buy and cook fresh food we have come to rely on pills! There has been a perceptible shift of emphasis to producing lifestyle-enhancing drugs for sale to the general public. Elderly males are being persuaded to take drugs for 'erectile dysfunction' and powerful, potentially dangerous, anti-inflammatory drugs are being sold as cures for the common cold. How widely will the new generation of drugs for Alzheimer's disease spread into the market and be used by all of us who think we are becoming a bit forgetful as we grow older? A glance at any newspaper or magazine will show just how far this dependence on drugs has gone.

SO WHAT IS ENVIRONMENTAL MEDICINE?

This chapter has been necessarily wide ranging. This is because as human beings we cannot separate ourselves from our environment; we are part of it and it is in everything we do. We have adapted to it over tens of thousands of years, but we also have enormous potential to change it for good or ill. As with drugs and food, environmental changes may have beneficial and adverse effects at the same time.

The good doctor learns to think of people in their environments, of illness as a relative failure of adaptation, and of the practice of medicine as a usually imperfect effort to enable ill individuals to return to better adaptation. Environmental medicine is not a specialty, it is an attitude of mind that sees individuals as part of their environment, being influenced by it and in turn influencing it. It should pervade the good practice of medicine.

8

Sickness absence

Elizabeth Wright

SUMMARY

- Assessing employees in relation to sickness absence forms a substantial part of the work of most occupational physicians. This chapter discusses the complex multifactorial aetiology of sickness absence and its importance from an economic point of view.

- Absence can be broadly categorized into short-term and long-term. It is important to distinguish between persistent, intermittent absence, which may not be linked with a consistent medical condition, and long-term absence, which is usually associated with significant illness, because the practical management of each differs.

- Control and management of all absence in an organization is the responsibility of managers, while the role of the occupational physician is to give impartial, independent advice to help managers make decisions regarding the appropriate management of individual cases. Employment legislation does permit employers under certain circumstances to discipline and dismiss employees for illness or absence, and ill-health may be deemed a fair reason for dismissal if it affects an employee's ability to perform the work they are employed to do.

- Where an individual is no longer fit for their job, or has residual disability, the occupational physician can advise on possible modifications to the job or, if this is not feasible, fitness for other types of work. This allows the employer to consider redeployment in a more suitable post or, failing this, ill-health retirement. Rehabilitation, ill-health retirement and employment of the disabled are discussed in greater detail in Chapter 9.

- People unable to work because of ill-health may be entitled to a range of State Benefits. Occupational physicians should be aware of the benefits available, where information may be obtained and how patients can access the system.

- Sickness absence tends to be lower in organizations where the personnel manager is involved with its management. The intervention that has the greatest impact on absence is probably the return-to-work interview, for both manual and non-manual employees. A history of previous absence is the most effective way of predicting future absence in any individual.

> • Primary prevention of sickness absence may be possible through organizational change, but a reduction in duration of individual absences can be achieved through prompt referral to the occupational health service (OHS) for assessment, and by facilitating rehabilitation initiatives to enable employees to return to work sooner.

INTRODUCTION

The health assessment of workers in relation to sickness absence forms a substantial part of the work of most occupational physicians and can be one of the most difficult elements. While the responsibility for controlling and managing sickness absence rests with managers, the doctor's role is to provide independent, impartial advice on individual cases to help managers to do so fairly and appropriately. As the occupational physician is employed by an organization, there may be difficulties in that employees perceive the doctor to be acting on behalf of their employer, and the managers expect this to be the case. Education at the outset of managers and employees in the role of the occupational physician and other aspects such as confidentiality helps to avoid any future misunderstandings.

Case history 8.1

A 38-year-old physical education (PE) teacher was referred to the occupational physician by her manager for advice on her fitness to return to work. The teacher had been on sick leave for almost a year. She attended her appointment accompanied by her husband. A diagnosis of progressive multiple sclerosis had been made 3 years previously and it was apparent that she had become very disabled, with marked ataxia which made it impossible for her to walk without a stick. In addition, she had been obliged to give up driving because of visual problems. It transpired she had been having difficulties teaching PE at a primary school for some time before going off work but had struggled on because she enjoyed her job. She was clearly unfit for her present post but was very keen to continue working in some capacity. The occupational physician advised the lady's employer that she was unfit to work as a PE teacher (there were no adjustments which could have been made to enable her to continue) but would be capable of part-time sedentary work, perhaps helping pupils with educational difficulties. Unfortunately it was not possible to find a suitable alternative job and the teacher was retired on medical grounds.

This case illustrates that in some cases it is very difficult to achieve rehabilitation after sickness absence, and therefore ill-health retirement is the eventual outcome. The principal outcomes of sickness absence are shown in Figure 8.1. The vast majority of employees return to work as usual after a spell of absence, but a few will be unable to do so because of residual impairment. Depending on whether the impairment is temporary or permanent, and on the nature of the job, it may be possible to rehabilitate these individuals back to their original employment, or to an appropriate alternative post. Employers should endeavour to keep people in work whenever possible through rehabilitation before considering other options such as ill-health retirement. Rehabilitation is discussed in greater detail in Chapter 9. While employers do have legal responsibilities to make adjustments to a job to accommodate people with disabilities, 'light work' is not often available and it may not be possible to make 'reasonable' adjustments. There is no onus on any employer to *create* a job for someone who is no

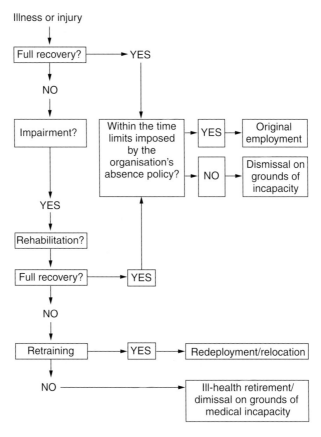

Fig. 8.1 *Outcomes of ill-health in relation to prospects for continuing employment.*

longer capable of their previous duties, even if they are suffering from a work-related injury or illness, although suitable adjustments are discussed in the next chapter.

Definition of sickness absence

It can be quite difficult to define sickness absence. It is basically non-attendance at work when the employee should be there, and which the employee attributes to sickness. It excludes absence that has been previously authorized, such as time off to attend a hospital appointment, or a relative's funeral, as well as absence for statutory reasons such as maternity leave. More unusual statutory reasons are suspension from work under the Ionizing Radiation Regulations or the Control of Lead at Work Regulations, when exposure limits have been exceeded.

Case history 8.2

A 23-year-old hospital domestic assistant had frequent uncertified absences since commencing employment 18 months previously. As her sickness absence was well above average for the department she was referred by her manager to the OHS for advice on her fitness for the job. Her most recent absence had been the previous week, when she had phoned in 'sick' for the third time in 1 month. In the referral letter the manager explained that current staffing difficulties were resulting in complaints from some of the wards, and the manager herself had been obliged to 'help out' on several occasions despite the fact she was struggling to cope with influenza. During the consultation, it emerged the young woman was a single parent with financial difficulties. In order to support her family she had another part-time job working as a barmaid in a nightclub and after finishing work in the early hours of the morning she was sometimes too exhausted to go to work later at the hospital.

This case shows that so-called 'sickness' absence may have important socio-economic or domestic causes. Moreover, individual perceptions of illness vary considerably, with the result that the presence of a mild or moderate degree of ill-health keeps some individuals off work while others decide to carry on. In this case the manager with 'flu was probably more unwell than the member of staff off sick. Although the majority of absence is the result of incapacity of some kind, there are also many other reasons that people decide to stay off work, such as family and social reasons, or difficulties in the workplace, for example bullying or dislike of the job.

It can be useful to consider sickness absence in a behavioural context. We all know that there are some individuals who are frequently absent, while others have very little time off sick. Minor illness may cause one employee to be absent from work, while another would never consider taking time off. Conversely, there are some employees with major health problems who will struggle to attend work long after others would reasonably have taken sick leave. This 'absence behaviour' is dependent on individual perceptions of health, first, whether illness is present or not, and second, whether time off work is reasonable. The latter will depend on both real and perceived views on the nature of their work and its effect on their ill-health, attitudes of work colleagues and management towards their absence, real or imagined fears about transmission of infection to others and concerns about financial or disciplinary repercussions if time off is taken. The term "presenteeism" is used to describe a situation where employees are reluctant to take time off work, even when unwell, usually because of fear of disciplinary action or financial penalty. This is becoming an area of concern for employers because of the impact an impaired worker has on productivity and performance of the overall organization.

ECONOMIC EFFECT AND COSTS OF SICKNESS ABSENCE

Over the past 50 years in the UK there has been a progressive rise in sickness absence, which has occurred despite improvements in the health status of the population and the availability of health care. The reasons for this are multifactorial and include socio-economic factors, such as a changing age structure of the population, an increasing number of women in the workforce, improved living standards and generally higher expectations of life. A similar trend has been noted throughout Western Europe and the USA. It seems that national absence rates tend to rise in affluent societies where there are more liberal attitudes towards medical certification and well-established benefit schemes. The costs of sickness absence are of great concern to industry and have far-reaching implications for the economy as a whole.

Case history 8.3

A hospital medical records department manager requested advice on the prospects of a future return to work of a 52-year-old member of staff, who had been off work for 6 months with 'stress and depression'. The medical records assistant had been attending the occupational health department over a period of time and had made a good recovery with antidepressants. The physician felt that she was ready to go back to work but when this was suggested the lady burst into tears and said she did not want to go back as she felt that her illness had been caused by stress at work. During the consultation she made it quite clear that she was not prepared to return to work under any circumstances. Her trade union representative had advised her not to resign from her post, so she would be remaining off sick for the foreseeable future.

What is the role of the occupational physician in this case? Although primarily acting in the best interests of the patient, the physician also has a responsibility to the employer to prevent abuse of the sick pay system, which is designed to assist those who are genuinely unable to work. This organization's sick pay provision was for 6 months at full pay, followed by 6 months at half pay, representing considerable costs over a year's absence. This employee had made it clear she did not intend to return to work and unless management action was taken she would receive a full year's sick pay, followed by a further period of notice on full pay plus holiday pay. How might this situation be resolved? Responsibility for managing absence rests with the managers but they need appropriate advice from the physician on which to base their actions. In this case the employee was prepared to consider redeployment. However, she did not wish to apply for any of the other posts that were available at the time and her employment was eventually terminated on the grounds of incapacity after 9 months absence. Employees are not (usually) entitled automatically to receive the maximum sick pay provision, and employment may be lawfully terminated before pay expires if there is no prospect of an individual returning to work.

This case illustrates the potential costs to organizations if absence is not managed. Not only do they have to provide sick pay but also they may have costs in relation to providing cover for an absent worker. The extent of sick pay provision varies between different countries, for example in Germany companies only have to pay the employee for the first 6 weeks for a specific illness, but after that illness insurance meets the costs for a period up to 72 weeks. Staff shortages may also place other employees under additional stress and this can result in low morale and poor productivity. The effective management of sickness absence can therefore result in considerable savings.

Most European Union countries collect data on absence from work, but as different methods of collection are used it is difficult to make direct comparisons; for example, in Denmark the first 2 weeks of absence are not counted, and there may be differences in the definitions of short-term and long-term absence. Bearing this in mind the following figures should be interpreted with caution. It has been suggested that there is a correlation between the generosity of member states' sickness benefit schemes and short-term absence. In 1991 expenditure on sickness benefits amounted to about 7% of the gross domestic product in Germany, the Netherlands and France, and 5% in the UK.

Figure 8.2 shows short-term and long-term absence for many European Union countries. The Confederation of British Industry (CBI) has been carrying out surveys on absence in the UK since 1987. The latest survey reported that in 2004 168 million working days, an average of 6.8 days per employee, were lost as a result of absence, a drop from 176 million in 2003. Despite the drop, the average cost of sickness absence

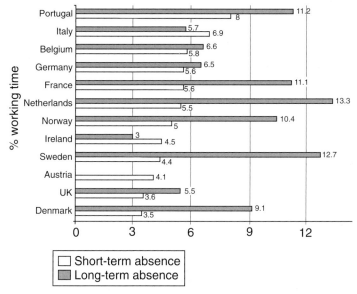

Fig. 8.2 *Levels of absence in the European Union 1998. (Source CBI, 2004, Who cares wins: absence and labour turnover.)*

per worker continues to rise, with an estimated total cost to UK employers of £12.2 billion annually. This figure represents only the direct costs of absence – wages for additional overtime or temporary staff and lost production time. If the indirect costs, such as lower customer satisfaction or poorer quality of product or services leading to loss of future business, are taken into consideration, the true costs to industry are likely to be considerably higher. Figure 8.3 shows the trend in absence levels in the UK.

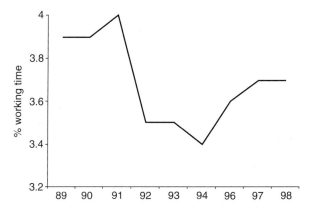

Fig. 8.3 *Trends in absence levels 1989–97 as a percentage of total working time. (Source CBI, 2004, Who cares wins: absence and labour tunover.)*

It is difficult to estimate the total number of working days lost as a result of sickness absence, but figures based on claims for sickness benefits in the UK suggest that in 1991 503 million working days were lost. The main reasons were:

Disorder	Million days lost
Musculoskeletal disorders	133
Cardiovascular disease	100
Psychological disorders	91
Respiratory disorders	35
Accidents	28

Source: *Social Security Statistics*. Government Statistical Service. London, UK: HMSO, 1992

These figures exclude absences of less than 3 days (which do not require certification in the UK) and absences of less than 8 days (which are self-certified), so the actual number will be very much greater: absences lasting 1–3 days account for approximately 15% of sickness absence.

MEASUREMENT OF SICKNESS ABSENCE

There are several reasons why an employer might want to quantify sickness absence. First, sickness absence can have a major economic impact on an organization and is therefore an important area for loss control. Measurement of the amount of absence, and the areas or employees most greatly affected, provides managers with the information necessary for effective sickness absence management. Most organizations that measure sickness absence use electronic payroll systems for data collection. Second, the identification of clusters of specific illnesses or conditions in certain types of workers or in specific locations in a workplace can be an indicator of possible work-related health problems requiring further epidemiological study; for example, high sickness absence levels in a specific department could be as a result of underlying difficulties such as bullying or harassment. Managers themselves can sometimes be the perpetrators. Finally, from the occupational physician's perspective, absence monitoring schemes encourage early referral of employees to the OHS, which is important for effective rehabilitation into the workplace.

Unfortunately there is no standard way of quantifying sickness absence, making comparisons between organizations extremely difficult. Some common ways are described below.

Absence is generally quantified in terms of **frequency** and **duration**, which are used to express the incidence rate and prevalence or severity of absence.

Frequency is measured in **spells** of absence, a spell being defined as an uninterrupted period of absence. Absence frequency rate is measured over a given time period, either a month or a year:

$$\text{Frequency rate} = \frac{\text{number of new spells of absence per year or month}}{\text{total number of employees}} \times 100\%$$

This calculation tells you the percentage of employees who are off over a given period of time but it does not tell you how long people are off for, or whether some people are off more often than others.

Duration of absence may be expressed in calendar days or working days. Many organizations prefer to use working days in order to calculate the costs of absence to the company; however, the use of calendar days may be more useful if comparisons are to be made with other studies of sickness absence.

The expected normal working days must be defined for any particular organization as they can vary from:

- calendar days – 365
- working days – 260 (based on a 5-day working week for 52 weeks) or 235 (taking average holiday entitlement into account).

$$\text{Mean duration of absence per employee} = \frac{\text{total number of days absence per year}}{\text{total number of employees per year}}$$

This tells you the average number of days off per employee but does not give any information regarding the proportion of long-term and short-term absences. The calculated average will be high because of the influence of a small number of absences of very long duration. Most absences in an organization last only 1 or 2 days.

Prevalence rates can also be calculated to identify days where absence is particularly high or low, or to monitor absence during epidemics. They can be calculated for a particular day or over a given period of time. Again prevalence rates are of limited value for measuring sickness absence in industry as they give no indication of the frequency or duration of episodes of absence.

$$\text{Point prevalence rate} = \frac{\text{number of employees absent on a day}}{\text{total number of employees who should be present}} \times 100\%$$

Another way of measuring absence is to calculate the number of days lost per employee over a given period of time:

$$\text{Period prevalence} = \frac{\text{number of people absent over a given time}}{\text{total number who should be present during given time}} \times 100\%$$

Severity rates, by comparison, are widely used in industry and can be expressed as the Lost Time Rate, which is calculated in terms of number of hours or days lost as a percentage of hours or days which should have been worked over a given period of time. This parameter is often used in industry to monitor performance and set targets for absence management. It can be calculated on a weekly or monthly basis, enabling comparisons to be made between departments of an organization. Its limitation is that it gives no indication of the proportions of long-term and short-term absence.

$$\text{Lost time rate} = \frac{\text{number of working hours or days lost per week or month}}{\text{total number of possible working hours or days}} \times 100\%$$

By now it should be apparent that a combination of different measurements of sickness absence is necessary to provide all the information you might need. The extent to which this information is collected varies a great deal from one organization to another.

BRADFORD FACTOR

In organizations where the majority of staff work in shifts or rotas, the disruption caused by frequent short-term absences is often greater than that caused by occasional long absences. The Bradford formula is a method of scoring an individual's absence that gives more weight to the number of spells within a given period than to their duration, so is useful for identifying persistent short-term absence. It can be used as part of a Sickness Absence Management Policy to monitor trends in absence and to set trigger points for management action.

It is calculated using the formula: $S \times S \times D$
S = number of spells of absence/year taken by an employee
D = number of days of absence taken by that employee in the same period

FREQUENCY DISTRIBUTION OF SICKNESS ABSENCE

While it is useful to calculate the rates described above to measure absence, it should be remembered that these are mean rates, and give no indication of the range of values that can be encountered when looking at individual records. In reality the distribution of sickness absence in the workplace is highly skewed. Many employees will take no spells of absence at all in any given year but a small minority will take many. In general, half the total time lost is caused by 5–10% of the workforce.

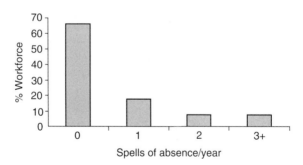

Fig. 8.4 *Distribution of absence spells in a workforce.*

CAUSES OF SICKNESS ABSENCE

Ill-health resulting in absence from work may be the result of work-related illness, such as occupational asthma, dermatitis, or upper limb disorders, or of mental or physical illness unrelated to work, or of a combination of the two; for example, work-related back pain causing secondary depression.

Work-related illness, which in the UK, for example, has been estimated to affect over 2 million people in one year, is theoretically preventable through effective risk management systems. The common occupational diseases are now musculoskeletal disorders, psychological problems, dermatitis and asthma, as has been discussed in

Chapter 2. Back pain and musculoskeletal disorders are by far the most common work-related illnesses in the Western world. A study by the UK Health and Safety Executive in 1995 estimated that 1.2 million people were suffering from a work-related musculoskeletal disorder, with 44% experiencing back pain alone. The Department of Health has estimated 11 million working days are lost annually due to back pain. The most common reason for work-related musculoskeletal problems is manual handling, followed by posture and repetitive work. The occupations most likely to be affected are coal mining, nursing and construction work.

Case history 8.4

A 34-year-old electricity linesman ruptured his biceps tendon while attempting to lift a heavy wooden pole at work. This is a physically demanding job involving the erection of overhead electricity lines (Fig. 8.5). Surgical repair was necessary and he was off work for the following 6 months undergoing physiotherapy. When subsequently referred to the occupational physician, there was marked muscle wasting and he was unable to extend the elbow fully. He was clearly unfit to return to his usual job but it was possible to find him temporary work in the office while he underwent further intensive physiotherapy. Just over a year after the accident he regained the full use of his arm and was able to resume his normal duties. He subsequently made a claim for damages against his employer.

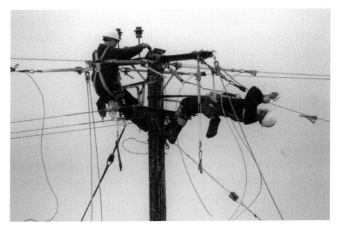

Fig. 8.5 *Electricity linesmen at work. Note the extreme postures adopted. Photograph courtesy of Dr E. Wright.*

Case history 8.5

A 58-year-old sewage operative was referred to the occupational physician for advice on his fitness for work. His duties included installation and repair of underground sewage pipes, a manual job involving heavy lifting, work in confined spaces and exposure to unpleasant human waste. He had not taken sickness absence but his line manager had noticed that he seemed to be having difficulty carrying out some of the heavier tasks at work, such as lifting manhole covers. The patient had undergone two hip replacement operations 4 years and 6 months previously, making an excellent recovery on both occasions and returning to work without any problems. His current complaint was knee swelling and pain that had become progressively worse over the previous 3 years. Assessment by an orthopaedic surgeon had been carried out and he was being managed conservatively with anti-inflammatory analgesics and, more recently, by steroid injection, which had been of limited benefit. On examination there was a restricted range of movement at the knee and he was unable to kneel or squat. He admitted that he had been struggling with certain aspects of his work for some time, but had hoped to be able to continue until normal retirement age. A report from his General Practitioner confirmed his severe osteoarthritis and he was subsequently retired on the grounds of ill-health.

Compare these two cases of work-related musculoskeletal conditions. With the linesman it is easy to establish that the injury was **caused** at work – an acute medical problem developed while carrying out a risky activity. However, it is much more difficult to demonstrate a link between occupation and common degenerative conditions like osteoarthritis, which develop over a period of time. Rather, in the case of the sewage worker, the heavy nature of the work was **aggravating** the condition. It is not unusual for older workers with these conditions to carry on at work, despite sometimes suffering severe discomfort, without taking time off. The problem comes to light when colleagues or a supervisor note the individual seems to be having difficulty undertaking certain tasks or that work performance is deteriorating. In the past it was often possible to find 'light duties' for such individuals, especially in the public sector, but current management practices tend to preclude this, so it results in increasing numbers of medical retirements, which consequently put a strain on pension schemes.

Mental health problems are the second most common work-related illnesses, estimated to account for 11% of work-related ill-health. The occupational physician is likely to come across a wide range of psychiatric and psychological disorders, from overt psychosis to post-traumatic stress disorder, depression, anxiety and stress-related illnesses. Litigation for work-related stress is on the increase, for example in the UK since the well-known case of *Walker v. Northumberland County Council* reported in the Industrial Relations Law Reports *(1995) IRLR 35.* Mr Walker was a social services officer responsible for four teams of field workers in an area where suspected child abuse was prevalent. The volume of work increased considerably and he suffered a mental breakdown. After 3 months of absence he returned to work, having been advised that he would receive more support, but this failed to materialize and he subsequently suffered a further breakdown. This led to his being medically retired by the Council. Mr Walker sued his employer for damages and the matter was settled out of court for £175,000. The following case is very similar.

Case history 8.6

A 43-year-old social work team manager who had been absent from work for 10 months with 'stress' was referred to the occupational health physician by the personnel manager of the Local Authority, seeking advice on his future fitness for the job and asking if he was fit to attend a disciplinary hearing. About a year previously serious concerns had been raised about his performance at work and a subsequent investigation deemed disciplinary action appropriate. The manager's explanation was that he had been under pressure for several years as a result of lack of resources resulting in an inability to provide services, which ultimately had led to criticism of his work. He was a conscientious person who often worked late and regularly took work home with him in the evening. Despite discussing his difficulties with his own line manager nothing had been done and when he was finally told he was being transferred to another post pending investigation of his work, he went on long-term sickness absence with clinical depression. After 10 months of treatment with antidepressants his health had improved to a limited extent; he was sleeping better but still had difficulty concentrating and was extremely anxious about the hearing. In his view he was unfit to attend and he could not envisage ever returning to work in the social work department.

This case is typical of a referral as a result of work-related stress and one that can be very difficult for the occupational physician to resolve. An individual states he has been under sustained pressure at work for a prolonged length of time. Ultimately his health has been affected, yet he has struggled to carry on at work rather than resort to taking sickness absence. Eventually something happens which is 'the last straw', in this case the disciplinary hearing, and he is no longer able to continue. One would expect that removal from the stressful environment and antidepressant treatment for 10 months would have led to recovery, but in this case worry about the impending disciplinary hearing was prolonging the ill-health. He was certainly not fit for work, but was he fit to attend a hearing? Provided an individual is capable of understanding proceedings it is generally better to attend and get it over with, rather than prolong events and continue to worry about possible outcomes. Will he ever be fit to return to work? This is a question often asked by managers but unfortunately without the benefit of a crystal ball can be very difficult for occupational physicians to answer. Most people with depression will fully recover in about 6 months, but where work is perceived as the underlying cause and there is no prospect of changing the working environment to improve the situation it can be much harder to rehabilitate an individual. In some situations where there has been long-standing pressure and the employee no longer trusts their employer or manager, it is often not realistic for them to return to the same job and run the risk of recurrence of their illness, and it is preferable to explore redeployment in an alternative post. Medical retirement is rarely indicated and the majority of cases would not meet the criteria laid down by pension schemes.

Most referrals for sickness absence will not be for work-related health problems, but for other illnesses that prevent an individual carrying out their duties or that impact on safety at work. The length of absence will depend on the nature of the illness and the requirements of the job; for example, a nurse with a prolapsed disc would find it more difficult to go back to work than would a secretary working in an office.

Case history 8.7

A 44-year-old electrician was referred after 4 months sickness absence. His manager was concerned about his future fitness for work with high voltage electrical equipment in a remote area where he worked alone and unsupervised. Prior to his absence an incident had occurred where he had disrupted the local power supply, resulting in damage to company property. It transpired he had developed an acute psychosis with paranoid delusions that his work was creating magnetic fields that were to be used as part of a global conspiracy. Following the incident he had been compulsorily admitted to a psychiatric hospital where his condition settled with treatment and was discharged a month later. When seen by the occupational physician he was taking regular medication, no longer exhibiting paranoid ideas and was keen to return to work. A report was obtained with his consent from his general practitioner. This revealed that over the previous 10 years the patient had experienced several hypomanic episodes, on some occasions exhibiting paranoia and requiring admission to hospital.

Safety of this patient, his colleagues and the general public was paramount in this case. The occupational physician advised that in view of the risk of recurrence it would be better to employ the man in a position where he would not have access to potentially lethal electrical equipment, and where he could be supervised. Fortunately it was possible to arrange this and he returned to work. As an additional precaution, his work colleagues were asked to keep an eye on him and report any changes in behaviour to his manager.

FACTORS AFFECTING SICKNESS ABSENCE

Within any organization it is apparent that there are some individuals who are off work frequently, while others have very little sickness absence. Why should minor illness cause one employee to be absent from work, while another attends? Clearly the medical condition alone cannot be the sole reason for absence, and other factors must be influencing the decision to stay off work.

The factors affecting sickness absence can be separated into three categories: personal, geographical and organizational. These are outlined in Table 8.1. It is notable that only a few of these are strictly medical.

Table 8.1 *Some factors influencing sickness absence*

Personal	Geographical	Organizational
Age	Region	Nature of organization
Gender	Climate	Size
Occupation	Social insurance	Industrial relations
Personality	Health services	Sick pay
Job satisfaction	Unemployment	Working conditions
Medical conditions	Social attitudes	Supervisory quality
Family responsibilities	Pension age	Environmental hazards
Journey to work	Epidemics	Labour turnover
Life crises		Personnel policies
Alcohol		Occupational health service
Social activities		

Personal factors

Personal factors are by far the most important, in particular, age, gender and occupational status. Sickness absence increases with age, but the pattern differs. Younger people tend to take more frequent spells of absence of short duration, particularly during the first few years of starting work. This relates to the period of adaptation from home and school to a work environment and new responsibilities. Older people tend to take fewer spells, but of longer duration, which reflects the greater likelihood of serious health problems with advancing age.

Numerous studies have demonstrated that women, particularly those in the reproductive years, tend to take more spells of absence than men. This is often attributed to the influence of social and domestic responsibilities, such as having to care for children or elderly relatives.

Occupational status is also important, higher rates of absence being reported in unskilled workers than in managerial or professional grades of staff. The CBI survey in 2004 estimated a UK annual average of 8.4 days' absence for manual workers compared with 6 days for non-manual workers. Relevant factors are dull, unrewarding employment with low status, which may also be hazardous, stressful and physically demanding. It may also be more difficult for a worker to return to work with, for example, a musculoskeletal injury, if they are employed in a manual occupation rather than an office job.

Job satisfaction, which depends on a number of different factors, will influence employees' motivation to attend work. Individuals who dislike their work and feel that their manager is ambivalent about their attendance are more likely to go off work with a minor ailment than those who enjoy their work and feel part of a team.

The presence of a medical condition ought to be the most important factor influencing sickness absence; however, this is certainly not the case. For any individual the decision to stay off work will depend on their own subjective view of their state of health and be influenced by other non-medical factors such as those described in this section. In practice it is usually the worker who makes the decision that he or she is unfit for work, rather than their doctor, although the latter will be called upon to provide the necessary certification.

Geographical factors

Geographical factors reflect the political and socioeconomic differences between countries or regions where an organization is located, and multinational organizations are well aware of differences in absence rates between different locations (see Fig. 8.2). Regional differences may depend on the type of industries in the area, the public sector and general manufacturing having higher rates than financial and professional services and the retail sector. Other relevant factors include the strength of the local economy and unemployment levels. This underlines that 'sickness absence' is not necessarily a reflection of 'organic disease' but is influenced by socioeconomic factors at a regional or geographic level and therefore the remedies at these levels are not medical ones. Similar considerations apply at a company level as considered below.

Organizational factors

Organizational factors are probably the most important external factors influencing sickness absence. The size of an organization, the way managers operate, sick-pay schemes and shift patterns all interrelate to affect the length of a spell of absence. Organizations that (in the UK) provide fully paid sick leave for 6 months followed by half paid leave for a further 6 months will know from experience that individuals will often return to work when full pay expires, irrespective of their health status. Absence rates tend to be higher in the public sector (9.1 days) than in the private sector (6.4 days), which could be linked to company size, as smaller organizations with fewer than 100 employees tend to have lower absence rates compared with those with over 5000 employees. The importance of organizational factors is emphasized by the report on the findings of a supplement to the 1990 Labour Force Survey on work-related ill-health that found that 57% of employees with stress/depression felt their illness was work-related (Davies and Teasdale 1994). Management style or perceived attitude can have a major influence on absence; where an individual feels valued and part of a team, morale and attendance improve. This is demonstrated by the following case.

Case history 8.8

A 26-year-old man who worked in the information technology department of a large organization was referred to the occupational physician by his manager because of eight episodes of absence lasting 1–2 days in the previous 6 months. The reason given was migraine headaches. The young man had a long history of migraine, which was inadequately controlled by his current medication. His headaches had been occurring more frequently over the preceding 6 months and he attributed this to inadequate ventilation at work. It transpired during the consultation that there had been a number of changes in his job, and he had been passed over for promotion. As a result he felt undervalued and demotivated at work. At his appraisal his manager had told him that his unsatisfactory attitude was one of the reasons he was unsuccessful in obtaining the post he wanted.

The occupational physician referred the young man back to his GP to discuss alternative treatments for his migraine. She also suggested that he had a frank discussion with his manager regarding the way he felt about his job. This took place a few weeks after the consultation, and helped the situation for a while. However, a year later he was referred again with further short absences. He resigned before being seen.

CATEGORIES AND MANAGEMENT OF SICKNESS ABSENCE

'Absenteeism' is characterized by short absences where a medical reason is usually given as an excuse but the underlying reason is usually non-medical. There can be a link with weekends, holidays or other times convenient for the employee and there may be reports of the employee undertaking inappropriate activities such as attending football matches or taking part in the local amateur dramatic production! This type of behaviour is a matter of conduct and managers should address this through appropriate disciplinary measures.

Sickness absence generally falls into one of two categories, short-term absence and long-term absence. There is no strict definition of either but short-term absence generally relates to spells lasting from a single day to a few weeks, while long-term absence relates to continuous spells lasting usually 6 weeks or more. In any organization the majority of absences will be repeated episodes of short-term absence, but the majority of lost working days will result from long-term absence of a few employees. The CBI survey previously mentioned reports that long-term absence accounts for 5% of cases but 33% of total lost working days annually. Both can be very disruptive, resulting in reduced productivity and additional pressure on remaining staff.

Short-term absence

In the UK a medical certificate is not required for absences of less than 3 days, although some organizations use their own forms for self-certification. Between 3 and 8 days a self-certificate is required (Form SC1) for Department of Work and Pensions (DWP) purposes so the individual can be paid Statutory Sick Pay (SSP), which is discussed later.

Generally short-term absence is a result of minor self-limiting illness, whereas long-term absence is more likely to be caused by a significant medical problem. In either case it is likely that non-medical factors will be contributing in some way towards the absence. The influence of non-medical factors tends to predominate in repeated short absences. Managers sometimes label individuals who take repeated spells of short-term absence as 'malingerers'. However, individuals rarely take time off purely to avoid work, and in these cases there is usually a combination of a minor ailment with other factors such as workplace conflicts or domestic responsibilities. Repeated episodes of short-term absence may occasionally be indicative of more serious problems such as substance abuse, a poorly controlled medical condition, such as migraine or diabetes, or even occupational disease, such as asthma.

Case history 8.9

A 23-year-old man was referred to the occupational physician with the following absence record:

Start date	Day	Finish date	Day	Reason	Duration
05/11/99	Fri	09/11/99	Tue	Viral infection	3
15/07/99	Thurs	16/07/99	Fri	Food poisoning	2
27/04/99	Tue	02/05/99	Sun	'Flu	4
04/11/98	Wed	08/11/98	Sun	Sickness	3
15/10/98	Thur	25/10/98	Sun	Muscle strain	7
12/09/98	Sat	18/09/98	Fri	Sickness	5
24/08/98	Mon	07/09/98	Mon	Hospital operation	11
12/08/98	Wed	16/08/98	Sun	Sore throat	3
01/08/98	Sat	02/08/98	Sun	Upset stomach	1
22/06/98	Mon	22/06/98	Mon	'Flu	1
10/06/98	Wed	14/06/98	Sun	'Flu	3
20/01/98	Tue	20/01/98	Tue	Sickness	1

His manager was concerned at the amount of time off the young man had taken over the previous year, 12 spells totalling 44 days, attributed to a variety of complaints. On a number of occasions since the previous November he had reported for work and stated that his GP had advised him that he had a condition which meant he should not speak to customers over the phone. As he worked as a customer services adviser in a call centre, a pressurized job involving spending most of the time on the telephone dealing with customer queries and complaints, the advice that he attributed to his GP in effect made it impossible for him to carry out his job. Initially he was transferred to another department on a temporary basis where he could rest his voice, but the manager noted that he had no apparent difficulty speaking to colleagues at work, and indeed had volunteered to work additional shifts in his normal job over the start of the new millennium, which attracted a high rate of overtime pay.

The manager felt this was inconsistent with a medical problem and eventually, on one of the occasions when he reported to work refusing to take calls again, the manager asked him to at least try for a couple of hours to see how he got on. At this point he became upset and anxious and had to be sent home. He was referred to the occupational physician for advice on finding a solution to the problem.

At interview it transpired that he had suffered from a viral chest infection which had resulted in a recurrence of childhood asthma. Because of his wheeziness and sore throat his doctor had advised him to rest his voice for a while, a sensible suggestion given his job. However, the young man enjoyed the challenge of his temporary placement in the office, where he was able to develop his computer skills and only used a telephone occasionally, and was using this medical advice to delay his return to his usual job. He had spent a number of years in the same post and was ready to move on, as the job was stressful and pressurized. In addition there was some uncertainty about his employment as a result of company reorganization. The frequent short spells of absence he had taken over the past year were not the result of any serious underlying health problems but were indicative of his job dissatisfaction. After liaising with the GP and manager concerned, the occupational physician was able to advise that the young man gradually take on his previous duties over the next fortnight and he returned to work. In addition it was suggested that the manager discuss his future career development with him. Initially his return to work was promising but later, like many of his colleagues, he was made redundant as the firm shed staff for reasons of 'efficiency'.

Cases of recurrent short-term absence are often harder to manage than long-term absence. This is because long-term absence tends to be caused by a significant medical problem, whereas short-term absences may be attributed to any number of unrelated ailments. Recurrent absence can, however, be indicative of an underlying health or substance abuse problem, or of an individual with work-related difficulties. One of the main aims of assessment by the occupational physician is to identify those with underlying problems who would benefit from some sort of intervention to improve attendance in future. Failure to identify these individuals could result in their being subject to the organization's disciplinary procedures and ultimately lead to dismissal.

Long-term absence

In cases of long-term absence the medical condition itself largely determines an individual's fitness for work but the duration of absence may be prolonged by non-medical factors beyond their control, such as delays in obtaining hospital appointments and waiting times for physiotherapy or surgery. In addition, the point at which the individual decides to return to work may be influenced by the type of job, whether management is perceived as supportive, worry about being able to cope, fear of further injury, or the fact that their sick pay has expired. It has been shown that the prospects of returning to work decline with length of absence. Approximately 70% of those off for a month will return to work, but only 20% of those absent for a year will do so. In the UK, absences of 8 days or longer require a medical certificate, provided by a GP (Med3) or hospital, if the individual has been an in-patient. The prognosis for return to work after long-term absence is illustrated by the following case.

Case history 8.10

A 45-year-old teacher was referred to the OHS after 9 months absence as a result of 'debility'. She was suffering from a depressive illness secondary to the death of her mother after a protracted terminal illness. Treatment with antidepressants had lifted her mood and she was sleeping better, her concentration and memory were good and she was starting to socialize again. The occupational physician felt that she was ready to consider returning to work part time, and that it would be beneficial for her to resume contact with her work colleagues, but when this was suggested she broke down and said she felt she was not well enough yet. On further questioning she revealed a number of potential difficulties at work, including a heavy workload resulting from having to cover for colleagues' sickness absence, dealing with difficult adolescents, and perceived lack of support from the head teacher, who had a reputation for being a bully.

A diagnosis of 'debility' or 'neuraesthenia' on a sickness certificate usually means an individual is suffering from an underlying psychiatric or psychological condition. Doctors may use these terms to disguise the diagnosis, as some individuals may not wish to reveal the nature of their illness to the employer. This lady was making a good recovery but had lost her confidence as a result of being off work for so long. It is worth noting that bullying in schools does not always involve the pupils. Following a meeting between herself, the human resources (personnel) manager and her line manager to discuss her working situation, she was persuaded to return to work on a part-time basis to refamiliarize herself with the workplace. She met her line manager weekly to discuss her progress and by the time she was reviewed at the OHS 6 weeks later, she was feeling ready to increase her hours and responsibilities. She had also spoken to other members of staff and they were considering making a formal complaint against the head teacher. Ideally this teacher should have been referred earlier as it might have been possible to get her back to work much sooner if she had received appropriate support. Active rehabilitation of employees following long-term absence is beneficial to both the individual and the employer and is discussed in greater detail in Chapter 9.

Table 8.2 summarizes the main differences between short-term and long-term absence.

Table 8.2 *Features of short-term and long-term absences*

Short-term absence	Long-term absence
Lasts a few days	Lasts weeks or months
May be recurrent	Likelihood of return to work diminishes with duration of absence
Employee usually self-certifies	Employee requires medical certificate
Usually result of minor self-limiting illness	Usually a significant medical problem
Influence of non-medical factors great	Non-medical factors can prolong absence
Can indicate more serious health problem or substance abuse	

MANAGEMENT OF SICKNESS ABSENCE

Within an organization the responsibility for managing and controlling sickness absence rests with management. Usually this is the line manager, with input and advice from a variety of sources such as the human resources (personnel) department, safety department and the OHS. Good channels of communication between everyone concerned are therefore essential for the effective management of individual cases, as well as for the overall policy.

Monitoring sickness absence

In order to manage sickness absence it is necessary to have comprehensive attendance records. Many organizations use electronic payroll systems, which can provide data to individual departments or managers regarding staff attendance. Basic data should include age, sex and occupational status, and details of each spell of absence, including duration and diagnosis. From these figures sickness absence indices of frequency (average number of absences per person per year) and severity (average number of days lost per person per year) can be calculated.

Having established a baseline, managers can then focus on those individuals who have higher than average absence, and take appropriate action under the organization's absence policy.

Sickness absence policies

Organizations operating sickness absence policies tend to have lower absence rates than those that do not. Such policies are usually drawn up with input from trade union and staff representatives, as well as managers, and should provide a framework for dealing with individual cases in a supportive and fair manner. An alternative and more positive title is 'Attendance Management Policy', which focuses more on keeping an individual in employment or assisting their return to work rather than tending towards punitive measures to deal with absenteeism.

Key elements of a sickness absence policy

A model policy on sickness absence should include the following:

- policy statement outlining the aims of the policy, to whom it applies and who is to be responsible for its implementation
- procedures for notification of absence
- monitoring and record keeping
- trigger levels of absence at which managers should take action (with guidance)
- actions to be taken for frequent short-term absence
- use of disciplinary action – circumstances under which it will be taken, procedures to be followed, outcomes if attendance fails to improve
- action to be taken for long-term absence
- procedures for referral to the OHS
- rehabilitation – duration, financial aspects, possible outcomes if rehabilitation is unsuccessful
- procedures for exploring redeployment opportunities
- financial aspects – income protection schemes, etc.

- ill-health retirement procedures
- procedures for dismissal on grounds of incapability
- guidance on return-to-work interviews
- the role of the human resources (HR) department – to provide specialized advice to managers regarding termination of employment, early retirement, rehabilitation and redeployment, disability, and substance abuse.

The CBI survey previously referred to compared the effectiveness of different absence management policies and practices in organizations that operated the policies and those that did not. The survey found that in general sickness absence was lower in organizations where the personnel manager was involved with its management. Policies that had the most impact on absence were return-to-work interviews, for both manual and non-manual employees, followed by pre-employment medical assessments for non-manual employees and provision of OHSs for manual employees. The practices with least impact on absence levels were attendance bonuses and increasing the length of time before sick pay became payable.

The role of managers

Most organizations monitor attendance in some way, and employees whose attendance is unsatisfactory are likely to be interviewed by their manager in the first instance. Many organizations have 'trigger' points for action when an individual's absence level reaches either the national average or a preset level in the company. This method allows managers to be seen to act fairly and consistently towards staff throughout an organization. Some examples of triggers are:

- three separate spells of short-term absence (2–7 days)in a 3-month period
- or two spells of long-term absence (>7 days) in a 12-month period.

The action taken by managers should differ depending on the individual circumstances of each case, and 'triggers' are not to be interpreted rigidly as special cases may need different action (as illustrated below). Short-term recurrent absence is likely to be treated differently from long-term sickness. In order to comply with employment law managers must be able to demonstrate they have acted 'reasonably', that is, they have taken into account the nature of the illness, the likely length of absence, the need to have the employee's work carried out and the circumstances of the particular case.

The first step is likely to be an interview with the employee to investigate the facts. The attendance record and the reasons for absence are reviewed to see whether there is a clearly identifiable medical problem or, alternatively, whether the absences appear to be the result of a variety of seemingly unrelated diagnoses. The employee's explanations must be considered before deciding what action to take. It may be necessary to obtain further medical information and this may be obtained from the employee's general practitioner, specialist or the occupational physician, with the employee's informed written consent. It is not appropriate for managers to pry into confidential medical matters and at this point referral to the OHS, if there is one, may be indicated. It is not necessary for every individual with unsatisfactory attendance to be referred for medical advice and managers should use their discretion. Where there is no indication of any underlying problem, there is nothing to be gained by referral in order to verify whether or not an individual has had a particular ailment once they have recovered and are back at work. However, it may be helpful for medical advice to confirm the presence or absence of any serious underlying problem in order for the manager to take the appropriate action.

Case history 8.11

A student nurse was referred to the occupational physician following 10 spells of absence lasting between 1 and 12 days, totalling 42 days over a 12-month period. The reasons given were 'tonsillitis'. The manager sought advice on whether there was any serious health problem and whether attendance was likely to improve in the future. The patient was somewhat unhappy at being referred and stated she had 'always had sore throats' and had been told nothing could be done. She managed her symptoms by having an odd day off and only seeing her GP if she felt she needed antibiotics.

What approach should the occupational physician take? The patient was currently asymptomatic and examination of her throat entirely normal. Having established that while she may have been having recurrent bouts of pharyngitis, there was no evidence of anything more serious, the physician needs to explore non-medical factors. Enquiry should be made into the job, shift patterns, difficulty with tutors or colleagues, secondment to other hospitals causing isolation, as well as social factors such as personal problems and alcohol or drug use.

The patient asserted she enjoyed her course and was having no difficulties academically; however, she did not get on well with the staff in some of the wards where she undertook placements. This was influencing her decision to stay off work with minor symptoms.

Where there is no evidence of any serious underlying medical condition to account for absence the physician should state this in a written report. This is not denying that the student has had genuine sore throats, or implying they are malingering, but is merely confirming the absence of anything serious that might be amenable to treatment. It may be helpful to advise the manager if there are personal or work difficulties in the background that might need to be taken into consideration in the management of absence.

Following receipt of a report confirming the absence of a serious medical condition, the most likely management action would be a further interview with the employee to set standards for attendance over a period of time. This is, in effect, the start of formal disciplinary procedures, and if the employee fails to achieve the standards set, the outcome ultimately may be dismissal on the grounds of unacceptable attendance. Employment legislation does permit employers to discipline and dismiss employees for illness or absence, and ill-health is potentially a fair reason for dismissal if it affects an employee's ability to perform the work they are employed to do. This is something that both employees and some doctors find hard to accept, particularly in cases where an individual has a genuine medical condition through no fault of their own, or they have been injured at work. It also brings to light the risks of conflict of interest when a local GP is also acting as occupational physician to a company employing patients registered with his or her practice.

Case history 8.12

A 32-year-old male clerical assistant with a 10-year history of Crohn's disease was referred to the occupational physician after being off work for 3 months with an exacerbation. The condition had been fairly well controlled in the past with Salazopyrin but symptoms had become gradually worse over the previous 6 months and consisted of frequent, uncontrollable diarrhoea up to 10 times daily, with accompanying abdominal pain. The young man had seen a gastroenterologist for investigation and was being treated with steroids. Although the condition had improved to a certain extent and he was having several 'good' days each week, it was not possible to predict which days he was going to be unwell and his symptoms meant he could not leave the house. Various solutions were considered, including relocating his workstation closer to the toilet facilities. Work from home was not feasible. The employer generously allowed him a further year off work in the hope his condition would improve but when reviewed by the occupational physician he was no better and was having financial difficulties as his sick pay had expired. He remained unfit for his job and was not well enough to be redeployed. His employment was subsequently terminated on the grounds of medical incapacity. Although seemingly harsh, this benefited him financially in that he received full pay throughout his period of notice, and for the annual leave he had been unable to take.

Not all employers are as sympathetic towards their workers and in this case the employer would have been justified in terminating employment sooner if operational difficulties were resulting from the individual's absence.

Sometimes even very short absences can be indicative of serious health problems that may warrant immediate action. In other words, the inclusion of trigger points for action in an attendance policy should not replace common sense and good judgement when there may be safety implications, even if associated with very little or no absence from work. This is clearly demonstrated in the following case.

Case history 8.13

A 35-year-old ambulance paramedic was referred to occupational health urgently by his divisional manager after 3 days off work with a 'dizzy turn'. The manager was concerned about his fitness to drive, as there had been rumours that he had in fact had a seizure. On questioning, the paramedic admitted that he had experienced some form of fit. His wife, who witnessed it, called an ambulance, and he had been admitted to hospital. Initial investigations were negative and he was discharged the following day, having been told, he said, that there was no evidence of epilepsy.

Examination by the occupational physician was unremarkable but in view of the uncertainty about the diagnosis it was recommended that he did not drive until further information was available from a specialist's report. He was reviewed a month later when the report was available. This confirmed that electroencephalograph and brain scan were normal, but the history was strongly suggestive of a seizure having occurred, perhaps secondary to alcohol consumption. Anticonvulsant therapy was not indicated. The paramedic was very anxious about the implications for his work. UK government guidance states that driving must cease for a year following a single seizure and, if public service vehicles are driven, 10 years must elapse before a licence can be restored. As driving was an integral part of the job this effectively meant the patient was no longer fit for duty. Redeployment in a non-driving capacity was not possible and his employment was terminated on the grounds of ill-health.

The aim of absence management is to facilitate return to work and keep people in employment as far as possible. Although disciplinary measures are used when appropriate and it is sometimes necessary to terminate employment, it is more usual for managers to be supportive towards their employees, and some will go to great lengths to assist in the rehabilitation or redeployment of staff. This is particularly so in cases of long-term sickness absence.

Case history 8.14

A 48-year-old engineering manager was referred to the occupational physician after an incident at work where he had walked out after a disagreement with his line manager. His doctor had subsequently signed him off sick with 'stress-related illness'. Having worked for the organization for over 25 years, he was having difficulty coming to terms with new working practices introduced as part of the latest company reorganization, and which were, in his opinion, unsafe. At interview he was extremely agitated and wanted to talk at length about a file he had brought with him containing correspondence relating to various issues at work. He had felt under pressure at work for several years and was becoming increasingly frustrated with changes in his workplace. In the past he had been a meticulous and conscientious employee who was rarely off work. There was no previous history of mental health problems and he was happily married with no domestic worries. His symptoms included insomnia, irritability, difficulty concentrating and tearfulness, suggesting depression. His general practitioner, whom he found very supportive, had commenced antidepressant therapy and referred him to a clinical psychologist. Unfortunately there was a long waiting list and he was unlikely to be offered an appointment for almost a year. After liaising with the manager and general practitioner, the occupational physician arranged referral to a private clinical psychologist, which the company had agreed to pay for. Over the following 6 months there was marked improvement in his health with cognitive therapy combined with medication. When reviewed he felt ready to return to work and a structured rehabilitation programme was arranged with his manager. During the first month the employee was supernumerary and was relieved of management responsibilities, which allowed him gradually to increase his hours while refamiliarizing himself with the workplace. Further training in operating procedures was provided and regular meetings with his line manager were held to discuss his progress. Over the course of the following 3 months he gradually took on full responsibilities again and when reviewed by the occupational physician was coping well.

This employee was very much valued by his employer, who was not only prepared to fund the cost of private treatment in view of the lengthy waiting list but to accommodate a period of rehabilitation to assist the employee's return to work. This not only benefits the employee but is also cost-effective for the organization if duration of absence is reduced as a result.

REFERRAL TO THE OCCUPATIONAL HEALTH SERVICE

Referrals to the occupational physician may be made formally, by managers in accordance with the organization's absence policy, informally, or by employees referring themselves. Sickness absence is only one of the reasons managers refer to the OHS, but it is generally the most common. A referral is usually initiated after a manager has interviewed a member of staff about their unsatisfactory attendance but can also occur if work performance is a cause for concern or if substance abuse is suspected. The timing of referral may vary. While it would be appropriate to wait for a couple of months before referring a school cleaner who had undergone abdominal hysterectomy, a bus driver off for a day with 'dizziness' should be referred more urgently.

Employees who have little personal experience of the OHS often have preconceived ideas about being referred. They may find it threatening, suspecting that the occupational physician is 'checking up' on them, or they may worry that they might find themselves deemed to be no longer fit for work. It is important that managers discuss the reasons for referral with the employee beforehand and gain their informed consent. Employees must understand that the consultation is confidential and that the role of the OHS is to be supportive and helpful. They must be told that a report will be sent back to the referring manager but that this will be confined to an opinion on fitness for work and no medical information will be divulged without the employee's consent. They also need to be advised of their right to see a copy of any report, which is now covered in the UK by the Data Protection Act 1998. Rarely, an employee refuses to give consent for a report, and in this situation they are normally advised that management will make their decision based on the information that is already available. This is not always in the individual's best interests and every effort should be made to encourage them to give consent. In practice, most employees are happy to agree if the reasons for referral are fully explained to them; for example, guidance from the Faculty of Occupational Medicine of the Royal College of Physicians of London suggests that written consent for assessment should be obtained from the individual before they are seen, although in practice many occupational physicians feel this is unnecessary, unless dealing with a particularly sensitive case.

Referral letters vary greatly in quality, from the briefest 'please see and advise' to lengthy correspondence giving not only all the relevant information, but the manager's personal views on the individual's problems or attitudes, plus hearsay from other members of staff! These types of letters are certainly helpful and very illuminating, but it should not be forgotten that employees may request a copy of the referral letter from the manager, nor that the letter may become evidence at a subsequent industrial tribunal or court case. Managers, as well as physicians, should be wary of making unwarranted comments. The ideal referral letter should contain the following information:

- **personal details:** name, address, date of birth
- **employment details:** job title, length of service, whether full-time or part-time, any particular hazards of the job that are relevant (a job description is usually helpful)
- **other relevant details:** difficult social circumstances, conflict with other members of staff
- **absence details:** dates and reasons over the previous 12 months, any pattern to the absence
- **reason for referral:** too much absence, poor time keeping, concerns about work performance, etc.
- **specific questions they would like answered:** is this person fit for work, likely duration of absence, is there anything that could be done to assist the employee to return to work, is medical retirement indicated, is the problem work-related?
- **any information regarding the employee's performance that may be relevant:** incidents at work, time-keeping, behaviour, change in personality
- **confirmation that the employee understands the reason for referral.**

The quality of the information provided is very important. Unless the referring manager provides enough background information and asks the right questions, they are unlikely to receive a medical report which provides them with the advice they need to manage the absence appropriately. The following referral letter is an extreme but genuine example of how little information some managers provide.

An unhelpful referral letter

Dear Doctor

XY   Maintenance assistant

I have received a long-term sickness certificate in respect of the above named and should be grateful if you would make the necessary arrangements to see him and provide me with a medical report on the likelihood of him returning to work in the near future.

Yours sincerely.
Manager

This letter fails to give any details of the duration of absence, the reason, or the type of advice the manager is seeking. Without the necessary information, the subsequent report may fail to provide the advice the manager requires. A standard referral pro forma for use by managers can be helpful to obtain basic information, with space for managers to provide additional information if necessary.

A helpful referral letter

Dear Doctor

Staff Nurse ZX date of birth 13/4/67

I would be grateful if you could review this nurse whom you saw earlier this year in relation to the personal problems she was experiencing. Staff Nurse X has now been on this ward for 9 months and she did seem to settle in quite well after her earlier difficulties. Recently, however, I have been approached by several of her colleagues, who were expressing concerns about her. She appears to be unable to focus on tasks, is easily distracted and disorganized. Her verbal reports are poor and she takes a long time to complete paperwork. Incidentally, staff have noticed that she avoids being in close proximity to others and sometimes smells strongly of menthol, although this may not be significant. She has had no sickness absence since her last review.

I have spoken to Staff Nurse X about my concerns and she has agreed to attend occupational health. I would be grateful if you could advise me whether you feel she has any problems which we might be able to offer help and support with, and whether she is fit to continue working on this busy ward.

Yours sincerely
Sister
Ward 10

Although this referral letter is quite brief it gives a good description of the way this nurse's work performance is affected. A number of clues to the possible underlying reason are mentioned and the physician will need to explore issues such as alcohol and substance abuse with the individual as well as any personal difficulties she may be having at or outside work.

THE ROLE OF THE OCCUPATIONAL PHYSICIAN

The role of occupational physicians in the management of sickness absence is sometimes not fully understood by managers or employees. While it is management's role to control sickness absence, it is the occupational physician's role to assess employees and provide independent and impartial advice to help managers make appropriate decisions regarding individual members of staff.

The primary responsibility of occupational health practitioners is to the individual employee, but they also have to consider the needs of the organization. Because of the potential for conflicts to arise because of these dual responsibilities, the occupational physician has to be careful not to breach accepted standards of medical ethics. Potential conflict of interest can arise where GPs are working in occupational health and they should endeavour not to see employees who are also patients registered with their practice.

While the occupational physician's role is to assess employees and provide advice to help managers make decisions, the physician has neither the right nor the authority to tell managers what to do. Equally managers are not bound to accept any medical advice they are offered but failure to follow appropriate advice could lead to difficulties at a later date if the case ends up at an employment tribunal.

Besides assessing the worker and workplace, the occupational physician may also process and interpret information from the patient's medical advisers and relay it to the employer, within appropriate ethical constraints. Their detailed knowledge of the workplace and understanding of the organizational structure and culture place them in an ideal situation to advise on fitness for the job and suitable rehabilitation.

ASSESSMENT BY THE OCCUPATIONAL HEALTH SERVICE

Assessing employees with sickness absence requires a holistic approach. The history is important, as is evaluation of social, domestic and emotional factors. Job-related factors such as poor interpersonal relationships should also be identified. It is essential that appointments be of adequate length to allow time to explore all these issues. Physical examination may be of limited benefit in some cases, particularly repeated short-term absence, but can help exclude underlying illness or substance abuse.

Defining the problem

The initial step in the assessment process involves defining the problem. The referral letter is reviewed to establish the reason for referral and to gather information regarding the nature of the job, absence record and certified reason for absence. A history is taken from the employee but it may be necessary to contact the individual's GP or specialist for more specific clinical details. This should be undertaken only with written informed consent, 'informed' meaning that the individual understands that the information will be used to advise on their employment, and that there could be implications resulting from this.

Assessing clinical and non-medical factors

Having taken a history and carried out a clinical examination to establish the nature of any medical problem and its effect on ability to work, it is necessary to explore the patient's personal circumstances and attitudes towards work in order to determine non-medical factors affecting the absence. A good way of assessing the presence of work-related difficulties is to ask someone whether or not they like their job. The reply is usually either strongly affirmative or else hesitant, giving an opportunity to explore any reasons for job dissatisfaction. The interview may also reveal other problems prolonging a spell of absence, such as a long waiting list for physiotherapy where it might be possible to liaise with the GP and expedite treatment, perhaps by the employer offering to pay for it privately.

Formulating a plan for managing the case

The next step is to formulate a plan for clinical management and the advice that will be imparted to management in the report. It is good practice to advise the employee regarding the nature of the content of the report at the time of the interview. They are entitled to request a copy but if trust has been established with the occupational physician many individuals do not ask for one, although some occupational physicians offer the worker a report routinely. It is paramount that medical confidentiality must be preserved and nothing should be written that might cause embarrassment at a later date.

Making recommendations

The recommendations made after assessment will depend on the employee's health and functional capacity as well as prognosis. Advice may be given on whether there is an underlying medical condition, the likely duration of absence, the likelihood of future absence, the need for modified duties on a temporary basis on return to work or the need to explore redeployment, retraining or ill-health retirement. Further detail on report writing is given later. Other recommendations that might be appropriate are carrying out a workplace visit, suggesting that risk assessment or environmental monitoring be carried out and advising on suitable personal protective equipment.

Communicating advice

Effective communication between the OHS and managers is crucial in order to manage individual cases. Meetings involving the employee, manager and occupational health department can be very useful to discuss the way forward, whether planning rehabilitation or discussing redeployment or the details of ill-health retirement. An added advantage is that joint meetings improve communication and prevent any misunderstandings about a situation. It may also be necessary to liaise with safety advisers, hygienists, personnel managers, and other members of the organization with interests in Health and Safety. The opportunity to inform the patient's doctor of any recommendations given should be taken as this helps to avoid conflicting advice being given to the patient, and thwarts the attempts of some patients to manipulate a situation to their own ends.

Occasionally a situation arises where there is a difference of opinion between the occupational physician and the GP. The most common reasons for this are the latter's lack of understanding of the job requirements (they may have to rely on the patient's description of the job) or their desire to support the patient, who may no longer wish to be employed and is seeking the most financially advantageous way of leaving.

Case history 8.15

A 29-year-old secretary was referred to the occupational physician with back pain. She had developed a painful back in the later stages of her pregnancy, had been on maternity leave, and had been due to return to work 2 months previously. She returned to work for 2 days only, during which she seemed well with no mention of back pain, and had shown photographs of the baby to her colleagues. Since being off again there had been reports of her carrying heavy shopping and the manager felt that her behaviour was perhaps inconsistent with the diagnosis. When seen by the occupational physician she was very smartly dressed, looked well and examination of her back was unremarkable. This was her first child and there were some difficulties with childcare because her husband worked away from home all week, their extended families did not live close by and she appeared to lack support. The physician's view was that she was fit to return to work and, giving her the benefit of the doubt, arranged a phased return to work. Steps were also taken to assess her workstation and ensure her chair was satisfactory. Despite this, the patient continued to hand in sick notes stating 'back pain'. With the patient's permission the occupational physician contacted the GP to discuss the case but the patient's absence persisted.

By this time the manager was becoming frustrated at the situation but unsure how to proceed as the GP and occupational physician appeared to hold conflicting views regarding fitness for work. The employer decided to follow the advice of their own medical adviser and the patient was given an ultimatum to return to work or failure to do so would result in disciplinary action. The secretary did return to work but was successful in her application for voluntary redundancy soon after.

Employers are not bound to accept the medical advice they receive and they might not be competent to decide between medical opinions. In situations such as this, which are rare, the view of the occupational physician is usually accepted on the basis that they are better informed about the demands of the job. Legally, precedent has been set establishing that employers are entitled to accept the opinion of their own medical adviser. Where doubt remains it may be advisable to obtain the opinion of an independent consultant.

Evaluating the outcome

Follow-up review appointments with the patient should be arranged to monitor progress and assess outcomes. Feedback from the manager regarding performance can be extremely helpful in situations where the patient's view differs from the manager's in this respect. The frequency of reviews will vary but in general should be less often than in general practice and once the individual has returned to work and is doing well there is no need for further follow-up.

MEDICAL REPORTS AND CONFIDENTIALITY

Occupational physicians are bound by the same rules on medical confidentiality as other doctors, and reports to referring managers can only include medical information with the consent of the individual. Reports to management are generally limited to statements regarding fitness for work or the functional capabilities of an employee to perform certain tasks. Managers are always keen to have as much information as possible so they can make decisions regarding absence management. It is important for the occupational physician to ensure that they have addressed all the questions posed in the referral letter, as well as addressing other important issues. Managers understandably dislike indecision, and while it is not always possible to predict future absence or the exact date of return to work, occupational physicians should try to give clear and concise advice as far as they are able.

It is possible to provide a great deal of relevant information in reports without breaching confidentiality. Guidance may be given on the following points:

- whether or not employees have health problems that affect their fitness for duties, that is, the capacity to attend work and to perform it safely
- the likely duration of any period of absence, or if it is not possible to be precise, the minimum expected period of absence
- whether the employee will be fit to return to full duties or whether limitations will apply
- the nature of any limitations and whether they are likely to be temporary or permanent
- what steps could be taken to assist an individual's return to work
- if an individual is not going to be fit to return to previous duties, the type of work they might be fit for, to allow managers to consider redeployment
- whether retirement on medical grounds is recommended
- the likelihood of future episodes of absence, their duration, and the period of time over which they are likely to occur
- whether the Disability Discrimination Act 2005 is likely to apply, and suggestions for any adjustments that management might consider
- whether the employee has a work-related health problem and ways this problem might be addressed
- whether the condition is reportable under statute, e.g. RIDDOR Regulations 1995 in the UK
- arrangements made for further review of the employee
- any additional information required from the manager either immediately or prior to the next review
- whether a meeting with the manager would be helpful
- whether a workplace visit or other steps to assess workplace risks would be appropriate
- whether any needs for training or other facilities or support have been identified that might benefit the employee when they return, e.g. in relation to manual handling.

Key points to remember

- Keep reports short, concise, well structured and relevant. There is a risk that lengthy reports may confuse the reader or provide inconsistent advice.

- As far as possible, be decisive when making recommendations, but be prepared to highlight important areas of uncertainty.
- In cases of alleged work-related ill-health, be careful not to confirm this unless you can substantiate your statement.
- Never write anything that you would not be prepared to have read out in court.
- Always answer the questions posed by managers in referral letters. If the referral letter has been poor, a valuable way to educate the manager as well as to help the worker is explicitly to answer questions that a good referral letter should have posed.

SICK PAY SCHEMES AND SOCIAL SECURITY BENEFITS

Although many steps have been taken to harmonize aspects of policy throughout the European Union, there is still a wide disparity of approaches in this area. A summary of UK benefits relevant to incapacity for work is shown in Figure 8.6.

The doctor has two roles in relation to the sickness absence process: a statutory role and an advisory role. The statutory role, normally that of the GP, is to provide medical certification to the employer or Department for Work and Pensions; the advisory role is to inform patients regarding the types of benefits for which they might be eligible. The occupational physician in particular should be familiar with the relevant benefits for incapacity for work, injury at work, occupational disease and employment of the disabled. Benefits for work-related injury and disease are covered elsewhere.

Employees who are absent from work on account of ill-health are normally required by their employer to provide a certificate naming the cause. At one time this certificate had always to be provided by a doctor, but self-certification is now acceptable for short absences up to 7 days. For longer periods a doctor's certificate is required.

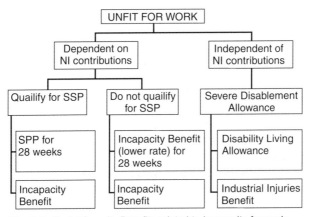

Fig. 8.6 *Social Security Benefits related to incapacity for work.*

Statutory Sick Pay (SSP)

In the UK the Statutory Sick Pay Act 1994 requires employers to provide a minimum amount of sick pay to employees who are ill and unable to attend work, for up to a maximum of 28 weeks. Most employees are covered provided they have paid sufficient National Insurance (NI) contributions. However, many large employers have their own schemes for providing sickness benefits; for example, the National Health Service in the UK generally pays full salary for up to 6 months and thereafter half salary to 12 months. For the very few low paid or temporary workers who do not qualify for Statutory Sick Pay, Incapacity Benefit is available from the Department for Work and Pensions.

Up until 1994 the UK Government reimbursed employers for most of the cost of Statutory Sick Pay; however, the costs are now largely borne by employers themselves, providing another economic reason for better management of sickness absence.

Incapacity Benefit

In 1995 Incapacity Benefit was introduced to replace the previous Sickness and Invalidity Benefits. Again, in order to qualify, employees must have paid sufficient National Insurance contributions. Incapacity benefit is payable to those whose entitlement to SSP has expired. This is normally after 28 weeks, but may be sooner if individuals are not entitled to SSP for some reason, or their SSP stops before 28 weeks. It is paid at three rates, the short-term lower rate up to 28 weeks, the short-term higher rate from 29 to 52 weeks, and the long-term rate thereafter. Incapacity Benefit is taxable.

Not all employees will qualify for Incapacity Benefit. There are two legal tests of incapacity used to assess claims for Social Security Benefits in the UK. The 'own work test' applies for the first 28 weeks of sickness, that is, claimants must be incapable of doing tasks they might normally be required to do in their **usual** job. After 28 weeks a different test is used to assess claims for Incapacity Benefit. This used to be known as the 'All Work Test' and it tests an individual's ability to perform certain activities, such as walking, sitting, lifting and carrying, etc., legally defined in the Social Security Act 1994. In order to qualify for Incapacity Benefit claimants need to be incapable of carrying out **any** work, not just the job in which they were employed. This leads to situations where, for example, a labourer with chronic back pain would be regarded as fit for other types of work, and denied benefit, although he remained unfit for his own job. At present a number of pilot schemes are in place focussing on ways of assisting the long-term sick back into employment. The UK benefits system is undergoing major review and further changes will be implemented over the next few years.

Case history 8.16

A 19-year-old administrative assistant was off work for 3 months with 'stress and anxiety'. Her boyfriend was in custody awaiting trial on drug charges, and as a result she had been asked to leave her flat by her landlord, who happened to be a relative of her close work colleague and flatmate. She was relatively new to the area and her own family lived 100 miles away. When seen at the OHS she had been treated with an antidepressant for 6 weeks and was beginning to recover from her reactive depression. Her personal problems were ongoing, in that she had to find alternative accommodation by the end of that month, and she had fallen out with her flatmate. Having only been with the company for 6 months her entitlement to Statutory Sick Pay had expired and her only income was Incapacity Benefit. This put her under some pressure to return to work when she was still having some difficulties with memory and concentration, and was anxious about continuing to work with her flatmate, who had told the other girls at work about her problems.

A meeting was held with her line manager who arranged for her job to be transferred to a different office. By liaising with her doctor and the Department for Work and Pensions it was agreed that she would return to work on a part-time basis and would continue to receive benefits as it was felt work would be 'therapeutic'. After a few weeks working part-time in her new job her health greatly improved and she was able to increase to full-time employment again.

In certain circumstances where a medical practitioner feels it would be beneficial for an individual to undertake some work, it is possible for them to return to work and continue to receive Incapacity Benefit provided they work no more than 16 hours per week and earn less than a stipulated amount. In this case an individual who is not fit enough to return to work on a full-time basis benefits from a gradual reintroduction to work, without financial detriment, avoiding further problems that might have arisen by returning full time too soon to a stressful environment.

PREVENTION OF SICKNESS ABSENCE

Pre-employment

In the past there was a widely held view among employers that routine pre-employment medical examination could ensure that only the fit and healthy, who would be unlikely to be off work, were employed. Pre-employment screening does have a limited place; for example, careful recruitment and selection processes can ensure employees have the prerequisite fitness for jobs with specific hazards, such as those requiring heavy physical effort or possible exposure to allergens. However, the best predictor of future absence is a history of past absence, and managers should routinely request this information when taking up references from previous employers. Many employees with chronic medical conditions such as diabetes or epilepsy actually tend to take less time off than do their healthier colleagues. In the UK, the Disability Discrimination Act 2005 makes it illegal to discriminate against people on health grounds unless their condition precludes them from doing the job or compromises safety. However, it is not discriminatory to ask questions pre-employment to ascertain disability and to assess the needs of applicants to ensure that those with disabilities are placed in suitable employment that is not going to have a detrimental effect on their health.

During employment

During employment sickness absence may be minimized by:

* preventing spells of absence occurring in the first place
* reducing the duration of any absences that do occur.

It should be clear by now that sickness absence has as much to do with socioeconomic factors as with ill-health in a workforce. At an organizational level, prevention of absence depends on identifying the underlying problems affecting morale in the workplace and tackling issues such as management style and culture. This is difficult and takes time, and employers often find it easier to provide facilities such as employee counselling schemes, access to aromatherapy, on-site fitness rooms, or unproven interventions such as teaching relaxation skills. This attitude may be reinforced by some government initiatives ostensibly focusing on improving health in the workplace, and many employers have taken part in these hoping that 'health education' will improve the overall health of their employees and result in reduced absenteeism. Evaluation of the effectiveness of these schemes is difficult and any subsequent reduction in absence levels may have as much to do with improved morale in a workforce who perceive their employer as 'caring' as any health improvement, although there are some studies that have demonstrated a reduction in absence.

A specific method of trying to prevent absence occurring is to offer influenza immunization to a workforce. Mass immunization is costly but there may be a case for immunizing key staff or those with medical conditions that put them at particular risk. Studies on the cost-effectiveness of influenza vaccination have shown conflicting evidence to date, but it may well have a justifiable place in some healthcare contexts.

Reduction in the duration of absence can be achieved in a number of ways and is one area where an OHS may make a significant contribution to an organization. Early referral to the OHS allows the individual's health and functional capabilities to be assessed fully and any non-medical factors contributing to the absence to be identified. Depending on the nature of the underlying problem the occupational physician can liaise with GP and hospital specialist as necessary, or explore ways of resolving any workplace issues with an appropriate manager. If an organization provides access to treatment either through a health insurance scheme or by providing counselling services or physiotherapy, prompt treatment may greatly reduce the duration of a spell of absence.

Prolonged absence from work can result in loss of confidence and skills. Anxiety about returning to work, particularly if work is perceived to have been the cause of the problem, can become a major factor in delaying return. By recognizing this, the occupational physician can provide support and arrange some form of rehabilitation to facilitate the return to work. This will be dependent on what is operationally possible in an organization, but it is usually possible to arrange a period of reduced hours or restricted duties for a few weeks. Some employers identify certain jobs that are particularly suitable for employees returning to work after illness or injury and initiatives such as this enable workers to return to work sooner than they might otherwise have done if they had needed to be fit for normal duties.

Where individuals are clearly unfit for their job, with no prospect of imminent recovery, the occupational physician should make a decision regarding fitness and advise the employer as soon as possible so that the possibility of redeployment can be explored if appropriate, or else arrangements made for medical retirement. This will be discussed further in the next chapter.

CONCLUSION

In managing sickness absence it is essential to use clear definitions and to collect valid data both at the level of the organisation and when dealing with the individual. Medical conditions provide only partial explanations for 'sickness absence'. Therefore the role of personal, geographic, organizational and other factors needs to be understood. Management, including prevention, of sickness absence is dependent on good policies and well trained managers as well as competent advice from the occupational physician.

9

Work ability and rehabilitation

Gillian Fletcher

SUMMARY

- Assessing fitness for work in terms of function, safety and performance is an integral part of the work of occupational physicians.

- This assessment may be undertaken prior to employment or following significant sickness absence and must be related to the tasks and working environment.

- Appropriate advice to management will include a programme for rehabilitation.

- A significant proportion of the working population has a long-term disability or health problem. This proportion rises with age.

- There are a range of services and specialist sources of advice for employment of the disabled.

- Where employees are no longer able to carry out paid employment they may be eligible for state benefits.

INTRODUCTION

The preceding chapter discussed the role of the occupational physician in the management of sickness absence. One of the most important aspects of the work of the occupational physician is the assessment of the functional capacity of employees and potential employees both before employment and on return to work after a significant illness. Following significant illness the functional assessment and assessment of the workplace will lead on to goal setting for the employee and liaison with and advice to management on an appropriate programme of rehabilitation to attain those goals. Successful rehabilitation into the workplace is likely to increase self-esteem and confidence as well as the monetary benefit. Employers should not discriminate against disabled people where this treatment cannot be justified. This applies to all aspects of employment and includes recruitment as well as during employment.

FITNESS STANDARDS FOR EMPLOYMENT

In assessing fitness for work the fundamental concepts are function, performance and safety rather than the nature of the underlying condition.

Case history 9.1

A 31-year-old man applied for a post as an accounts assistant. He had cerebral palsy and had reduced function of his right arm as a result of spasticity. Although able to stand to transfer from his wheelchair to bed, he was unable to walk. The job required him to be able to enter figures for wages and he needed to be able to use a filing cabinet. Using his own wheelchair he was unable to access the top drawer. He needed to have access to all three drawers to complete tasks easily. He was provided with a wheelchair that rose to an appropriate height and an adapted keyboard. With these adaptations he was able to complete the full range of duties. His underlying medical condition, of course, remained unchanged.

Concepts and definitions

It is important that there is a clear understanding of what is meant by the different terms used in describing the sequelae of injury or illness. In 1980 the World Health Organization proposed the following international classification of impairment, disability and handicap (ICIDH).

Impairment is a change in normal structure or function resulting from a disease, disorder or injury. It encompasses any loss or abnormality of a psychological, physiological or anatomical structure or function. The disturbance is at the level of the 'organ', e.g. loss of a limb, hearing or sight. The result is a structural disablement.

Disability is any restriction in performing or lack (resulting from an impairment) of ability to perform an activity, e.g. behaviour, mobility, communication, memory. As a functional disablement it should be seen as a continuum in terms of severity, ranging from very slight to severe. This has importance in relationship to employment, as progression of the disability may require further modifications and adaptation of the workplace to allow continuing employment.

Handicap is a disadvantage for a given individual resulting from an impairment or disability that limits or prevents the fulfilment of a normal role for that individual. That role may be in relation to a particular environment, e.g. work, and the consequences may be cultural, social, economic and environmental. They may be manifested as: physical, in relation to independence; social, in respect of integration; and economic in relation to self-sufficiency. Handicap is a restrictive disablement.

The above definitions are illustrated in the following examples.

Case history 9.2

A 55-year-old woman developed severe osteoarthrosis of the hip. Objectively, the impairment was reduced joint movement. This caused the disability of being unable to stand for any length of time, to walk any significant distance, climb stairs or drive. She was handicapped by being unable to continue her work as a district nurse.

Case history 9.3

A 63-year-old joiner working in ship refitting developed angina. The impairment was reduced cardiac function. This resulted in the disability of only being able to walk short distances and being unable to climb ladders or lift heavy objects. His work required him to be able to carry out these tasks, so he was occupationally handicapped by being unable to work. He underwent a coronary angiography which confirmed the anatomical impairment of narrowing of the coronary arteries. After a wait of 6 months he was admitted for coronary artery bypass grafting. The impairment of reduced cardiac function improved and this was confirmed on exercise testing. He had good exercise tolerance and was free from angina. In addition he had a long history of recurrent depression. Although his cardiac function had improved he had a recurrence of his depressive illness. He was offered rehabilitative measures such as part-time working or working in a small group. However, he was unable to return to work and was retired on grounds of ill-health.

The definitions apply equally to mental health problems and are not restricted to physical disorders.

Case history 9.4

A 40-year-old planning engineer had experienced recurrent episodes of mania and depression from the age of 25 years (impairment). This resulted in difficulty in relationships with work colleagues and in dealing with stressful situations (disability). Although he was able to work in a small working group he was handicapped occupationally by being unable to take managerial responsibility and unable to be involved with outside contractors or potentially confrontational situations. He was placed in a small working group on an office-based project without tight deadlines. His psychiatrist referred him to a psychologist to work on a one-to-one basis on stress management. With these measures he was able to work effectively, although with a more limited range of work.

ASSESSMENT OF THE WORKER

Functional assessment

Table 9.1 lists 13 recognized functions that contribute to disability, that is, the restriction or lack of the ability to perform an activity in the manner or within the range considered normal for human beings, regardless of the pathological process.

In occupational assessment and rehabilitation attention must be directed towards assessing those functions that will have a direct bearing on the ability to return to employment. The following case histories illustrate the relevance of the various functions in relation to work.

Physical abilities (locomotion, reaching and stretching)

This case history illustrates the assessment of locomotion and reaching and stretching.

Case history 9.5

A 23-year-old kitchen porter had suffered with chronic osteomyelitis of his foot for 8 years, resulting in bone erosion and a limp. As a result of continuing infection he had undergone a below-knee amputation.

Table 9.1 *Functional assessment of disability*

Functions	Parameters
Locomotion	Walking, climbing steps/stairs, bending and straightening, balance
Reaching and stretching	Degree of forward, sideways or upwards movement
Dexterity	Holding, gripping, turning
Seeing	Distance/near
Hearing	Perception of sound, tinnitus
Continence	Bladder and bowel control
Communication	Being understood, understanding others
Personal care	Able to feed, dress and wash
Behaviour	Conduct, treatment of others
Intellectual functioning	Memory, concentration
Consciousness	Fits/convulsions
Nutrition and digestion	Dietary requirements, timing of meal breaks
Disfigurement	Amputation, burns, cosmetic

Following his below-knee amputation he was fitted with an artificial leg. Approximately 1 month later he was seen by the occupational physician, who had already established with the personnel manager and the kitchen supervisor that every effort would be made to rehabilitate him back to work, although both managers were highly sceptical of achieving a positive outcome.

In practical terms he was able to demonstrate that he could climb steps and stairs and had sufficient stability to achieve good balance, which enabled him to twist and turn, reach and stretch. He did not yet have sufficient stamina to enable him to weight-bear or be physically active for any length of time. This was partly because of the continuing adaptation of the stump to the socket of his artificial limb. However, mentally he was very apprehensive about returning to work. He perceived himself as 'disfigured' and a freak and was unsure of the reaction of his colleagues. He was also worried about being pressurized into returning to work within a defined time limit.

This initial assessment was of the opinion that he would be able to return to work, with the minor reservation that he might experience irritation of the stump as a result of the heat and humidity in the kitchen, but that more time was required to allow his stump to adapt. He returned for a further assessment 1 month later. During the interval he had been visited at home by both the personnel manager and kitchen supervisor. This visit improved his self-esteem, particularly when they stated that he was a valued member of the team and also removed any fears of being pressurized into undertaking any jobs before he felt confident to do so. He had also increased his own confidence in his abilities by decorating an elderly disabled neighbour's house.

At the second assessment he was full of confidence in his abilities and an individual rehabilitation scheme was implemented. He returned to work for 3 hours on 2 days a week during a quiet period. He was not allowed to lift kitchen equipment or to push trolleys. He was allowed to do any other task that he felt capable of performing. In fact he operated the dishwashers, washed up manually and prepared vegetables, with a colleague doing any necessary lifting. His confidence increased and after 2 weeks he requested an increase in his hours. Over a period of 4 weeks his hours were gradually increased to full-time but he remained on restricted duties. At this time he only had minor stump irritation and he asked to extend his range of tasks. He started loading food onto trolleys and delivering the trolleys to wards nearest the kitchen. Four months after his return to work he was working as a normal member of staff and was fully integrated into the workplace.

Dexterity

Fine movement of the hand and the ability to grasp and manipulate objects is an important function for many jobs.

Case history 9.6

A 40-year-old firefighter lacerated his left forearm in a fall at home. This resulted in impairment through damage to his median and ulnar nerves with, subsequently, a complete degeneration lesion of his ulnar nerve at the site of the injury. This was confirmed by electromyographic studies. Clinically, there was wasting of his interossei and lumbrical muscles and loss of sensation along the medial border of the forearm and the fourth and fifth fingers. Nerve regeneration was detectable after 4 months.

He regained full movement of his left wrist and, in spite of loss of abduction and adduction in his fourth and fifth fingers, his disability improved in that he developed the functional ability to grip tools and manipulate equipment. The sensory loss in these fingers remained. A practical assessment of his functional capabilities on the fireground was undertaken satisfactorily and he returned to full duties.

Seeing

Sight is an important sense for many tasks and standards may be set, for example for driving. For work involving reading, aids may be available for visually impaired people (see Specialist services in employment for the disabled, page 248).

Hearing

For certain positions the ability to hear and localize sound is important, both for the safety of the employee and the ability to perform their role.

Case history 9.7

A 23-year-old firefighter sustained a severe head injury in an unprovoked assault. The outcome was total and permanent unilateral deafness and tinnitus. He was retired on health grounds from active work as a firefighter. He was given assistance in approaching a local college for retraining in a different career.

Firefighters are considered to need bilateral hearing to enable them to localize sounds, instructions and warnings.

Continence

Loss of continence due to an illness or operation often leads to a loss of confidence. Members of the occupational health team must be able to give practical advice to help the employee as illustrated below.

Case history 9.8

A 35-year-old countryside ranger underwent an ileostomy for ulcerative colitis. When assessed 3 months postoperatively he was starting to adjust psychologically to the ileostomy. Physically he was feeling well but was concerned about the facilities for changing the ileostomy bag if this should be necessary at work. He worked from a building in the middle of a country park where there was a shower available in the event of the bag leaking. An appropriate bin was provided along with polythene bags. The physician checked that the local authority considered this waste as normal domestic refuse. He returned into work and gradually increased the length of walks on patrol duties. He was monitored by the occupational physician and gradually increased his range of duties. He did not carry out the heavier tasks of using a sledge hammer or chainsaw until 6 months after return.

Communication and disfigurement

Case history 9.9

A 55-year-old surgeon had a total laryngectomy and block dissection for carcinoma of the larynx, resulting in considerable cosmetic disfigurement. He subsequently developed oesophageal speech.

At assessment, he related that he had already seen a small number of long-standing patients on an individual basis and now felt confident that his disfigurement was not a handicap and also that he could communicate adequately both face to face and over the telephone. This was confirmed by the occupational physician. As he still lacked physical stamina, a rehabilitation programme in relation to a reduced work schedule was implemented. He started working three sessions a week initially in the out-patients department. He was not on the on call rota. He had started to increase his range of duties to include operating when sadly he died suddenly 6 weeks after returning to work.

Personal care

With developments in renal dialysis and the introduction of continuous ambulant peritoneal dialysis (CAPD), patients with renal failure whose renal function is maintained in this way may be able to return to work providing they are not significantly impaired by chronic anaemia.

Case history 9.10

A 30-year-old nurse on CAPD was assessed before returning to work in the endoscopy department. The facilities to change the equipment at work were provided together with the necessary time allowance. Although she had a significant anaemia she felt she could cope with the demands of the job, and it was arranged that her ability to continue working would be monitored jointly by the renal and occupational physicians. She was able to remain in full-time work until a donor kidney became available, at which time she underwent successful renal transplantation.

Behaviour and intellectual functioning

Behaviour and intellectual functioning is one of the most difficult areas to assess in relation to ability to return to work, and one where knowledge of the intellectual requirements of the job and the importance of interpersonal relationships is essential. Disability may be idiopathic, for example Alzheimer's disease, may result from self-inflicted damage, such as abuse of alcohol or drugs, or may be the consequence of a head injury (which may or may not be work related) or of exposure to neurotoxins such as solvents.

Case history 9.11

A 28-year-old man was employed as a sales assistant in a department store. He was involved in a road traffic accident on his motorbike, which resulted in a fracture to the base of the skull and a compound fracture of the right tibia. He required ventilation for a prolonged period in the intensive care unit and was transferred to a rehabilitation unit for head injuries. Early contact was made with the occupational therapist but because of the severity of the injury plans regarding his return to work could not be made until 10 months after the original accident. During this period he had a grand mal seizure and was started on medication. He wanted to return into his original post. He came into the department on several occasions with the occupational therapist for familiarization. He started working a 2-hour sessions twice a week. Initially he did not use the till and he was closely supported by colleagues and was restricted in not climbing ladders in the stockroom. His hours of work were gradually increased and he was retrained on using the till. Unfortunately his performance at work started to cause concern. He had difficulty in learning about any new stock and difficulty in completing the supporting paperwork to transactions correctly. At his request he was moved to the shoe department. Although he managed well initially, there were occasions when he fitted the left shoe to the right foot, or vice versa. Again there were difficulties in learning about new stock. With his agreement he was moved to a different area dealing with customers' parcels. Unless supervised continuously, he tended to wander out of the department and had difficulty in filing the parcels in the correct order. He was moved to the goods area where he priced goods. Here there were difficulties with him failing to price goods correctly.

Managers within the departments had consistently given support and additional training. He had been referred to a specialist agency to see if supported employment is appropriate to give an increased level of assistance. A post then became available in the area where employees left bags for collection in the evenings. The number of tasks was limited and the post had a high level of supervision. He was able to carry out the full range of tasks and did not require any assistance from supported employment.

This case illustrates the difficulty of assessing function after head injury. Objective psychological tests do not correlate precisely with function in the workplace and therefore supervised work placement assessments have an essential role to play. It also illustrates the patience of some employers in finding appropriate placement for employees with disabilities.

Consciousness

The assessment of someone who has had or who has the potential to have fits or convulsions will depend on the existence of any primary cause, for example tumour, and its treatment, the response to and compliance with anticonvulsant therapy and the requirements of the job.

Case history 9.12

A 40-year-old firefighter, whose individual role included driving fire appliances, had a brief episode of neurological symptoms, which included a transient hemiparesis and altered facial sensation. The putative diagnosis was an intracerebral bleed but cerebral angiography showed no obvious cause such as a berry aneurysm. The firefighter had no further clinical symptoms and his neurological abnormalities completely resolved within 2 weeks. Magnetic resonance imaging 6 weeks later showed a small area of scarring at the site of the presumed bleed. He was referred to the occupational physician for assessment. His employers felt he was no longer fit for employment in the Fire Service. Physical examination was entirely normal and he was anxious to return to work.

The occupational physician had to balance, on the one hand, his excellent personal health and, on the other, a duty of care to the public and himself in respect of the small possibility of the development of post-traumatic epilepsy. The risk was estimated by his consultant neurologist as less than 5%. Expert independent neurological opinion was sought so that there was no bias related to personal care of the patient. The occupational physician was advised that freedom from fits for 12 months from the date of the original episode would place the risk of having a fit in the future at no greater than a fit occurring for the first time in a member of the general public.

The firefighter was very antagonistic to the occupational physician and provided letters from his specialist to support his immediate return to full duties. The occupational physician remained firm in the opinion that a period of 12 months should elapse from the time of his intracerebral bleed before he could return to full duties. The firefighter remained free of any episodes of altered consciousness or unconsciousness during this 12 months and was able to return to full duties.

Attitude

Those who have had a life-threatening illness or operation may feel that, having cheated death once, the most must be made of the rest of their life. Although thorough clinical assessment following rehabilitation may confirm physical fitness to return to employment, mentally the patient may not be prepared to accept any possible risk, particularly if it is felt that the original precipitating factor for the illness was work related. A common example is a high physical demand or 'stress' in relation to myocardial infarction. Although persuasion by the occupational physician may be initially productive in that the employee returns to work, this outcome might not be sustained.

Case history 9.13

A 62-year-old male domestic assistant in a hospital sustained a myocardial infarction. He made an excellent recovery and, after assessment at 3 months post-infarction, he commenced a rehabilitation programme with restricted duties and shortened working hours. By 6 months post-infarction he had resumed normal, full-time duties. At 9 months post-infarction he requested to see the occupational physician and asked to be considered for ill-health retirement. He gave a history of minor aches and pains but no significant disability and then said, 'I don't feel I should be working after a heart attack. I have had one chance and it is time to take life a bit easier'.

What would you do?

The occupational physician, after again reassuring him that his symptoms were not indicative of angina and offering him a further cardiological opinion, discussed with him, with the consent of his manager, the option of shorter hours and a lighter programme of work, similar to that which he had undertaken during his rehabilitation programme. However, none of these options were acceptable. He made it clear that he had already approached his primary care physician who was willing to furnish him with sickness absence certificates for the duration of his sick pay entitlement. At his age and with his past medical history he would be highly unlikely to obtain further employment and so he was retired, rightly or wrongly, on the grounds of anxiety secondary to his myocardial infarction.

ASSESSMENT OF THE WORK

For the purposes of assessing fitness for work and or for rehabilitation at work it is essential to assess the work itself. There is an immense breadth and variety of physical surroundings, mental and physical tasks carried out and skills needed in the workplace (see also Chapters 4–6).

Work demands

Assessment of work demands includes the physical demands involved in lifting, carrying, pulling or pushing loads. The frequency of the action and the height a load is lifted will alter the demand. Recovery time will depend on the timing and length of breaks. The total length of the shift will affect the daily physical demands.

Case history 9.14

An employee who worked wrapping a protective covering around reels of finished paper approached the personnel department of a paper mill. He was currently signed off his work and he had recently had investigations for chest pain. The investigations included an angiogram. Following assessment by the cardiologist and cardiothoracic surgeon he was told that he would benefit from a triple bypass operation. Unfortunately the waiting list was around 6 months and further delay seemed likely when an increase in cases of influenza stopped any planned admissions. The operator was frustrated by being off work and was concerned that his sick pay would finish before he could return.

His ability to return into work depends on an assessment of his cardiac function and how this matches with the physical demands of his work. The workplace visit showed that his work was on the level and involved moving reams of paper from the finishing machine. The paper was then shrink-wrapped before moving it for weighing. The reams were then moved off the scales to the cutting department. The weight of the reams was between 60 and 70 kg. The work used a unpowered roller truck. In a 12-hour shift around 40 reams were wrapped and weighed. The work was done standing and there were three breaks lasting a total of 90 minutes. Each time the paper was moved, inertia had to be overcome, which involved a considerable physical effort. His normal work rotation involved night as well as day shifts. The workplace visit allowed a detailed assessment of the tasks and the physical environment, including slopes and the condition of the floor, in a way that could not be achieved by reading a job description.

The assessment of his work was that it was heavy manual work and that it was detrimental to his health to restart work prior to the bypass operation.

Physical environment

Simple adjustments to the physical environment can make a big difference to the prospects of an employee returning into work, as the following case history illustrates.

Case history 9.15

A 42-year-old social worker was referred to the occupational physician during a period of prolonged absence. A background medical report from the primary care physician stated that she had been diagnosed with insulin-dependent diabetes mellitus 10 years previously. The condition was well controlled by twice daily insulin injections until she had an acute exacerbation of rheumatoid arthritis. This had involved shoulder, hip and the small joints of both hands and feet. She had been unable to draw up and inject her own insulin. However, upon switching to second-line treatment for the arthritis her joint condition improved and the inflammation in the joints had settled. When she initially met with the occupational physician the level of pain was reducing and with this her mobility and concentration were improving. However, she became fatigued easily. She worked in an office that was on the second floor. There was no lift in the building. In addition the catchment area contained many second- and third-floor flats that had no lifts. Visiting clients in their own homes was an essential part of her work as many clients were frail and elderly and unable to attend an office for interview.

The social worker returned to work, starting on two mornings a week. For her return her office had been moved to the first floor. Her caseload of clients was carefully chosen so that they lived in ground- and first-floor flats and were less likely to present with crisis situations. With these adjustments she extended her hours to working four mornings a week and followed by increasing her daily working hours by an hour each day each week. She worked up to her normal working hours within 6 weeks of her return. The long-term goal is relocation to a ground-floor office with a catchment area of single-storey houses or flats with lifts.

Temperature

Cold

A number of jobs require work to be carried out in either cold or hot temperatures. Workers may be required to assist clearing snow and ice or to work in refrigerated warehouses. There will be employees with a limited number of medical conditions, either because of the nature of the condition (e.g. Raynaud's disease) or because of treatment (e.g. beta blockers for hypertension), who will be at increased susceptibility to cold.

Heat

Humans depend on maintaining body temperature within a narrow band around 37°C. The main mechanisms of achieving this are by increasing bloodflow to the skin and by sweating. Hyperthermia develops when the body's capacity to lose heat cannot match the total body heat load. In extremes of heat, heat exhaustion resulting from cardiovascular insufficiency brought about by dehydration and insufficient fluid intake and salt depletion may develop. This is a medical condition with a high mortality. The main preventative measures are outlined in Chapter 4. However, specific advice regarding fitness for employment for individuals with predisposing medical conditions such as gross obesity, diabetes mellitus, impaired sweat production and cardiovascular disease will be needed. Certain drugs such as tranquillizers, beta blockers and diuretics may alter the response to heat.

Shift work

Many posts require shifts outside accepted normal working hours. Employees with certain medical conditions such as insulin-dependent diabetes mellitus, asthma or peptic ulceration may find it harder to adjust to work involving shifts. The occupational physician will need to advise on whether shift working is advisable, as illustrated in the following case history.

Case history 9.16

A 53-year-old man was asked to start taking his turn for night shift in a pharmaceutical firm. The employee approached the occupational physician with concerns about his fitness to work night shift. He had been diagnosed 6 months previously by his primary care physician as being hypertensive. He had been commenced on a single daily dose of beta blocker. The blood pressure was satisfactory on examination. There was no evidence of any end-organ damage. He had no other significant medical history. Although 24-hour working had commenced 3 years previously, he had been excused his previous turn as his wife had been unwell. She was now fully recovered. He felt that he adjusted poorly to night shifts and really dreaded the thought of starting them.

Was there sufficient medical evidence to recommend that he did not work night shift?

His treatment regimen would not need to be adjusted and his reluctance to participate in the night shift predated his illness. With his permission management were approached to see if he could participate in a shorter period of night shifts and to use this time for him to train another operator with his particular skills.

Chemical exposures

Statutory exposure limits (see Appendix) are set at a limit to protect the health of workers. Workers with a pre-existing medical condition such as asthma might be at risk of increased symptoms at much lower levels of exposure to irritants such as sulphur dioxide. There may also be difficulty in wearing some types of respiratory protective equipment for employees with markedly reduced respiratory function. The response in these instances should focus primarily on reducing exposure at source, as described in Chapter 6. Chemical exposure is also illustrated in Case history 9.28.

Work equipment

All jobs require tools or other specialized equipment. The simplest is a pen for writing, progressing to complex computers and large pieces of earth-moving equipment. Work equipment may be responsible for specific symptoms such as hand–arm vibration syndrome. Carpel tunnel syndrome is also reported with the use of equipment that transmits vibrations to the arm. Carpel tunnel is also a common condition in middle-aged women. The following case illustrates an approach to rehabilitation in a lady with carpel tunnel syndrome.

Case history 9.17

A 45-year-old school cleaner was referred to the occupational physician after managerial concern regarding her fitness to continue in employment. The background medical report stated that she had recently had an operation to her right wrist to release compression of her carpel tunnel. On meeting the physician she gave a history of typical symptoms of median nerve compression, such as tingling of the second and third finger at night which had completely resolved following operation. The history predated her using mechanical cleaning machinery. As symptoms had fully resolved, management was advised that she was fit to continue to use mechanical cleaning machines for up to 1 hour per day. She was advised to report any recurrence of symptoms to her manager and to have formal health surveillance annually. The health surveillance would consist of a symptom questionnaire and examination of the function of the hands annually to detect any deterioration in function.

Psychological aspects

The psychological aspects of work concern the interaction of the person and his or her psyche with the work environment and other external influences. The effect these interactions have on emotional reactions, cognitive functioning (i.e. thinking, concentration, memory perception and creativity) and the integration of the person with the environment can be used as a measure of stress. These aspects of work are far harder to measure than those of the physical environment as they are subjective. The levels of perceived stress will vary both between individuals performing the same tasks within an organization and also vary with time within the same individual. On starting a new post, many tasks may require the employee to work to full capacity. With increasing familiarity the employee will feel more competent and confident in a wide range of tasks and be ready to take up new challenges. If these were all presented on the first day of employment, the familiar symptoms of anxiety, increased heart rate and doubts in abilities would be likely to ensue.

Good employment practices and management of organizational issues will reduce the causes of stress. Prior to start of employment it is important to identify the psychological as well as physical demands of the post and for these to be highlighted in the job description. People should be selected according to competence-based criteria. Appropriate training needs to be provided and clear goals defined. Frequent feedback on performance will enable job-related concerns on both sides to be addressed.

FUNCTIONAL ASSESSMENT AND EMPLOYMENT

The assessment both of the functional abilities of the employee and assessment of the workplace are appropriate at different stages, such as at the commencement of employment and where the health of the employee has led either to sickness absence or to difficulty in carrying out the full remit of the job.

Policy at commencement of employment

An employer should have a clear policy regarding employment that addresses the needs of all job applicants, including those with medical conditions and disabilities. Within the

United Kingdom, for example, there is now a statutory requirement for an employer to make reasonable adjustments to allow a disabled person to commence employment (see Employment of the disabled, page 241).

Assessment prior to employment

The primary purpose of the pre-employment medical assessment is to ensure that the subject is fit to undertake the work effectively and without risk to their own or others' health and safety. The medical assessment for fitness to work is matching the health requirements of a post with the health status and fitness of the applicant.

The health requirements may be statutory, such as driving licence requirements for heavy goods or passenger service vehicles. The standards may be led by the industry, for example, guidelines for the medical standards of fitness for offshore work drawn up by the Medical Advisory Committee of the United Kingdom Offshore Operators Association, or there may be no specific guidance. Employers need to set fitness standards for a variety of reasons. In order to be competitive an employer needs employees who are able to attend work on a regular basis and perform their work efficiently. The employer has a general duty under the Health and Safety at Work Act to ensure, so far as is reasonably practicable, the health, safety and welfare at work of all his employees. In assessing fitness for employment, consideration must be taken of risk to both the mental and physical health of the employee.

Case history 9.18

A 27-year-old man with cerebral palsy applied to work in a retail warehouse. He had reduced peripheral vision. He was able to meet the physical requirements of pushing loaded cages, and was assessed as fit to work in the area where goods were moved by hand. To ensure his own safety he was not allowed to work in the carpet warehouse, where there were frequent movements of a forklift truck with a protruding carpet boom. There were concerns about the suitability of employing him in this type of environment, particularly with regard to his perception of risk and his ability to move goods safely. The employer agreed to employ him under the Job Introduction scheme (see Employment of the disabled, page 241). Within this scheme he had a job coach who initially worked with him at all times. Over the first few weeks he demonstrated his ability to work safely and efficiently. The level of support was reduced as his confidence grew and he was eventually able to work independently.

The employer also has a duty to protect persons other than his employees. He is required to conduct his undertaking in such a way as to ensure, so far as is reasonably practicable, that persons not in his employment who may be affected thereby are not exposed to risks to their health or safety. This is illustrated in the following case history.

Case history 9.19

A man of 65 years of age applied for a post as a school crossing patrol guide (SCPG), helping children to cross the road.

The candidate declared on the pre-employment questionnaire that he had reduced vision in his left eye resulting from an eye injury many years previously. There had been deterioration in the vision in his right eye for the previous 2–3 years.

He was assessed by the occupational physician and, with his consent, a background medical report was requested from his primary physician. This stated that only light and dark could be perceived by the left eye and that the cause of deteriorating vision in the right eye was macular degeneration. The local authority had made an earlier decision to set the visual standard for SCPGs. The reason for this was that it was acknowledged that the local authority had a duty of care to the school pupils that were assisted by SCPGs. The visual standard was set at the same level as for driving a car. On objective testing the candidate's vision failed to meet the required standard. The manager was advised that the applicant had reduced vision below the required standard and made the decision not to employ him.

The assessment should also consider any medical condition that may make it difficult to carry out the required tasks. The next case looks at the detailed assessment of the work and links it with the assessment of the client.

Case history 9.20

A 39-year-old woman applied for a post as a social worker linked to a paediatric ward. She had previously worked as a social worker with a different authority. Her pre-employment health declaration stated that she had previously had otosclerosis, which had resulted in a hearing loss. As this may have affected her ability to communicate with clients she was assessed by the occupational health physician. At the assessment the applicant was able to communicate without difficulty with the physician using hearing aids. She recognized she had difficulty in hearing where there was a high level of background noise. The applicant explained that she always let clients know of her hearing problem and moved to a quiet area for interviews. For case conferences with other professionals she also always advised colleagues of her difficulty and sat where she could see their faces. In addition she had been provided with an amplifier for the telephone and a personal T-loop system for small group work. The occupational physician tested that her ability to communicate on the phone was satisfactory. Although the condition is likely to be progressive, reports confirmed that there had been only minimal deterioration in the preceding 10 years. The physician advised that the applicant was fit to commence employment without any additional adjustments.

This case history also exemplifies how important it is to ascertain exactly what the job entails. This can be done by obtaining detailed job descriptions and by discussing the post with the line manager. It may include a visit to the workplace and a field test of specific abilities or a structured job simulation exercise.

If there are any restrictions on employment, these must be stated clearly and be as precise as possible, as is illustrated in the next case.

Case history 9.21

A 49-year-old woman applied for a post as a sales assistant in a department store. On her job application she declared that she suffered from epilepsy. She was initially interviewed by the occupational health nurse. The prospective employee had grand mal epilepsy with a fit frequency of about once every 2 months. She did not have a warning aura. The position applied for was in ladies' fashions. The stockroom had a high ceiling and required employees to climb ladders to reach the stock. The manager was advised that she was unfit to climb ladders and that it was advisable for her to use the lift rather than the stairs or escalator. In addition, reassessment was recommended prior to a change in departments. This was to avoid an unsuitable placement in such departments as china and glassware, where the employee would be at greater risk of injury and the employer at risk of damage to stock. These were considered as reasonable adjustments by the employer and she commenced employment.

Policy on rehabilitation in the workplace

Successful rehabilitation into the workplace is likely to improve the self-esteem and the financial position of the employee. It is therefore probable that it will lead to improvement in health. In the wider context it avoids people becoming dependent on state benefits. Personnel managers and line management need to have a clear policy on rehabilitation and their obligations, both statutory and as an organization, to the employee. Although additional resources may be required, these need to be offset against the potential costs of a retirement pension and the hiring and training of new employees.

The following definitions are used to describe the process of rehabilitation:

- **Rehabilitation** is the process of helping individuals to maximize their psychological and social capabilities to cope with life, after they have, in some way, been deprived of their former capabilities.
- **Medical rehabilitation** encompasses all activities that will enable the person to live independently. It will incorporate the skills of various healthcare workers, for example, doctors, nurses, physiotherapists, occupational/speech therapists and psychotherapists, and techniques such as reconstructive surgery and the use of technical aids. Both physical and mental activities must be encouraged at an early stage and be appropriate to the physical and mental capacity of the patient.
- **Occupational rehabilitation** describes the activities to enable a person to gain or regain the skills for employment. These activities may be workplace orientated and/or provided by outside agencies such as the the Disability Service Team in the United Kingdom (see Employment of the disabled, p. 241).

Resettlement defines those activities that enable a return to the previous employment or redeployment following the acquisition of any relevant new skills.

Advice on rehabilitation

The process of assessment is similar to that of the pre-employment assessment. It involves assessing the abilities of the employee and matching them to the job requirements. Management should be encouraged to provide information to the occupational physician to assist with this assessment and to formulate the questions they wish to have answered. These questions are likely to be along the following lines:

- Will a return to work pose a risk to health either to the employee or to others?
- Can the employee return to full hours and duties? If not, which rehabilitative measures are likely to be successful?
- Will further training assist return?
- Are there any other treatment options that are likely to improve function?
- Can the employee return to full hours with reduced duties? If so, can the duties that the employee can manage be specified?
- Can the employee return to full duties at reduced hours? What is likely to be the most appropriate way to increase hours?

- Can the employee return to reduced hours and reduced duties? Will full recovery be possible? What is the likely timescale?
- Will avoidance of specific chemical or physical exposures at work allow a return?
- Is alternative work likely to be possible – indication of appropriate tasks and hours?
- Would supported employment (see Employment of the disabled, page 241) be an appropriate option?
- Is the employee unable to give effective service in any available post?

Goal setting for occupational rehabilitation should commence as early as possible during recovery. It should not be seen as a sequel to medical rehabilitation but, wherever appropriate, as proceeding in tandem. By setting the goals at an early stage there is likely to be an increase in morale and a decrease in apathy and boredom. Where there is an occupational health service, liaison should commence at an early stage between the occupational health physician or nurse, the personnel and line managers, the employee and the doctors involved in the treatment of the employee. Discussions can take place regarding the possibility of rehabilitation – the agreement to develop and participate in a programme may be influenced by a number of factors, including outstanding litigation and compensation claims. Previous work satisfaction and level of performance will be important in motivation to return to work.

Case history 9.22

A 52-year-old man worked as a community education worker. He was involved in a road traffic accident, which caused disruption of the left brachial plexus and resulted in complete paralysis of the left arm and continuing pain. Work involved leading a youth group and taking a leadership role with community groups. Discussions with the personnel manager and the employee showed that the employee had found work difficult for a number of years. The accident had led him to become more introverted and reticent to meet new people. After visiting the workplace it was apparent that he would be unable to cope with the additional impairment of loss of use of the left arm and of confidence. Retiral on grounds of permanent incapacity was recommended.

In organizations or small industries where there is no occupational health service, the primary care physician may find it helpful, with his patient's consent, to approach directly the personnel or line manager and discuss the possibilities for an early, phased return to work. On the other hand, the patient who is a 'key' worker may be approached by his manager with proposals as to how an early return to work may be facilitated.

As in most aspects of the practice of occupational medicine there must be a detailed knowledge of the job requirements, which will include information from the line manager, job description and the description from the employee. A workplace visit will clarify the nature of the work and the physical surroundings.

The decision of primary importance is whether a return to work would cause harm either to the employee or to other employees or to others. If there is a risk, the likelihood and severity of harm should be quantified. The degree of harm should be considered as to whether it is likely to result in temporary or permanent disability. The determinants of rehabilitation are illustrated in Fig. 9.1, while the options and pathways for rehabilitation are shown in Fig. 9.2.

The following is an example of an assessment where, unfortunately, the outcome was that the employee was unfit to work.

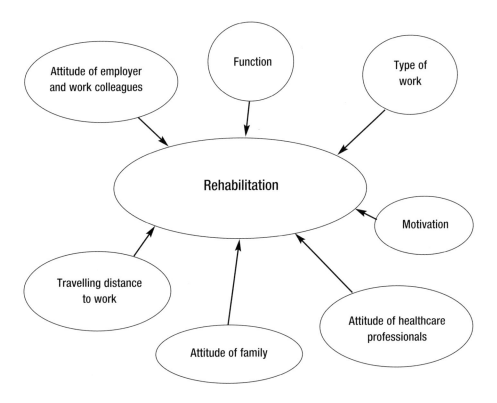

Fig. 9.1 *Determinants of rehabilitation.*

Case history 9.23

A lady who was employed as an SCPG was referred following long-term sickness absence. At interview she admitted that her absence was because of an alcohol problem. She gave permission for a report from her primary care physician. This confirmed that she had a long-standing alcohol problem, which had recurred and was resistant to treatment. The lady was adamant that she was now fit to resume her duties as an SCPG. Information from the line manager was that she worked unsupervised at a road junction escorting primary school children over the road.

The occupational physician assessed that she was at risk of causing major or even fatal injuries to both herself and the pupils if she came to work under the influence of alcohol. The lady strongly disagreed with this advice. In line with good occupational health practice a second opinion was obtained from another consultant occupational physician. The second occupational physician was in agreement with the opinion of the first consultant that the risk of major injury to herself or school children was sufficiently high to exclude her from work.

The manager made the decision to dismiss the employee. While reasonable adjustments should always be pursued, this case illustrates that there are circumstances where the safety aspects make dismissal the only option.

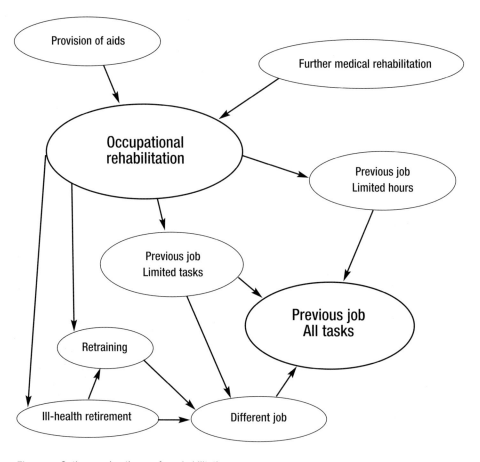

Fig. 9.2 *Options and pathways for rehabilitation.*

Further improvement

Is the employee fit to return into work and to perform the full range of duties? If this is not the case, what are the measures that are likely to enable a return to work?

Further treatments

The occupational physician should be prepared to give an opinion on whether there is further treatment that is likely to be beneficial or if the medical condition is likely to improve spontaneously. This would include psychological treatments and possibly further occupational therapy or physiotherapy. This is illustrated in the following case history.

Case history 9.24

A 54-year-old teacher of information technology approached the personnel department after a 6-week period of sickness absence for advice about medical retiral. The secondary school teacher enjoyed teaching and felt he worked in a school with a supportive headmaster. Following two recent bereavements he had noted himself becoming increasingly anxious. He regularly cycled to school but had found himself experiencing symptoms of chest tightness unrelated to exercise. He found concentration difficult and had difficulty in getting to sleep at night.

Different treatment options were discussed with him and referral to a clinical psychologist was arranged. Cognitive behavioural therapy was started and with this his confidence improved. He was able to restart teaching and after a short period on reduced hours was able to resume his normal duties.

Graded return to work in terms of hours

If the graded return is to normal duties, management are usually able to accommodate reduced hours for the initial period of return. Whether the pattern of hours is of whole days with rest days between work days, or of daily work with shorter hours, will depend on practical factors such as travelling time to work and the availability of lifts. In most cases the employee will be able to return to full contractual hours approximately 4 weeks from starting. Unless the employee is able to manage at least two 3-hour sessions a week, it is unlikely that he or she is ready to restart a rehabilitation programme. It improves confidence and morale when the level is achievable without undue fatigue. This reduces the risk of the employee needing to take further time off work. At levels below 6 hours a week it is difficult to rebuild skills and confidence. Some benefits systems do present the possibility of therapeutic work, which enables an employee to remain on benefits while working for a few hours each week. This was illustrated in the above case history.

Graded return to work in terms of duties

Case history 9.25

A metallurgist working in ship refitting was involved in a road traffic accident where he was catapulted from his motorbike when it was in collision with a car. He received treatment for a fractured tibia. Although he complained of pain in his wrist, this was not X-rayed for over a month. During this time he noted decreased pronation and supination of his wrist with a reduction in grip strength. His tasks normally involved laboratory work and taking samples on board ships. The latter part of his duties involved climbing up and down ladders to move from one deck to another in ships undergoing refit. On his return to work he was able to undertake safely the full range of laboratory work but would have been at risk of falls if he had attempted to work afloat. Following an orthopaedic operation he regained full function of his right wrist and he was eventually able to resume full duties.

Case history 9.15 illustrates a combination of adjustments in both hours and duties.

Extra training

A telesales assistant (see Case history 9.34) raised with her manager difficulties in using the computer and concerns that she was working more slowly than others. The manager arranged extra training. Unfortunately because of the underlying health problem this was not successful.

Caseload reduction

Sometimes, although an employee can carry out all tasks, these can only be accomplished at a slower pace as is illustrated below.

Case history 9.26

A secondary school teacher aged 56 years was absent from work following a cataract operation to her right eye. Although a synthetic lens had immediately been inserted, she was waiting for new glasses and had concerns about how long it would take her to read and mark pupils' work. In addition, during her time off there had been curriculum changes. Physically the operation was minor and she felt able to sustain a full day's work without difficulty. The head teacher was agreeable to her returning to work full-time but reduced the number of classes she was taking for the first 4 weeks. The additional time allowed longer for correcting work and for familiarization with the new curriculum and preparation of course work. After 4 weeks she was able to resume her full teaching role.

Increased management feedback

Prolonged sickness absence, particularly with mental health problems, often leads to reduced confidence and increased anxiety at the thought of returning to work. An open management style with positive feedback allows the employee's confidence in his or her own abilities to increase.

Case history 9.27

A records clerk had been absent from her work for 3 months. Prior to her sickness absence she had felt increasingly tired and had lost confidence. She found both personal criticism and criticism of her work very hurtful. Her primary care physician diagnosed a depressive illness and treated her with antidepressant medication and arranged for psychological assessment. The clinical psychologist took her through a programme of cognitive behavioural therapy. With this she was able to recognize the negative attitude she had developed towards her own abilities. For her return to work she talked with the personnel manager regarding her concerns about return. In a joint meeting with the employee, line manager and personnel manager the difficulties about feedback were discussed. The line manager agreed to regular meetings and assured the employee that any difficulties about work quality would be addressed at an early stage. When the employee was reviewed after return to work she was confident and had received positive feedback regarding her work. Her general self-esteem had improved and she felt better able to cope with minor criticisms.

Avoidance of specific chemical exposures

In some cases a specific work exposure leads to ill-health. A successful return to work will require either further control or avoidance of the exposure.

Case history 9.28

A 30-year-old quality assurance chemist referred himself to the occupational health department with a skin rash. The facial rash was consistent with contact dermatitis. As the chemist worked with a number of different opiates he was referred to a dermatologist for patch testing. Patch testing confirmed an allergic contact dermatitis to morphine and diamorphine and advice from the consultant was to avoid exposure to opiates. For his return to work he moved into a different area of the business that excluded him from work with opiates.

Redeployment

Redeployment is an option that should be considered when an employee is unable to return to their own work, even with reasonable adjustments, without risk to their own health or the safety of others.

Case history 9.29

A printer aged 40 years was employed in a retailing concern printing notices and price labels. A workplace visit showed that he used a number of printing inks. Solvents such as dichloromethane were needed to clean the rollers. He developed dermatitis and contact testing was carried out in the dermatology department. The patch testing showed no specific allergies. He was given full instruction in skincare and received appropriate treatment via his general practitioner. However, although the skin condition improved while he was away from work, it continued to deteriorate when at work and he remained with marked thickening and cracking of the skin, particularly on the tips of the fingers.

As all the preventative measures failed to show any improvement, the decision was made to redeploy him before the condition became a chronic one. He moved reluctantly from his post in printing into display which involved preparing shop window displays. His work involved no contact with solvents. Over the following 6 weeks his skin condition improved and remained in good condition. However, he found adjusting to his new work difficult. Previously he had the status of working in the management corridor and now his workshop was in the sub-basement. He had enjoyed the autonomy of working as the only printer whereas now he had to adjust to becoming a member of a team. Despite his initial reservations the redeployment was successful.

An employee may have difficulty in adjusting to a new post even where there is a positive health gain. The decision will be harder where there is a loss of earnings.

Ill-health retirement

To be told by an occupational physician, general practitioner or hospital consultant that consideration should be given to retiring on health grounds can be one of the most depressing, morale-sapping statements that a patient hears, even if it has been anticipated. The subject should not be raised until it becomes overwhelmingly clear that either the patient's health will preclude a return to the previous employment, for example, persistent exertional dyspnoea after myocardial infarction, or that the work environment will continue adversely to affect the patient's condition, for example in the case of occupational asthma when there are no opportunities for exposure control or redeployment within the organization. However, having made the recommendation, it is very important for the doctor to maintain a positive attitude and, having decided what the patient cannot do, begin to concentrate on what can be achieved and what skills there are to offer, which may not only be work related but have developed in connection with hobbies and leisure activities. The patient must be aware of the facilities and scope of the services offered by the statutory agencies and how to access the system.

Case history 9.30

A 45-year-old painter developed pain in his cervical spine which was referred to both arms and was associated with intermittent paraesthesia and numbness in the left arm, in the C6/7/8/TI distributions. These symptoms were elicited during an annual health assessment, which was undertaken as part of a voluntary health surveillance scheme for members of the works department. The painter had not complained voluntarily as he was afraid of losing his job.

Examination by the occupational physician revealed pain in the cervical spine with disability manifest by limitation of movement, weakness of the extensors of the forearm together with decreased grip strength. Impairment was confirmed by radiographs of the cervical spine which showed the presence of degenerative disc disease. He was referred for physiotherapy with resulting improvement in his symptoms and resolution of his neurological signs.

Six months later his symptoms returned. He requested to see the occupational physician who, on questioning the painter, also elicited a history of dizziness which was clearly associated with rotation and extension of his cervical spine. He did not want a further period of sickness absence. With the cooperation of his managers it was agreed that his work would be restricted so that he would not be allowed to paint ceilings or high walls and, in addition, he would be allowed time to attend for physiotherapy. However, on this occasion, the severity and frequency of his symptoms progressed and he accepted that sickness absence was inevitable. Further X-rays showed progression of his degenerative disc disease and subluxation of the vertebral body of C6 on C7. He was referred for specialist advice.

After several lengthy discussions with the neurologist, neurosurgeon and occupational physician, he decided to agree to cervical fusion, knowing there was no guarantee that it would enable him to return to work as a painter. Assessment, 6 months following surgery, showed partial success in that he was pain free and had no neurological deficits. However, he lacked the cervical mobility that was necessary to enable him to fulfil his job description. There were no opportunities for relocation within the organization.

He was referred, by the occupational physician and with the general practitioner's agreement, to the specialist disability employment adviser (DEA) while the papers were being processed for his retirement on health grounds. The DEA advised him that the best use of his skills would be to set up a small business. He was placed on specific courses to teach him the necessary practical management skills. Six months following his retirement he contacted the occupational physician to say that he was self-employed, having started a business as a painter and decorator, and had employed a young lad to undertake the physical aspects of the work that were beyond his own capabilities.

During the often lengthy assessment process it is important that morale and confidence are maintained. This can be achieved by suggesting participation in voluntary work, which will not adversely affect benefit entitlement.

Case history 9.31

A 45-year-old firefighter was retired on medical grounds with chronic lumbar back pain associated with degenerative disc disease. He had associated depression, being very despondent and feeling that he was 'on the scrap heap'. Talking to him revealed that his hobby was bird watching. He found that this was compatible with his back condition and provided him with relaxation and temporary abatement of his depression. He was encouraged to approach the warden of the nearby nature reserve to see whether they could use his knowledge and interest as a voluntary warden with the freedom to come and go as he pleased depending on his mood. The warden was delighted to have extra help; the ex-firefighter became increasingly involved and his depression resolved; he was eventually appointed, when a vacancy arose, as a full-time employee.

Employment of the disabled

A proportion of people of working age will have an impairment that handicaps them in terms of employability. The proportion rises with age; for example, the Labour Force Survey undertaken in the United Kingdom during the summer of 1999 reported that 11% of people aged 20–29 years had a current long-term disability or health problem compared with 31% in those aged 50–59 years. The impairment may be congenital or acquired through injury (occupational or non-occupational) or illness. There is little objective evidence to show that disabled persons have above-average sickness absence. On the contrary, many disabled employees are strongly motivated to overcome their disability and attendance rates are frequently better than average. Disability does not equate with ill-health nor necessarily with sickness absence.

When assessing medical fitness for work it is important to assess the degree of any associated loss of function and any resulting disability or handicap. The assessment may include receiving reports from the general practitioner or specialist. This is particularly relevant for mental health problems. The capabilities of the person with the disability should be compared to the job requirements. In Great Britain the Disability Discrimination Act 1995 states that discrimination occurs when a disabled person is treated less favourably than someone else, for reasons associated with their disability, but where the action cannot be justified. This includes the process of employment. Providing there is a good match between the job and the person's abilities there is no evidence that there is an increased safety risk either to themselves or to other employees. Communication with the employee, line manager, personnel manager and occupational health department is essential to identify placement needs. Any restrictions should be precisely stated and based on firm foundations. The following case histories show how adjustments, either through altering job responsibilities or through the provision of extra facilities, can permit the disabled to carry on in employment.

Case history 9.32

A 35-year-old lady applied for a post as a home help. On her pre-employment questionnaire she declared that she had suffered from schizophrenia for a number of years. With her permission a report from her consultant psychiatrist was received. This confirmed that she had suffered from schizophrenia for a number of years requiring admission to hospital and had a tendency to mood swings. He felt that she might have difficulty in relating to elderly clients. The occupational physician saw her for assessment. She appeared well at interview. However, the post was for relief cover at weekends and would be completely unsupervised. The occupational physician assessed that she was unfit to work in an unsupervised post with vulnerable clients who may themselves have unpredictable behaviour. The report stated that she was unfit to work alone with vulnerable clients. The personnel manager was informed that she could be fit for supervised posts working in a different position such as cleaning.

Case history 9.33

A consultant radiologist developed multiple sclerosis at the age of 35 years, shortly after his appointment. The disease followed a slowly progressive course until, 20 years following onset, he was having difficulty, due to weakness, in walking round the hospital site, attending ward rounds and lectures. His balance was impaired and he was restricted in the extent of patient screening that could be safely undertaken. The physical fatigue also affected mental functioning, particularly in terms of concentration. After much persuasion by the occupational health service he agreed to investigate the use of a wheelchair. This provided limited benefit in increasing his range of mobility and, thereby, lessening his mental fatigue. Subsequent technical developments made available an electric tricycle (Fig. 9.3). This greatly extended his range of mobility, allowing him to attend ward rounds, clinical meetings and lectures, conserved his physical strength and thereby lessened mental fatigue and its associated effects.

Disabled people find it harder to gain employment; for example, disabled people account for nearly one-fifth of the working-age population in the UK, but only about one-eighth of all people in employment. This means that there are 6.5 million people in the UK with a current long-term disability or health problem that has a substantial adverse effect on their day-to-day activities, or which limits the work they

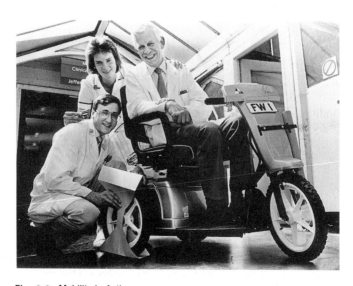

Fig. 9.3 *Mobility in Action.*

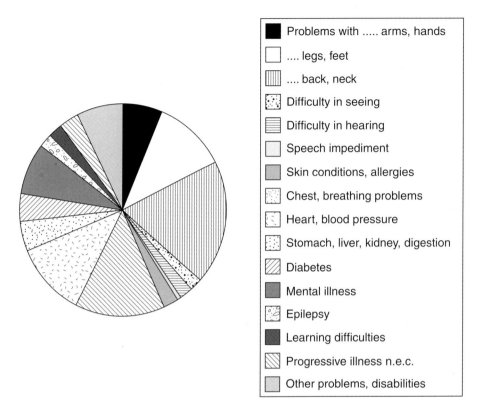

Fig. 9.4 *Main disabilities as highlighted in the Labour Force Survey of summer 1999.*

can do. Figure 9.4 shows the distribution of disability according to the UK labour Force Survey. As previously stated, the proportion of the population with a disability varies with age and there are some geographical changes, although this may be associated with differences in the age profile. Employment rates vary markedly with the type of disability. High employment rates are achieved with conditions such as diabetes, skin conditions and hearing problems. However, around 75% of people with mental illness and over 60% with learning difficulties are out of work and on state benefits.

Disability within the European Union

Throughout the European Union there is concern that the gap between the disabled unemployment rate and that of other workers has grown in recent years. Structural changes in the labour market, with an increased emphasis on intellectual ability, advanced education and adaptability mean fewer job opportunities for people with the double disadvantage of impairment and limited education and skills. In addition, if disabled workers lose their jobs through firms downsizing there are few prospects of regaining employment or moving to new careers. Countries within the European Union have ratified the International Labour Organisation Convention concerning Vocational Rehabilitation and Employment (Disabled Persons). Statistical comparisons between different member countries are difficult as limited data is collected by the member countries. Each member state has its own system for defining disabled people. The total unemployment rates vary fivefold between the lowest and highest member states. Throughout the Union proportionately more men and women with a disability are employed in agriculture, construction, health, personal and other services. Low numbers are employed in manufacturing, distribution, finance and education. A higher proportion of disabled people are in low-skilled occupations.

The specific legislation of the member countries regarding disability varies considerably. This will be illustrated by looking at the different policies of four member countries, namely, Denmark, Germany, Spain and the United Kingdom.

DENMARK

Danish legislation does not give a definition of disability. The aim of Danish policy is to provide each individual with the means to live as normal a life as possible. It is designed to integrate people with disabilities into work and the community on equal terms with others. Registering disabilities is discouraged because this action assumes that it is possible to categorize and confine disabilities and conditions to a specific definition.

The Ministry of Labour set up a fund in 1996 to pay for special education, on-the-job training, course upgrades and vocational training. In addition, specialized work tools and technical aids to assist in the workplace are funded. The fund also assists individuals and organizations working to improve the integration of people with disabilities into the workforce. Businesses are encouraged to accept more responsibility to integrate people with disabilities into the workforce. Five different types of institution exist in regard to training and employment.

1. Vocational centres, which assess working capacities and provide vocational training and retraining.
2. Vocational training institutions, some of which specialize in people with disabilities.
3. Individual sheltered employment in specially designed workshops. Public funds of up to 50% of the minimum wage may be available. To qualify, the individual must have made one or more attempts to be rehabilitated without finding employment.
4. Sheltered workshops, which allow people with disabilities to carry out some form of work.
5. Special day centres, which provide social skills training and preparation for sheltered workshops.

The transition from school into employment is overseen by 'Curators' who teach young people with disabilities from the age of 13 years and are responsible for vocational preparation. In addition, they are available to the young person and the family during the transition to training or employment.

In Denmark people with disabilities are entitled to financial, practical or social support on the basis of need, not according to the disability itself.

GERMANY

In 1974 Germany passed the Severely Disabled Persons Act. This provided protection against dismissal for individuals with disabilities assessed as being over 50%. In addition, the Act required all employers with 16 or more employees to reserve 6% of positions for people with disabilities. If this did not happen, a compensatory levy was paid to the Government. This levy was used to subsidize sheltered workshops, residential homes and special projects in addition to being used to give individual subsidies.

The result of the scheme has not been entirely successful. Only 15% of eligible employers met the quota. There appears to be a reluctance on the part of employers to hire individuals who are protected against dismissal. Dismissal of a disabled person has to have advanced approval from the Regional Assistance Office. People with disabilities have, however, been successful in entering employment in small firms not covered by the quota. Subsidies are available to a firm once the firm has hired a person with a disability.

The Act also requests that enterprises employing five or more disabled persons elect a 'trustworthy person'. This person is requested to:

* stimulate hiring of more people with disabilities
* provide assistance and advice to co-workers with disabilities
* encourage the appropriate assignment of employment for people with disabilities
* advise the company on avoiding redundancy among disabled workers
* help to ensure a healthy and secure working environment with reduced risk of injury.

Research has shown that where a trustworthy person is appointed, the enterprise is more likely to continue hiring people with disabilities.

There are programmes targeted at the young unemployed who are experiencing difficulties in the transition from school to work. Priority areas include improving cooperation between schools and vocational training institutions and developing non-profit training and placement agencies with national employment services. Specially trained vocational counsellors facilitate the transition from school to employment.

For people with disabilities unable to work in the open labour market there are sheltered workshops. These offer both work and training and are subsidized by the government. In addition, supported employment offers training and employment in businesses. Job coaches ensure that the type of support is tailored to the needs of the person with the disability. People with disabilities attend specialized training centres for vocational assessment. The assessments usually take approximately 60 days and the results are used to design rehabilitation plans.

The Vocational Rehabilitation Act 1974 states that vocational assistance should include all forms of assistance that are necessary to sustain, enhance, generate or restore the capacity of the individual eventually to earn his own income through employment.

SPAIN

The 1978 Constitution guarantees the right of all Spanish citizens to work and seek full employment and explicitly recognizes the rights of people with disabilities. The 1982 Act on social integration stated that the first aim of the employment policy is to integrate workers with disabilities into the normal system of employment. Where this is not possible they will be incorporated into sheltered employment. With this policy 60% of disabled workers are employed in private enterprises and less than 3% in public administration. People with disabilities receive similar benefits to other disadvantaged groups such as unemployed youths. To enhance integration, a programme of special measures such as quotas, protection against dismissal and incentives for employers has been set up.

Businesses employing over 50 people must ensure that 2% of staff comprise individuals who have registered their disabilities with the employment office. Unfortunately many do not register their disability for fear of being discriminated against in finding work. This leads to the quota not being met. However, as in Germany, people with disabilities often find work in small firms not covered by the quota system.

Once in employment the government can provide protection against dismissal. Workers acquiring a disability during employment are entitled to re-employment in the same firm. If the worker regains full capacity, employers are required to reinstate them to the original post.

There is a grant for employing a person with a disability which extends over the first 3 years of employment. There are also reductions to social security payments and grants for special adaptations to the workplace.

Sheltered workshops provide remunerated employment for people incapable of working under normal conditions. During the 1990s, supported employment programmes were developed as an alternative to sheltered workshops. Some large companies have developed their own initiatives for the creation of services for people with disabilities.

Young people with disabilities are encouraged to participate in mainstream education and training programmes. Counsellors play a vital role in the transition from school to training or employment. Training for disadvantaged adults, for example, people with disabilities and immigrants, is available and can last from 3 months to 3 years. Further legislation stipulates that vocational rehabilitation can be made available in firms. This requires a special contract between the employer and the person with the disability.

In 1994 an employment plan was published for people with disabilities. This advised promoting employment of people with disabilities in the private sector. It recommended improved training and education for people with disabilities, with less attention on benefits and more initiatives to adapt working environments, for example with wheelchair access, enhanced transport.

UNITED KINGDOM

Historically the Disabled Persons (Employment) Act 1944 originated from the need to make provision for people disabled in the Second World War. The measures included in this Act were a register of people with disabilities. Employers with more than 20 employees were required to employ a quota of 3% of people with registered disabilities. Assessment, rehabilitation and training centres were also set up. During the 1970s and 1980s it was realized that the quota and registration systems were flawed. A wide-ranging review was commissioned in 1988, which was published in 1990 as a Consultative Document *Employment and Training for People with Disabilities*. This led to the introduction of the Disability Discrimination Act, which came into force on 2 December 1996. This repealed the previous definition of disability, quota, registration and designated employment provisions of the 1944 Act. The new Act gives a broad definition of disability as a mental or physical impairment that has a substantial and long-term adverse effect on a person's ability to carry out normal everyday tasks. The Act and associated guidance defines that a substantial adverse effect is something that is more than minor or trivial. It is a long-term effect that has lasted at least 12 months or is likely to last at least 12 months. A condition that may improve but has the potential to recur will also be considered as having a long-term effect. Other than for spectacles, the effects of artificial aids or medical treatment should be disregarded. Therefore conditions such as diabetes and epilepsy, which may have relatively little effect on day-to-day activities, are covered by the Act. The occupational physician should, if relevant, be able to give an opinion on the likelihood of progression of the disability and the potential need for specialist equipment or modification to the working environment. In the case of employees suffering a progressive condition, the Act will apply as soon as symptoms are experienced, even though their condition is not yet serious enough to be defined as a disability using the functional criteria.

For an impairment to affect day-to-day activities, it must do so in one or more of the following categories:

- mobility
- manual dexterity
- physical coordination
- continence
- ability to lift, carry or otherwise move everyday objects
- speech, hearing or eyesight
- memory or ability to concentrate, learn or understand
- perception of the risk of physical danger.

A person only needs to be impaired in one of the above categories to be considered disabled. Some conditions such as addiction or dependency on alcohol, nicotine or any other substance are specifically excluded from coverage under the Act.

The Act states that discrimination occurs when a disabled person is treated less favourably than someone else, for reasons associated with their disability, but where the treatment cannot be justified. With regard to employment discrimination can occur in all aspects of everyday working arrangements. This includes the areas of recruitment and retention of employees, promotion and transfers, training and development, the dismissal process and access to benefits provided by the employer. Employers are also required to consider reasonable adjustments to the workplace and/or to the employment arrangements which would otherwise have overcome the disadvantage encountered by the disabled person.

Many occupational physicians feel that the Act has given a legal framework to good occupational practice in relation to both the initial employment and subsequent rehabilitation of disabled people.

Local Education Authorities are required to make statements regarding planning the transition of young people with special educational needs from school into employment. Training is provided through Training and Enterprise Councils in England and Wales and through Local Enterprise Councils in Scotland. Around 19% of adults and 6% of young people commencing training have a disability.

In higher education there are no specialist institutions for students with disabilities. It is the responsibility of each institution to make decisions about admissions to courses. The provision of learning support and physical access to buildings is also a responsibility of the individual institution.

Young people aged 18–24 years with a disability who have been unemployed for 6 months or more are included in the New Deal for Young People. Under the scheme participants may have a job with an employer or a placement with a voluntary organization or a place on an environmental taskforce.

In addition there are a number of schemes that give incentives for employers to employ people with disabilities of working age.

Specialist services in employment for the disabled

People with a disability and seeking employment are initially assessed by the DEAs, who can be contacted through the local Job Centres. They are members of the Disability Service Teams. Disability Service Teams (formerly known as Placing Assessment and Counselling Teams) can advise employers on employing the disabled (Fig. 9.5). The specific schemes currently available in the United Kingdom are as follows.

1. **Access to work.** This scheme provides practical help and advice to disabled people. It is aimed at paying towards the extra employment costs resulting from disability. Some examples of the assistance that can be given are:

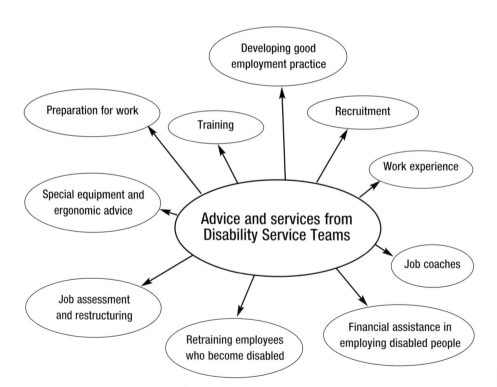

Fig. 9.5 *Specialist advice available for employers on employing disabled.*

- a communicator at a job interview for people with a hearing difficulty
- a reader for someone who has a visual impairment
- a support worker who may give assistance either at work or travelling to work. A job coach may support someone while they familiarize themselves with a job
- extra costs of travelling to work such as adaptations to a vehicle, taxi fares or other transport costs
- specialized equipment such as magnified computer screens or text screens or amplifiers for telephones
- alterations to the working environment such as installing specialized alarm systems or lifts.

For instance the amplifier for the telephone and the individual T-loop system used in meetings for the social worker described in Case history 9.20 was provided by the Access to Work Scheme.

2. **Job introduction scheme.** This scheme gives financial assistance to recruit a person who is disabled to test whether the job is suitable for them. The Disability Service Team gives support during this trial period. This was illustrated in Case history 9.18.

3. **Supported employment.** This is available to people with a severe disability who are unable to obtain or retain a job in the open market. At present these can be in subsidized workshops or with a host company. Funds are held by 'sponsors' who are either Remploy Ltd, a local authority or a voluntary organization. In a host company the person will work alongside other employees. Special adaptations to the workplace or equipment may be provided by the Access to Work Scheme. The employee may remain employed by the sponsor (e.g. Remploy) or become/remain an employee of the host company. Under either circumstance the host company pays for the actual work undertaken by the employee, with a contribution being made by the sponsor. The current trend is away from sheltered workshops into supported employment with host employers. Currently in the UK 22 500 people are in supported employment. The case history below illustrates one such case.

Case history 9.34

A 40-year-old lady had worked with a retailing organization for 15 years. During this time she developed low back pain which had resulted in a number of prolonged absences. She had recently moved into a department mainly involved in telephone sales. She presented to the occupational health nurse with symptoms of poor concentration, broken sleep, feeling anxious and tearful. She felt she had difficulty in learning the computer skills for her new job. The occupational health nurse found that the manager had recognized the difficulty and had arranged extra training and had also reduced the pressure of calls on the employee. Unfortunately neither of these steps was successful. The job was assessed and the conclusion reached that no further modifications were possible that would be likely to make a return to this post successful. With the employee's agreement she was redeployed to a clerical post.

Unfortunately, despite a slow introduction to the new post and an appropriate level of support, the employee's symptoms of anxiety and poor sleep returned. The occupational physician was concerned that there might be an underlying learning difficulty that accounted for the problems encountered in new working environments. The employee was therefore referred to the occupational psychologist with the local Disability Service Team. Shortly after this assessment the employee developed visual problems, which resulted in a referral first to an ophthalmologist and then to a neurologist. A computerized tomography scan of the brain showed enlarged ventricles. A diagnosis of hydrocephalus was made and further tests including a lumbar puncture were performed. At this point the employee was given objective tests of numeracy and spelling. These showed she was functioning at about 50% of accepted levels for open employment. The low back pain restricted her moving into a normal retailing position. Also during this period a lumbar puncture showed the presence of an IgG-specific oligoclonal band and a diagnosis of multiple sclerosis was made by the neurologist. The occupational psychologist advised that she would be eligible for a supported employment. A suitable post was identified that did not require keyboard skills, had easy access to a toilet and the work could be seated. The employee had made a successful move to this post and the funding for supported employment was organized.

This case history illustrates the value of objective testing in understanding the reason for this lady's difficulty in achieving satisfactory performance at her work. The level of support that she required in her work was substantial and above the level normally accepted as reasonable for an employer to make. Supported employment has allowed her to remain in employment while giving financial support to the employer to engage someone else to carry out the tasks she is unable to do.

However it is unrealistic to expect all work placements to be successful, as is outlined below.

Case history 9.35

A 25-year-old man with learning difficulties was employed by a local authority as a cleaner. He had started work under the Job Introduction Scheme. He worked well and applied for a full-time post when one became available at a different venue. The venue was further from his home but as he could already drive this was not a major problem. He started working well but over the months his attendance at work fell. He was referred to the occupational physician for assessment. A report from his general practitioner confirmed that he did not have an underlying illness to account for his poor attendance. It transpired that he no longer felt that cleaning work was suitable for a man and did not understand his obligation to attend work under these circumstances. A representative from the sponsoring organization met with the personnel manager, the line manager and the occupational physician. It was agreed that it was unlikely that any adjustments to the current post would be successful. It was decided to offer him an alternative placement in a more male environment where he would be working as part of a team. He turned down this offer and the sponsoring organization undertook to help him find alternative employment.

Members of some disability organizations believe that the Disability Discrimination Act is in itself discriminatory in that it divides people with disabilities from other members of society. It remains to be seen if it will be more effective than the previous quota system in giving appropriate job opportunities to people with a disability.

Future prospects

The European Commission published a paper in September 1998 entitled Raising Employment Levels of People with Disabilities. This acknowledges that, throughout the community, employment levels are 20–30% lower in people with a disability. Changes in the labour market, such as the disappearance of manual posts involving repetitive work, have an increased effect on people with elementary skills and learning difficulties.

Disability and employment is on the agenda of most of the Member States. The aims will be to try to reduce the skills gap by modernizing education and training systems and equipping workers to be able to take advantage of new job opportunities. On the positive side new technologies may open up job opportunities which disabled people have been excluded from until now.

The approach should aim at giving people appropriate skills to work, re-engineering work tasks so that they can be performed by people with different abilities and providing appropriate support. It is important to this strategy that people with disabilities see themselves as employable and that defining themselves as unable to work is not a prerequisite for obtaining support.

BENEFITS

Throughout the European Union there are concerns about the number of people out of the job market and relying on benefits. The number of people on incapacity or long-term benefit has doubled in the past decade and now numbers 1.75 million in the United Kingdom alone.

For example, in the UK the benefits outlined below are available. The conditions for the benefits do change and an employee should be encouraged to seek advice from the Benefits Agency and/or the local Citizens Advice Bureau to check eligibility for different benefits.

Statutory sick pay

Statutory sick pay is a non-contributory benefit and is paid to an employee who has been sick for 4 or more calendar days in a row and earns enough to pay Class 1 National Insurance Contributions. It is paid for up to 28 weeks at a time or for periods with less than 8 weeks between them.

Incapacity benefit

Incapacity benefit is a contributory benefit and is payable to people who are sick or disabled and have been incapable of work for 4 or more days in a row and are not entitled to Statutory sick pay. Incapacity benefit is based on a person's incapacity for:

- work in their normal occupation for the first 28 weeks of incapacity (the own occupation test)
- all work from the 29th week of incapacity (the 'all work test').

Medical certificates are only required to cover incapacity until the person has passed the 'all work test'.

Work preparation programme

The work preparation programme aims to assist people with disabilities to increase their employment prospects by improving their readiness, job finding skills and techniques. It can provide work experience when necessary. It provides modular, flexible programmes provided by an external provider and pays an allowance for this.

Industrial injuries disablement benefit

Industrial injuries disablement benefit is a non-contributory benefit that is payable only to employees who become disabled or develop a prescribed disease (see Appendix 1). The payment dates 15 weeks from the date of the accident and is normally only payable for a disablement of 14% or more. The decision takes account of an opinion of a doctor in the medical services. If eligible, it is payable from 15 weeks after the date of the accident or onset of the disease.

CONCLUSION

Occupational physicians have an opportunity and responsibility to work with management to ensure appropriate placement regarding medical fitness of employees both before and during employment. A supportive attitude to rehabilitation from management assists return to work and often reduces the length of sickness absence. A continuing challenge to all involved in employment is to encourage the employment of disabled people in posts that match well with their functional abilities.

10

Health promotion in the workplace

SUMMARY

- Health promotion in the workplace must start with the correct assessment of risks to health arising from work, communication of information about them, appropriate control measures and empowerment of the workforce to contribute to these processes. Thus health-promoting activities should be part of a needs-based strategy that controls work-related risks as well as addressing other means of maintaining health and well-being.

- The workforce is not a randomly selected captive audience to whom health promotion approaches designed for the community can be simply applied.

- Health promoting activities also arise opportunistically out of many individual contacts with workers.

- Strategies regarding smoking, alcohol and other substance abuse should recognize the mixed occupational, lifestyle and social implications of such substance abuse or misuse. In addition to an explicit policy, there should be consultation, education, individual counselling and other support.

- In relation to the reduction of psychological stress, lasting improvement is more likely if organizational causes of stress are identified and dealt with rather than by focusing exclusively on individual behaviour.

- Influencing dietary habits and encouraging weight reduction and exercise are laudable aims, especially in parallel with health protection measures.

- Inappropriate screening does not promote health and may foster unwarranted anxiety. It is no substitute for the good practice of preventive occupational medicine.

INTRODUCTION

The purpose of this chapter is to consider practical aspects of the promotion of health among the working population. It takes into account the special opportunities and difficulties associated with the workplace context. Promoting health in the workplace is part of World Health Organization (WHO) and European Union policy as well as that of probably all its member states. The WHO has defined health as a state of complete physical, mental and social well-being and not merely the absence of disease or infirmity. The following cases illustrate some common issues and misconceptions.

Case history 10.1

A firm manufacturing fine tools embarked on, and publicized, a health promotion exercise. This included offering a wide range of high fibre, low fat meals in the staff canteen, providing exercise facilities, and classes to help in stopping smoking. Many executives and some other office staff but few manual workers took advantage of this. Most employees still brought in their own lunches or went out for chips and beer at lunchtime. Few employees who did not previously engage in physical exercise started to do so as a result of this programme. In the meantime, some employees in parts of the firm continued to suffer from noise-induced hearing loss and tinnitus. Others had occupational diseases of the skin from exposure to cutting oils and other agents. One developed features of 'hard metal' lung disease. These were often first evident during their attendances at the Occupational Health Department or when referred by their general practitioner (GP) to hospital out-patient specialists. A clear strategy and mechanism for preventing many of these cases or managing their consequences was lacking. Most workers viewed health promotion as implemented by the firm with considerable scepticism and even resentment at what some perceived as rank hypocrisy.

At best the firm had viewed its workforce as simply a random sample of the community from which it is derived, and in respect of whom community-based initiatives on diet, exercise and smoking could simply be imported. At worst they were negligent of their primary responsibility to recognize and prevent occupational disease. Clearly, before beginning to assess priorities for preventive medicine in a workplace certain important considerations need to be understood; the failure of preventive action can often be traced back to neglect of one or more of the work-related factors discussed in this book. Occupational risks to health may be substantial, but at the same time very remediable in terms of cost effectiveness.

Sometimes, pursuing policies of health promotion that bear no specific relation to the workplace in question can be a convenient path of least resistance for all concerned – employers, employees and occupational health departments. Thus for employers this pursuit presents an image of doing something while not opening any cans of worms. Employees feel that something is being done for their health that would not have a bearing on their employment prospects, while occupational health departments may be pleased to find a health-related issue that enjoys the support both of employers and employees. This can be particularly true in an adverse economic climate, because employers might avoid anything that could increase costs and reduce productivity and competitiveness. At the same time employees might be wary of occupational health activities, which they might perceive as reducing job prospects for the workplace as a whole, or for individuals, in a climate of unemployment or of reducing overtime work. Thus a consensus commitment to some form of health promotion that is aimed at individual lifestyle rather than at workplace risks can appear an attractive soft option, and relatively risk-free or inexpensive compared to some of the measures described in this book or to a pay rise!

Moreover it is essential to consider the ethical aspects. Thus a strong case can be made that it is only ethical to engage in heath-related issues if they are built on good health and safety practice and that it would be unethical to claim to be promoting health in the workplace when ignoring valid interventions to reduce risks to health from work. In other words the first and foremost legal and moral responsibility of the employer is to reduce occupational risks to health and not those pertaining to the community as a whole. All employees are expected to fulfil the terms of their contract of employment and as most of them do this to various degrees their activities at work will follow similar patterns. However, beyond this, the extent to which each will participate in health promotion is influenced by many complex factors that are outlined or illustrated later.

A simplistic attitude on the part of well-intentioned health promoters might not be needed for those in the workplace who are already motivated in pursuing a healthy lifestyle and at the same time might exert no influence on the others who remain indifferent. Employees who perceive that the conditions of their job exert an important adverse influence on their health, safety or well-being are not likely to be responsive or sympathetic to health promotion attempts that explicitly or implicitly ignore these concerns.

Health promotion in the workplace should thus aim to develop an environment that promotes health in all its modalities (physical, mental and psycho-social). In order to achieve this broad aim it seeks to:

- educate and inform employees and employers in the risks to health arising from work and other factors
- influence the attitudes and hence the behaviour of employees and employers in relation to the promotion of their health and the health of others
- provide and empower workers with the opportunity to exert more control over their work, and in particular their work environment, as it relates to health
- provide professional support, facilities and assistance to fulfil the above aims.

Social and public perceptions, based on limited risk-based information, may influence priorities for protecting the health of the workforce by assuming that what is good for the community in general must be good for the workforce 'captive audience' without taking the special risks and needs of the workforce into account.

Case history 10.2

An award scheme was established for firms based in a large area in order to afford recognition to those that had fulfilled certain criteria for 'health at work'. The criteria were heavily based on evidence of lifestyle interventions, such as dietary measures, exercise facilities, smoking cessation and stress health management classes. A few large, high profile companies pursued the scheme but the majority of, usually smaller, companies (which employ the majority of the working population) were indifferent to the scheme. A large company employing thousands and with a turnover of hundreds of millions of pounds was assessed by a body which had developed the award scheme and qualified for a prestigious trophy on the basis of having fulfilled a number of the criteria. The company then experienced a work-related fatality. It was later prosecuted, found guilty of negligence, and felt compelled to return the award.

Occupational health and safety issues are often poorly addressed by many such award schemes, either being completely absent from the criteria or dealt with by self-certification of compliance with the law or by absence of impending prosecution. Moreover, does a national award scheme spending large sums of money to present some form of award to a few large and well-resourced workplaces represent the most cost-effective use of limited resources? For example, in the UK approximately 2 million people in any one year believe that they experience ill-health that has been caused or aggravated by work. The little objective scientific study that has been carried out appears consistent with these figures. Most of these people are employed in small industries. Would it not make more sense to allocate resources for education and enforcement for the majority, rather than investing it in presenting poorly targeted prizes to the minority?

Health promotion interventions determined by senior policy makers and filtered down through the ranks might not earn the support of an often suspicious workforce. Indeed patronizing attempts to predicate from on high may alienate a proportion of the workers. Those health promotion exercises that start by informing workers effectively, involving debate and common deliberation, are more likely to achieve their aims.

Case history 10.3

A well-intentioned manager in a large National Health Service hospital decided to introduce a programme of health promotion. A detailed policy was worked out, based on his concept of what the workforce needed, and included action on smoking, healthy eating, exercise and stress management. A committee was then established to set the wheels in motion and implement the policy. This included union representatives. Many members of the committee not only smoked but also considered themselves experts on stress management. The meetings of the committee, taking part against a background of management–union dispute with respect to NHS reorganization and redundancies, became a stage for argument about provision of recreational facilities, time off work for counselling and places for smokers to smoke! Resentment was then expressed that workers had neither been informed nor consulted on fundamental issues such as musculoskeletal ill-health and stress. The project came to an unsatisfactory end when the manager was himself declared redundant.

WORKPLACE NEEDS

As with most of the methods described in this book, a thorough assessment is a crucial first step before embarking on any intervention. Such an approach should avoid many difficulties encountered in the cases described above, and should obtain more positive results as illustrated below.

Case history 10.4

A trained occupational physician was appointed in a part-time capacity for a chemical firm that had previously employed the services of a GP. In the first few sessions many employees walked in quietly, waited to be weighed and then rolled up their shirt sleeves for their yearly blood pressure measurement and blood test. The new physician then discovered that it had been the practice for production workers to have a 'full medical' with a yearly estimation of liver function tests and full blood count.

On an initial site visit by the occupational physician, many respiratory and cutaneous hazards were evident but none for which blood tests would have been required as a form of health surveillance. The occupational physician spoke to workers individually, found out about their jobs, their lifestyles, their general health and their attitudes to it. Most employees welcomed the opportunity to sit down and be listened to. A minority complained to their union representatives and hence to the factory manager that 'the new doctor had stopped the blood tests'. The physician explained the reasoning for abandoning the tests to the factory manager, and asked for the opportunity of participating in safety committee meetings, where he explained the reasons for taking detailed occupational histories, and the limited value of blood tests in that particular context. This was paralleled by regular workplace visits by the physician and by occupational hygiene advice on reducing risks at source.

The workforce and management accepted that the more important work-related risks were now being assessed and accorded the priority that they deserved. The spontaneous consultation rate increased, concerns about health in relation to work or other factors were more openly addressed, both within the clinic and the safety committee, which became better attended by safety representatives and senior managers. On average one new health-related issue was placed on the agenda for each meeting and discussed following a short presentation by the physician. Discussion thereafter was generally fruitful, resulting in an agreed plan of action on both occupational health and lifestyle issues.

Health education is aided by a forum such as a safety committee, which allows employee participation and gives an opportunity for the occupational physician to hear of problems and give advice. Thus it becomes clear that issues raised by workers as individuals or expressed collectively are taken seriously, freely discussed and then progressed as part of an open health promotion strategy. Involvement with workers' representatives should be early and active and not merely an afterthought to help in carrying it through.

Case history 10.5

An employer in a large service organization sought the advice of an occupational physician for the purpose of launching a healthy workplace strategy. The personnel officer tabled various suggestions including changing the balance of food available in the canteen together with appropriate labelling, weight reduction and 'stop smoking' classes, exercise facilities, mammography, cholesterol and cervical screening. The physician reviewed various sources of information and found that the employer was doing very little to facilitate employment of disabled employees or to rehabilitate its own employees when off sick, even when disabled by their work. In fact managers were tending to press for premature ill-health retirement in many cases without attempting to alter the work to rehabilitate the workers. Health surveillance in relation to skin and respiratory hazards of occupation was scanty, while a disproportionately large resource was devoted to initial health assessment of job applicants. Many employees and some managers were very ignorant of the health risks arising from their work or on the means of reducing these risks. First aid provision was less than that required by law. The physician pointed out the contradictions between the professed aim to promote health and the plethora of ideas to modify lifestyle on the one hand, and the many shortcomings that he had found regarding health protection in relation to work.

As these case histories show, before the physician endorsed what had been the common practice, information relevant to health in relation to workplace hazards was sought. The findings led to the conclusion that the employers probably had the wrong priorities. It may be very tempting for health professionals to address a single issue, or a set of health promotion related issues, in isolation when asked to do so. However, they should exert their professional skills and judgement to view the whole picture and to give balanced advice on the basis of this. It should be borne in mind that apart from obvious differences in age and gender between the workforce and the general population there may be important differences in health status and in attitudes to health and safety. Thus because of various selection processes on appointment and during employment, employees may be healthier as a group than age-matched and gender-matched counterparts from the same social and geographical background. Salaried, white collar employment would generally be more likely than waged, blue collar employment to favour recruiting employees with healthier prospects. More hazardous jobs such as construction, especially if without security of tenure, might be more likely to attract employees willing to accept higher risks to their health and safety, and this culture might be reinforced by peer pressure within the workplace. All these factors need to be considered when prioritizing action in relation to groups of workers or individuals.

OPPORTUNISTIC HEALTH PROMOTION

Opportunistic health promotion for the individual employee can be a very powerful instrument despite permeating the workforce slowly. Consider the following case.

Case history 10.6

An accounts clerk presented to the occupational physician complaining of sore feet and wondering whether he had athlete's foot. The physician explained that such complaints would not normally be dealt with in the occupational health department but agreed to examine the feet on the understanding that further management would be undertaken by the GP. The feet were slightly swollen and the webs between the toes macerated. The employee jokingly conceded that he had slept in his shoes and socks. Further enquiry and examination revealed a substantial alcohol intake (of the order of 5 units per day), heavy smoking, symptoms consistent with chronic bronchitis, poor dietary habits, unsatisfactory oral hygiene and moderate obesity.

The physician enquired in detail about the patient's habits but in a non-judgemental way and provided answers to the patient's questions that followed the detailed clinical assessment. The patient then asked for the physician's advice on diet, smoking and rational alcohol consumption. This was provided verbally, backed up by health education literature, target setting and a review appointment with the occupational health nurse. The GP was consulted and agreed to this plan. Over a period of a few months the patient's alcohol consumption fell to about 14 units per week, his weight was restored to normal, he stopped smoking, and resumed attending the dentist. His feet improved with basic personal hygiene and without specific treatment.

While the above approach can only deal with a small proportion of a workforce it has a high chance of succeeding. The employee/patient has spontaneously asked for assessment and advice, which is then objectively provided. The employee knows that the assessment need not be accepted nor the advice necessarily followed, but having presented with this in mind is more likely to follow it. The employee's attitude is positive from the start and is likely to remain so provided a patronizing attitude is not adopted and the option of self-determination remains. Such an attitude can slowly but surely infuse a workforce.

Imparting of knowledge is an important prelude to influencing attitude and hence behaviour. Clearly a collective approach as in Case history 10.4 will reach a large number of people readily but an opportunistic one-to-one approach as in Case history 10.6 is more likely to have longer-lasting benefits for the individual.

SUBSTANCE MISUSE AND ABUSE

Having discussed assessment of the need for health promotion and the different approaches to introducing it, this part of the chapter will deal with some specific issues in more detail. Substance misuse and abuse can have widespread implications for the individual, family, society and the workplace; for example, tobacco smoking can influence the health and safety of fellow workers; alcohol and other substances can impair performance at work and safety in driving or operating machinery. These matters are therefore rarely purely individual lifestyle issues.

Tobacco smoking

Smoking in the workplace is a very important health and safety issue because of its influence on the health of non-smokers as well as smokers, on general well-being, and on fire hazards and transfer of toxic substances to the mouth of the individual. Most smokers are aware that tobacco smoking can seriously harm their health. Many of them would like to stop if they had the opportunity to do so. The working community can be an important peer pressure group, and the right culture and support can help in reducing the prevalence of smoking (although if the culture favours smoking and there is inadequate alternative support, smoking habits are often fostered). Therefore the workplace can be a crucial setting for reducing the scourge of tobacco smoking. Furthermore, there is now good epidemiological evidence of the risks of passive smoking, and debate about this issue in terms of health and safety at work is leading employers increasingly towards non-smoking policies.

Case history 10.7

A bus driver had been employed for several years by a company that permitted smoking on board, long after the epidemiological evidence of the harmful effects of inhaling tobacco smoke was available. He had never smoked and yet he developed cancer of the bronchus. He sued his employer, arguing that his cancer was, more likely than not, caused by his passive inhalation of side-stream tobacco smoke at work. The case was settled out of court by the bus company paying a substantial sum to the driver.

This case history illustrates the dilemma faced by employers when faced by a vociferous group insisting on freedom to smoke and an equally forceful lobby demanding unpolluted air. The recent evidence, accepted increasingly by courts and tribunals, that passive smoking may cause fatal disease now tips the balance firmly in favour of the introduction of non-smoking policies. There is also an increasingly large lobby of individuals with asthma who find that passive exposure to smoke causes worsening of their symptoms. How, therefore, does one reduce tobacco smoking in the workplace? Consider the following example.

Case history 10.8

A health authority had decided that it wished to set an example in relation to health promotion in the workplace. It decreed that as from a specific date, all smoking by staff was prohibited on its premises, and disciplinary proceedings (which could lead to dismissal) would be instituted against any staff member caught flouting the rule. A female domestic assistant who had smoked all her life found that all of a sudden she could not do so. Even most of her official breaks were not long enough for her to change into her outdoor clothing and go and smoke outside the premises. She resigned her job but promptly instituted proceedings alleging constructive dismissal.

What went wrong? Put yourself in the position of employees of different persuasions and analyse the situation. Clearly the smokers felt that they could not accept such a sudden imposition. They neither had the time to come to terms with it nor an alternative smoking zone for their breaks. However, what about the non-smokers? They had not been made adequately aware of the risks of passive smoking and, except for the few who were appreciably upset by their colleagues smoking, were therefore not particularly concerned with, nor necessarily supportive of, the policy. Moreover some of the employees, especially those active in trade unions, felt that in this, as in any other issue directly affecting habits and practice in the workplace, the management should have consulted with the workforce. Lack of consultation was an 'infringement of workers' rights' no matter how apparently worthy the cause was. An organization that wishes to promote health through the reduction or abolition of tobacco smoking in the workplace should therefore do the following:

- encourage and engage in debate on the issue, for example in safety committees
- inform all concerned about the evidence of the risks associated with tobacco smoking
- achieve a consensus between employers and employees on both a time schedule for implementation of the policy and its rules, and also the facilities to be provided to help employees give up smoking
- provide and publicize appropriate stopping smoking groups and clinics, with a balance of professional support and self-help
- give adequate notice of changes – say of the order of 3 months
- provide clearly designated smoking areas for employees who wish to continue smoking, during their breaks, after implementation of the non-smoking rules. In a number of workplaces the designated smoking areas are even outside the building – desirably with some limited degree of shelter and comfort.

Some firms may feel that the above is too complex or difficult to handle without the advice and support of external agencies. Help for firms that wish to implement non-smoking policies is available from a range of public, private and charitable health promotion organizations.

Alcohol abuse

Even more than tobacco smoking, misuse of alcohol or other substances can have implications with respect to work. Thus, it can harm the patient directly, it can increase safety risks for the patient and workmates, and can lead to reduced performance and absenteeism at work. All firms should have a policy in relation to alcohol and other substance abuse and the physician should advise on it.

Case history 10.9

A 55-year-old supervisor was referred for the first time to the occupational physician because she had been abusing alcohol, had become intolerable to work with, and was performing very poorly. Her manager said that her colleagues would no longer carry her and that they had got to the end of the line. He requested that she be retired on the grounds of ill-health or that her employment be terminated on the grounds of incapacity; as far as he and her workmates were concerned they were not ready to accept her back at work. The occupational physician made further enquiries and found that the worker's alcohol problem had been known, and had caused some difficulties at her work, for at least 5 years. Mean red cell corpuscular volume and serum gamma glutamyl transaminase level were both elevated to a level consistent with significant chronic alcohol abuse.

This was a case of too little and too late. The alcohol policy, as well as providing for general education about the health risks of alcohol, should make early intervention the rule. It should guarantee confidentiality for the victim and reassurance that so long as the policy and advice are followed, the firm will allow sickness absence for the problem to be dealt with. Earlier referral to the occupational health department could have permitted the worker to have recognized her problem and curtailed her alcohol consumption sooner, and her colleagues would not have been driven to the limit of their endurance.

The occupational physician said that the referral should have been made years previously and that the function of the occupational health service (OHS) was to assist in rehabilitating workers with alcohol problems. The manager reluctantly agreed to accept the worker back at work after a period of sickness absence during which a rehabilitation and monitoring programme was agreed in conjunction with her and an alcohol counsellor. Unfortunately after her return to work in a supernumerary and monitored capacity her alcohol abuse did not improve. Despite repeated warnings she continued to drink heavily, mainly on her own. She was abusive to her colleagues and customers and tried to deceive and manipulate both the physician and the counsellor. After a final disciplinary hearing she was dismissed.

Case history 10.10

A 47-year-old porter was formally referred to the occupational physician because of his alcohol problem. He had been noted to be late for work and hung over on some mornings, usually after payday or after a weekend off. Sometimes he came back late and smelling of alcohol after lunch breaks. His manager had given him a formal warning but said that he would support him provided he followed professional advice and showed reasonable goodwill and signs of improvement. The physician found that the worker lived alone, his only close relative being his mother; he socialized with a group of friends who drank heavily; he had no understanding of the relative alcohol content of different drinks and measures. Until the formal warning by his manager he had not realized how noticeably poor his performance had become, and he was particularly shaken by the prospect of losing his job. The physician reviewed the alcohol history in detail, at the same time taking the opportunity to explain the alcohol content of various drinks. The porter was given a diary in which to record his alcohol consumption every day and was reviewed at frequent intervals by the physician or nurse. During the counselling he acknowledged the role of peer pressure in fostering his drinking habits and followed the physician's advice to change his circle of friends. This took some time but was eventually achieved. About 9 months after the original referral, the worker, his manager and the physician were in agreement that he no longer had an alcohol-related problem, that he was a valued member of the workforce and that no further follow-up was needed, although, like other workers on that site, he was aware of the availability of the OHS for advice and support at any time should he need it.

Involvement of the workforce directly or through their representatives in development of substance abuse policies is a strong factor in its subsequent success. From the above case histories, it should be clear that in implementing an alcohol policy for the workplace, the following points should be considered.

- An explicit statement should be made that alcohol abuse can be and is a recognized problem in that workplace, but one that the employers and employees are committed to resolve.
- Information and education should be available on the risks associated with alcohol abuse, on their recognition and on rational, safe drinking practices.
- Clear rules should exist on whether, where and when alcohol drinking at work (including breaks) is allowed, and on summary disciplinary rules (e.g. about drink and driving).
- Explicit routes and mechanisms should be clear, including both self-referral and formal management referral of employees who may have an alcohol-related problem, for help by the occupational health department. This has to be accompanied by availability of sickness leave, and of job security. These would continue to apply so long as the individual complied with the specialist advice given.
- Appropriate professional support should be available for counselling employees and, where necessary, following formal referral, giving progress reports to the managers. Depending on the available occupational health staff training, resources and expertise this professional support may vary in its provision between the occupational health department and outside specialists or agencies.
- There should be a forum for monitoring, reviewing and improving the workings of the alcohol policy.
- Training should be available for managers and staff representatives on the implementation of the policy, such as on how to raise the issues, the role of occupational health, the OHS and other agencies, and the importance of confidentiality.

As with other legal aspects of employment, the absence of a policy on a crucial issue such as alcohol could mean that any dismissal in relation to alcohol might automatically be deemed unfair without even necessarily getting as far as judging the merits of the individual case.

Drug abuse

In many respects, the same principles concerning prevention and rehabilitation apply to drug abuse as to alcohol abuse. However, drug abuse can sometimes pose greater difficulty in recognition and management, especially because of the wide diversity of harmful agents and the range of occupational circumstances in which they may present. Moreover, the illegality of much drug-taking adds a special dimension, at least from the point of view of managers.

Case history 10.11

A 26-year-old nurse was referred to the occupational physician because of doubts about her fitness for work. No specific details were identified in the referral letter, although, on enquiry, the physician was told that she concentrated poorly, seemed to forget instructions that she had been given, and was slow in her work. On history taking and physical examination no cause for concern could be found and the physician reassured the nurse and her manager accordingly, but expressed a readiness to review her on request if necessary at a later date. About 9 months later the nurse was suspended from duty having been caught stealing benzodiazepines and other drugs from the ward. During disciplinary hearings it was claimed that she had become dependent on drugs after having been given anxiolytics when she was younger following the death of a parent. Extenuating circumstances were accepted and she did not lose her job. She was eventually rehabilitated in collaboration with a psychiatrist.

This was a near-miss situation in so far as the worker's job and career were concerned, and in the circumstances she was fortunate not to be dismissed or even reported to the police for theft. If the environment had been such as to encourage the worker to have sought help on her own accord, or if the physician had suspected the diagnosis and asked the correct questions, she might not have come within a hair's breadth of damaging her well-being for life through disgraceful dismissal from her job as a nurse. As with smoking and alcohol abuse, the abuse of drugs should be on the workplace agenda for health. Information and counselling should be to hand. However, there are some work circumstances in which possession of certain substances or biological evidence of their consumption constitute automatic grounds for summary dismissal, for example in pilots. In these situations the monitoring and enforcement should not be associated with the function of the OHS, because this could hinder the effectiveness of that service in contributing to health promotion in the workplace.

Case history 10.12

An occupational physician was appointed to a firm that manufactured controlled drugs. The firm had a policy, stipulated in the contract of employment of each worker, that possession of one of those drugs would result in instant dismissal without notice. In order to enforce this, workers could be searched without warning and some white-collar employees were constituted into search teams for either gender. The physician discovered that the nurse had been assigned to a search team although had never been called to participate in one – indeed no search had been carried out within recent memory. The physician advised the factory manager that it was inappropriate for occupational health staff to participate in what was a purely disciplinary and enforcement role, while at the same time attempting to engage in health-promoting activities, including availability for confidential counselling. The manager accepted this and the nurse was removed from the roll of search team members.

Similar considerations to the above would apply in the case of urine testing for drug abuse in conjunction with a disciplinary policy; this is not the responsibility of the occupational physician. The issue of drug testing in the workplace can be a very thorny one, and probably no advice given here could be guaranteed to provide the best answer for all individual circumstances. A useful guide is to work back from the purpose of the screening programme. If the purpose of the programme were to identify workers who were abusing drugs and then to take disciplinary steps such as dismissal, the situation would be analogous to that of a police force breathalysing for alcohol. In other words there is a strong case for this activity to be undertaken by the company as part of its security arrangements, completely independently of the OHS. However, if the company policy is detection of drug abuse, regarding it, like alcohol abuse, as remediable, then the OHS should have an important role to play in facilitating rehabilitation, although disciplinary steps may still be needed if this fails. Where the occupational physician has control over the use of tests that determine the presence of toxic agents or their effects on the body, these tests may have an important role if used in confidence, with the worker's knowledge and informed consent.

STRESS

Perhaps unsurprisingly, 'stress' is a subject that appears as widespread in this book as it is in the workplace. Probably more than any other manifestation of ill-health, it is of multifactorial aetiology with occupational, domestic and constitutional factors being involved to varying degrees. Often it is viewed as a workplace issue that is ripe for health-promoting interventions. It has been defined in a number of ways and the range of stress management techniques is even wider still. Essentially what most people understand by 'stress' is a physiological or psychological response to external stimuli that goes beyond what is accepted as normal. Perhaps 'strain' would have been a better word and an analogy with a rubber band is appropriate. Limited external stresses produce a response, a 'strain', which beyond a certain point becomes disproportionate and beyond the capability of the elastic properties of the subject. In the prevention of stress there are two poles of attitude. The prevailing one is usually to focus on individual behaviour by support and advice, to help in coping with the stress. The second is to alter or reduce the outside stressors so as to reduce the stress. While not dismissing the former, the doctor in industry should concentrate, and focus employers' and employees' attention, on the latter. This is, however, often easier said than done, because of the multifactorial nature of stress and of the relative inflexibility of organizations.

Case history 10.13

A 53-year-old computing officer came to consult the occupational physician after her manager had informally suggested that some form of counselling or stress management advice might help her. The employee was tense, anxious and distressed because she had found progressive difficulty in keeping up with increased work demands. The unit was scheduled to merge with another and she was uncertain of the consequences that this might have on her employment. She had some slight difficulties with vision because of severe myopia and a retinal detachment which had been treated, but this in itself was not a major problem provided she could work at her own pace. Her manager later said that she had become increasingly withdrawn into simple repetitive tasks while allowing a backlog of important requests to accumulate.

The physician expressed the opinion that an adequate and sustained improvement in her well-being would best be achieved by a change in her work plan and responsibilities. This was difficult to arrange but she was eventually given responsibility for the induction training in keyboard skills and basic computer training for new members of staff. This was a fairly circumscribed job with a steady and relatively predictable load, well within her skills, and resulted in continuing useful employment and well-being. A few years later her duties were changed again because of a reorganization and she developed an anxiety neurosis. This, together with some worsening of her vision, prompted premature retirement on grounds of ill-health.

Case history 10.14

A senior manager telephoned the occupational physician and sought a consultation away from their usual workplace. He complained of headache, heartburn, anxiety and tiredness, and of difficulty in falling asleep. He said that he had noticed increased irritability with close colleagues and family, and that his libido had decreased. He had reached the conclusion that his symptoms were stress related. There had been many changes in the organization, including the introduction of productivity targets expected of his unit, and he had to transmit these stresses and expectations to his juniors. This placed him in internal conflict. Together with a number of his peers he was uncertain about the consequences of reorganization, in which it was rumoured that one or more of them would be made redundant. Physical examination was normal. Further discussion permitted him to identify various occupational stressors, over which unfortunately neither he nor the physician could exercise significant influence, especially as he did not wish any other people to become involved.

The physician's reassurance that the symptoms were not an indication of some other underlying pathology provided some relief. The value of coping strategies such as allocating specific time and place for work and domestic activities was discussed and the physician provided him with further written information relating to other sources of advice.

The above cases illustrate some of the common occupational stressors that may affect even the most senior employees in an organization. Sometimes individual employees are reluctant for their particular issues to be taken up by the physician in a way in which they might be identified and possibly labelled as 'not coping'. However, the physician can progressively build up a picture of the health of the organization after seeing a number of workers with common problems. Retrospective review of the case records of the other employees from the same workplace might identify others with similar mental symptoms, and sickness absence patterns may be worse than the norm. On the next workplace visit the physician could probe the organizational structure, bearing in mind the important determinants of stress illustrated in Figure 10.1.

Diplomacy and communication skills are then invaluable and essential tools. The physician should suggest to the senior manager that sickness absence and problems with performance generally might yet worsen. A responsible and open-minded manager should be willing to explore the organizational determinants of stress and try hard to remedy them. Such an approach is more likely to result in lasting benefit to the workers and the organization than the hiring of a stress consultant to lecture on individual coping strategies.

One model sometimes used as a means of controlling workplace stress is the control cycle model, which addresses the problem in terms of four stages:

1. accept that many employees are experiencing problems of stress at work
2. identify the stressors, the extent to which people are exposed to them, and their potential harm to health
3. design and implement reasonable and practicable stress intervention/control measures
4. monitor and evaluate these interventions, reappraise the whole process and begin again.

Different people vary in their responses to outside factors, be they psychological or otherwise, and therefore exhibit different degrees of vulnerability. As stated in Chapters 5 and 6, the role of the physician in relation to the workplace is to help

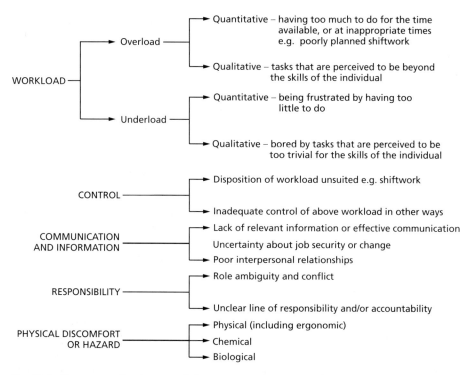

Fig. 10.1 *Some occupational causes of stress.*

ensure its safety, as far as is reasonably practicable. However, many difficulties present themselves. Thus with agents such as noise and respirable dust, it is generally the case that the more there is, the worse it is for everybody, while on the other hand, psychological stressors may affect different people in opposing ways. For example, tasks such as in information technology, which require a specific but limited degree of skill and knowledge, might be stressful to an employee who is set in their ways and habits and is finding difficulty with coping. It could also become stressful to a keener, motivated employee who easily masters the skills, but for an opposite reason, in that this individual may become frustrated at not being able to progress and use his or her initiative and control over the programmes being dealt with. Although Figure 10.1 has listed a range of occupational stressors, the reader should also consider causes of stress that are not included there. Thus unemployment is a very important direct cause of stress, while indirectly the fear of losing one's job is a similarly serious stressor. Moreover, physical ill-health, family and other social problems, especially lack of support, can add to occupational factors in provoking or exacerbating stress reactions.

DIET, WEIGHT REDUCTION AND EXERCISE

There is good epidemiological evidence that diet is an important determinant of health. Some characteristics of the Western diet appear to be associated with an increased risk of coronary heart disease and cancer of the large bowel and probably other diseases such as asthma and diabetes. However, there is still some scientific debate on issues such as recommending an increase in the proportion of polyunsaturated fats in the diet. In general, it would be appropriate for the occupational physician to offer the following advice:

- reduce the total fat and oil in the diet with particular reduction of animal fats (in meat or in dairy products) with a relative preference to vegetable oils and fish oils
- encourage high fibre plant foods such as beans, other vegetables and fruit
- maintain an adequate intake of protein of vegetable and animal origin (but relying on fish, lean meat and low fat dairy products)
- reduce overall intake of high energy foods, especially reducing intake of refined carbohydrates and alcohol.

Obesity is associated with an increased risk of some diseases, notably coronary heart disease, although there is probably not a direct causal link between the two. Moreover, in individuals suffering from back pain and other musculoskeletal complaints or other conditions affecting exercise tolerance such as certain heart and lung diseases, reduction of weight to the normal range can bring about a welcome improvement in symptoms.

Appropriate exercise undoubtedly improves well-being and increases the cardiovascular, respiratory and muscular limits of tolerance to further activity. There is increasing evidence that appropriate exercise may reduce morbidity or mortality from, say, coronary heart disease. Generally speaking, graded isotonic (kinetic) exertion is a preferable activity because it does not impose a sudden strain on the musculoskeletal or cardiovascular system. The redesign of jobs and work practices, discussed for example in Chapter 6, in order to reduce cumulative or acute musculoskeletal injury can complement exercise programmes by providing work that is safer, involves less load but more appropriate movement in manual handling. While some workplaces do provide exercise facilities on site, and these are to be welcomed, they should come low down on the list of priorities after all reasonably practicable means have been employed to make the workplace safe. In promoting health through altering lifestyle factors such as exercise, diet and hence body weight there is always the prospect of ending up preaching to the converted. However, as with 'stop smoking' campaigns, workers in peer groups can help each other attain common goals.

In relation to exercise, these goals have to be set in a manner that is consistent and integrated with workplace issues; for example, policies should be in place to encourage employees to walk, cycle or at least use buses, trams or trains to travel to work, and not merely sidetrack these issues and provide staff with access to exercise facilities. Correspondingly, for staff who have a sedentary job, a better approach to improve well-being and perhaps even productivity might be to allocate frequent short breaks during the day rather than to engage in 1 or 2 hours of vigorous 'workout' at the end. Nevertheless, as exemplified by Case histories 10.5 and 10.6, a campaign approach should be paralleled by an opportunistic individual approach, in parallel with other health improving measures, notably health protection at work.

SCREENING FOR NON-OCCUPATIONAL DISEASE

'Screening' for non-occupational disease is an important subject that should prompt various questions such as:

- screening for what?
- why?
- at what cost?
- who?
- what can be done if the result is positive?

Unfortunately 'screening' can become a bandwagon with a momentum of its own regardless of whether the essential criteria for scientific validity have been fulfilled. This is particularly true for diseases that are emotive or common, like cancer (e.g. breast, cervix) and coronary heart disease.

Case history 10.15

A 50-year-old security officer presented himself to the occupational health department asking whether a 'cholesterol test' might be on offer. He did not have any cardiac or vascular symptoms, although he complained of 'heartburn' which was relieved by antacid tablets. His father had died at the age of 64 years from pneumonia against a background of chronic lung disease, while his 75-year-old mother was alive and well with no history of cardiac disease. He had smoked at least 15 cigarettes a day since his early twenties and drank an average of 10 pints of beer per week. He was normotensive and not overweight, and the rest of his physical examination was normal. The relevance of various lifestyle risk factors in general and particularly with regard to his lifestyle was explained by the occupational physician. He accepted that his smoking history presented a higher risk than that which might be related to blood cholesterol level alone. Cholesterol measurement was not pursued as a first line but he resolved to attempt to stop smoking, to ensure his alcohol drinking remained under control, and to engage in regular exercise. He succeeded in reducing his smoking considerably, although not in stopping altogether. Having done so he was encouraged to see his GP for further review.

Employees who seek advice about screening tests believe that these are proven markers for health risks and that, implicitly, knowledge of these may help reduce their risks. The health professional should listen to the employee and seek to understand the motivation behind the request, and then proceed to assess all the health risks and place them in a logical order of priority. This should be followed by advice about reducing risks that are well recognized and which are important for the individual, before dealing with those that are speculative. Thus for instance, in Case history 10.15, the issue raised initially was that of cholesterol screening, while the first logical step should have been to stop smoking.

Anxiety resulting from false or misleading positive results, and adverse effects of the management which may follow, are sometimes inadequately catered for when balancing the risks and benefits of screening.

Case history 10.16

A 32-year-old executive was found to have positive dipstick screening test for haemoglobin in his urine in the course of a routine medical examination in industry. A repeat test was also positive and he was referred back to his GP with a letter indicating the results of this. A further urine test carried out by the GP was followed by a referral to a urologist, intravenous nephropyelography and cystoscopy. He was told very little about the purpose and the results of these tests. Besides the physical discomfort, he and his wife were very anxious about the proceedings and the implications. Eventually he was told that no abnormality had been found and he remained physically well although with the anxiety that he might have had something that had been missed.

So-called 'executive medicals' are widely practised in some sectors of industry. They probably do not constitute a cost-effective way of promoting health at work, and one wonders whether they are more of a status symbol whereby the recipient can demonstrate to colleagues how highly he or she is prized by the organization. They may be viewed as an extra 'perk' of the job, while occupational physicians widely justify them in terms of allowing unhindered access to the boss's ear!

Various reports, mainly from North American companies, have suggested that initiatives to improve lifestyle coupled with health screening appear to reduce the medical bills for which the firms are responsible. However, there are hardly any well-designed and executed scientific studies that have measured their effectiveness in the workplace in terms of either improved health or improved productivity.

CONCLUSION

In conclusion, employers must be expected first and foremost to take all reasonably practicable steps to avoid harming the health of their workforce. Insofar as the risks from work are concerned, there is a legal and moral obligation to do so, which also makes economic sense. Health promotion has an important role to play in the workplace, but it should be based on a thorough needs assessment that is targeted and specific, so as to avoid providing attractive but expensive wallpaper for the few, rather than the sorely needed bricks and mortar for the majority. It may be economically reasonable, as well as of benefit to the community as a whole, to aim to reduce general health risks, once the primary work-related objectives have been met. Regrettably, all too often firms embark on screening programmes that bear no relation to the prevention of work-related ill-health, and neglect simple and obvious means of assessing and controlling serious health risks from occupational hazards in their workplace.

11

Quality and good practice in occupational medicine

SUMMARY

- The delivery of quality in occupational medicine requires essential skills from the physician for the purposes of recognizing, managing and preventing work-related ill-health. However, complementary skills are also required, including the capacity to assess the occupational health needs of the workforce, to solve relevant problems and to communicate effectively at all levels. Moreover the occupational physician should deliver a service built on a sound and timely evidence base, in an ethical manner.

- Good practice in occupational medicine is primarily a responsibility of the individual physician. However, it is difficult for this to succeed in isolation. It should be reflected in equally good practice within the occupational health service. Likewise the management of the workplace and the attitude of the workers and of society at large are an essential context within which good occupational health practice should flourish.

- At all levels, audit and other methods of evaluation and assurance of structure, process and outcome are essential to achieve and maintain high standards of occupational medicine practice, of occupational health service delivery and hence of the health of the workforce.

INTRODUCTION – WHAT IS MEANT BY QUALITY IN OCCUPATIONAL MEDICINE?

First we need to consider what is meant by 'quality in occupational medicine'. Case histories may help to illustrate how perceptions of quality vary, and how some of these may be misconceived, both by 'experts' and by the workers and employers (or 'clients' as they are often termed nowadays).

The first case history illustrates the different perceptions of quality assurance experts and of occupational physicians.

Case history 11.1

An occupational health service (OHS) had its quality assessed by two groups of external reviewers for different purposes. The first was as part of a quality assurance exercise involving most of the company, and the second was by two occupational physicians assessing the service for the purposes of training specialists in occupational medicine. For the first purpose, the OHS was initially prepared for certification by employing experts to advise on the quality management systems that should be in place. Then it was formally audited externally for the purpose of ISO 9000 certification. This was successful and the OHS was awarded a 'Quality Assured' certificate, which was proudly displayed and which was used to impress prospective 'clients'. Subsequently the OHS was subject to the 'peer review' by occupational physicians appointed as assessors to determine whether a particular position within the OHS was suitable and could be approved for the purposes of higher specialist training of occupational physicians. Both assessments were wide ranging in different ways. However, by way of example of the issues raised, this case history will focus on one aspect of many: health surveillance for respiratory sensitizers (because this was an acknowledged risk for some categories of workers looked after by the OHS).

In the first assessment, the ISO 9000 auditors had been satisfied that the quality systems were present and 'assured' but at the subsequent visit, the specialist occupational medicine assessors had serious reservations.

What were the reasons for this? Was it that some assessors were 'doves' and others were 'hawks', or were they looking for different things? In other words, were there different perceptions of quality, and if so which were appropriate?

The ISO 9000 'Quality Assurance' lay assessors had determined that there were systems to ensure that employees on the list deemed to warrant health surveillance were called for health surveillance at the right time, and that measures were in place to ensure that none were missed out. They were also satisfied that the regimen was in place for servicing and recalibrating the spirometer as recommended by the manufacturer and that certificates of servicing of the equipment by an external agency were available for inspection. Even the height scale was regularly recalibrated and certified 'in case wear and tear of the carpet resulted in an inaccuracy in measuring height, and hence in calculating predicted lung function and in the interpretation of the observed lung function'. On the other hand the specialist occupational medicine assessors were concerned as to whether there was an appropriate and effective policy to assess and to control exposure at source, and asked what criteria were used to determine which categories of employees needed health surveillance, and whether maintenance workers, casual labourers or outside contractors might have been missed. Bearing in mind that an appropriate questionnaire is a more sensitive means of detecting occupational asthma than periodic spirometry, they were somewhat disappointed to find that a validated questionnaire was not in use, but merely a form with very limited headings for recording 'history, physical signs, lung function tests, conclusion, doctor's signature and date'. Therefore, by their criteria this would not have been an ideal environment in which to train a medical specialist.

Which interpretation of 'quality' would you consider the most relevant for the purposes of respiratory health surveillance? Do you think occupational asthma is more likely to be missed or misdiagnosed if suitable sensitive and specific questions are not asked, or if the height scale on the wall misreads by a couple of millimetres? Clearly the perception of the lay auditors had not necessarily been consistent with the best practice of occupational medicine. They had audited that which they understood and which they could audit (calibration and maintenance of machines) but not the right thing which mattered – a sensitive health surveillance strategy and technique. This is not to state that the quality assurance experts had got it all wrong – ensuring that all targeted employees are assessed and assessed promptly was certainly a laudable part of the quality management system. However, they had misinterpreted what all the right things were. Thus, although they ensured that what was being done complied with what was stated in the policy, they did not address whether the policy itself was right. To establish 'the right things' in the practice of occupational medicine, it is essential to review the needs, the evidence base for fulfilling these, and thence to establish a policy and guidelines designed to achieve a high standard of practice.

> Workers and their employers may also have misconceptions as to the purposes, needs for and quality of services provided by occupational physicians. Thus in the workplace described in Case history 10.4 in the preceding chapter the once-yearly 'medical examination' and full blood counts and liver function tests had been unquestionably perceived and accepted by workers and their managers as the best practice. The reassessment of the needs and hence of the service provision of this company is a good example of the decision making that is essential to achieve maximum effectiveness and efficiency in the delivery of occupational health.

Perhaps one could argue that the employers and employees were not best informed nor necessarily well placed to determine 'quality' or 'good practice' in occupational medicine, at least without some guidance in translating their implicit expectations and demands into justifiable needs. On the other hand, perhaps the occupational physicians concerned should have communicated better. The assessment of needs, effective communication and evaluating quality will be expounded further in the rest of this chapter.

ASSESSING NEEDS FOR OCCUPATIONAL HEALTH SERVICES

Assessment of needs for OHS delivery is one of the first steps that a physician in industry should undertake when starting a new employment. The subject is only covered in outline here, but by way of example, Case history 10.4 will be pursued further.

Case history 10.4 (continued, see page 256)

> As has been discussed earlier, there clearly was redundancy in the universal yearly non-specific medical exams undertaken by this chemical manufacturing firm. In addition to the part-time general practitioner (GP), it employed a full-time occupational health nurse and a safety officer. A small number of the employees were trained as general first aiders. Finally, glaring gaps were evident in the capacity to assess and advise on the control of occupational and general environmental exposure. The part-time GP was replaced by a part-time trained occupational physician. The nurse was retained on a part-time basis but first aiders were given additional training specific to the hazards of the jobs undertaken in the workplace. Steps were taken to train from within the staff and/or recruit staff members to fulfil the func-

tions of an occupational hygienist and of an environmental analytical technician. The blanket provision for blood tests on process workers was stopped and replaced by targeted health surveillance – for example measurement of cholinesterase activity in those process workers exposed to anticholinesterases, respiratory health surveillance for those exposed to respiratory sensitizers, and so on.

Although this is but one example, the principles can be applied to a wide range of workplaces. For example a large retailing company might feel it necessary to employ an ergonomist to assess and advise on the reduction of risks from handling of goods, operation of checkouts, etc. Trained occupational health nurses might then conduct the bulk of the OHS work.

In delivering an OHS to a workplace or group of workplaces, a number of sequential steps are essential. These are summarized in Table 11.1 (and most are amply described in previous chapters).

Table 11.1 *Essential steps in delivering an occupational health service*

Determine the demography of the workforce (age, gender, education and social background)
Assess the work-related health risks
Determine the needs to prevent ill-health and to promote health
Determine the needs to recognize significant exposure or work-related ill-health
Determine the needs to manage ill-health, and to rehabilitate workers (whether because of occupational ill-health or not)
Consider the options to fulfil the above needs by way of structures (including staffing, training, facilities and policies) and processes (preventive, clinical, managerial, educational) to fulfil these needs
Discuss, select and agree the best option.
Implement the chosen option for service delivery
Audit:
  (1) structure
  (2) process
  (3) outcome
Continue improvement on the basis of the above

However, even if occupational physicians and other OHS staff do their level best, success is only assured if all stakeholders ranging from employees to employers, healthcare workers in different spheres, politicians and other policy formers pull in the same direction. Thus the prime responsibility for delivering a healthy workplace must lie primarily with the employer. This should involve the partnership of the employees, and be underpinned by good professional advice in the relevant disciplines of occupational health and safety. In other words, an outstandingly good occupational health team in an organization where health and safety is not a high priority will have as much influence on occupational disease or injury as an excellent hospital would have on cardiac or respiratory disease in a society with a high prevalence of smoking.

DIFFERENT MODELS FOR OCCUPATIONAL HEALTH SERVICE DELIVERY

In practice, even though companies may have objectively identical needs, these are not always translated into identical provision of services, policies and processes. The context is therefore often determined by political, social or cultural factors beyond the physician's control. A variety of models for occupational health delivery exist in different countries or even within the same state. In some there is emphasis on multiple routine examinations or surveillance, while in others the approach is much more targeted. In certain countries, 'occupational health services' offer facilities in common with those offered in primary medical care or general medical practice elsewhere. Thus there are historical, cultural, national or legal reasons or other precedents that strongly influence the process; for example, a firm in France might engage a physician to conduct medical examinations routinely on all the employees, whereas the same firm in the UK might adopt a more targeted and limited approach; a firm in the Netherlands might employ an occupational physician solely to deal with matters of the influence of work on health or health on work, whereas in the same firm in Finland a physician might also undertake the role of a general medical practitioner.

Although it is not easy to classify methods of delivery of occupational health into rigid categories, it is possible to indicate some special features which may characterize the mode of delivery:

- a 'holistic' model; especially exemplified in Finland where 'occupational health' is very much an industry-based service providing a full range of primary healthcare functions, such as general medical practice, physiotherapy, etc.
- an inspectorate/prescribed regulation type of service characterized, for example, by the French system whereby rigid medical examinations and other assessments are explicitly laid down in detail
- a consultancy/advisory type system exemplified by the Netherlands where companies seek advice on specific issues ranging from occupational hygiene through to sickness absence management.

There are two main dimensions along which such an OHS can develop and deliver. They both need to be undertaken – in an ideal world simultaneously, but resources might dictate that one starts before the other.

1. The service can emulate the classical pattern of healthcare delivery, that is, starting with individuals who perceive they have problems, and who are then assessed and managed competently. This will need to be underpinned by adequate provision of information, and confidence building. An individual's assessment would be pursued in a number of ways. Initially there would be intervention for secondary protection of the individual, and their rehabilitation. This would be followed by intervention to reduce the risks to colleagues in the workplace. Thence, as a continuation of the 'ripple', there will be positive implications for the employer, the community as a whole, other workplaces within the same sector and so on.
2. The second pole of approach involves a systematic workplace-based needs assessment followed by appropriate delivery. Needs assessment should first be directed at a community level to determine priorities such as small and medium enterprises, or a particular sector of employment. Once the overall priorities are set, the workplaces in question would require an individual specific needs assessment to determine what advice or intervention is specifically suited out of the overall package that was made available.

These two poles are both essential and complementary.

Thus dealing with individuals can serve as a useful way of identifying sentinel cases to indicate that particular sectors or workplaces have problems. Correspondingly, a needs assessment that addresses a workplace as a whole, and that intervenes without a 'victim-based' approach will build confidence and will catalyse the presentation of individual problems.

A further layer of complexity is added by the range and detail of functions carried out by different occupational health and safety professionals. These may vary between countries and also between individuals in the same professional discipline. These differences may be reflected in job title but are often less overt; for example, in one context functions that might be undertaken by an 'occupational hygienist' or by an 'ergonomist' might as well be undertaken by a 'safety engineer'.

The service would have to be competent in its capacity both to advise in terms of ascertaining and managing cases of ill-health, and in their prevention. It must provide an easy and equitable access. It must integrate all the important stakeholders, contributors and beneficiaries in the context of health and work. It must also be integrated with the extant provision of healthcare generally.

In any case, however the OHS team is constituted, or however the service is provided, a cardinal feature of a good occupational health professional or a good OHS is the capacity to recognize and 'diagnose' organizational dysfunction; this has to go beyond merely recognizing that there is a problem and extend to ranking the determinants of the problem. These can range from an organizational/management structure, the personality of some people in authority, or a vicious cycle of a self-perpetuating negative culture – which is probably the most difficult to 'treat'.

In general, especially within the European Union, the trend is to strike a balance between supranational regulation and national enforcement on the one hand, and a free-market based OHS delivery on the other hand. Companies may choose to engage outside advice and assistance even when they have their own 'in-house' occupational health professionals. Outsiders may bring in a breath of fresh air and offer a perspective that is perhaps less blinkered or they may have particular skills. Sometimes, however, companies recruit outside agencies in order to be seen to be undertaking a discreet intervention, regardless of whether it is necessarily important or effective, and only as long as it does not generate embarrassing ripples in other areas.

Various models of fulfilling OHS needs of the community are being tested, as exemplified below.

Case history 11.2

Within a number of general medical practices in a city, a number of healthcare workers were aware of patients frequently presenting with apparently work-related ill-health. The need for more active investigation of these patients and understanding of their problems was recognized. However, there were clear limitations on the time and skills of the primary healthcare team. Therefore an occupational health project was set up in which primary healthcare workers with training and experience in occupational ill-health took occupational histories from patients, and provided relevant advice to them and to the GPs, as an adjunct to the services provided by the primary healthcare team.

By way of comment on this example, one clearly welcomes attempts to help to collect good detailed occupational history as described in Chapter 1, and to take steps to assess and review workers' risks as described in subsequent chapters. All measures to improve their awareness and that of managers of occupational ill-health in primary care, or in hospital practice, are clearly assets to the community. This extension of medical practice can work both ways; for example, in some countries or contexts the OHS provides primary medical general care. This is not the case in the UK system but as mentioned earlier does occur in other countries, such as in Finland, or amongst medical services provided by expatriates of major companies working abroad, usually in the developing world. Moreover, as illustrated in Chapter 10, in some cases the OHS is assuming a greater role in the prevention of, or screening for, an occupational disease. However, it is essential to ensure that the steps to widen the provision of healthcare and offer the best quality service and extensive choice do not result in a paradoxical situation. It would be ironic and regrettable if the OHS shifted its focus to dealing with ill-health that is not specific to occupation, at the expense of the primary role of preventing, or otherwise managing work-related disease; while at the same time this burden is shifted to the health service in the general community, which can at best 'pick up the pieces' for the unfortunate individuals, while not usually being in a position to prevent ill-health in the wider workforce.

PROBLEM-SOLVING SKILLS AND EVIDENCE-BASED OCCUPATIONAL MEDICINE

So far this chapter has outlined needs assessment and delivery at the overall strategic level, that is, the needs of the organization and its workforce. The next layer at the operational tactical level lies in developing evidence-based policies. Thus to remain with respiratory health, the same example as in Case history 11.1, it is clear that to achieve quality in occupational medicine, the first step has to be to determine the question(s) that need(s) to be answered. This is followed by a search for the information through a review of the evidence, and thence determining the best way forward. Thus in the context of respiratory sensitization, relevant questions in the order in which they are commonly posed might be:

- how do we prevent sensitization?
- can we prevent it by worker selection, or in other ways?
- how do we detect sensitization?

While space does not permit a detailed scientific review of the relevant evidence on this particular subject, Table 11.2 exemplifies a possible summary of evidence and the respective derived guidelines.

A further example of the application of an evidence base to the practice of occupational medicine is illustrated in the next example.

Case history 11.3

A review of outstanding sickness absence cases in a small healthcare establishment showed that many employees were off for prolonged periods complaining of back pain. Many were being advised by their GP to rest, others were awaiting further investigation or physiotherapy or until they were pain free before returning to work. The occupational physicians acknowledged divergences in practice between themselves as well. They needed answers to explicit questions, especially regarding the assessment of cases and the degree of bed rest or of mobilization that was indicated. They resolved to follow the principles of evidence-based medicine (Sackett *et al.* 2005). The patients (and problems) were clearly identified as workers complaining of back pain. The main interventions that needed to be

Table 11.2 *An illustration of how an evidence base can lead to derived practice guidelines*

Scientific evidence base	Derived practice guideline to ensure quality
The degree of exposure to sensitizers is a very important determinant of the risk of adverse health effects	Systematic hazard identification is needed together with steps to substitute sensitizers, e.g. latex antigen, and in any case measures to reduce personal exposure
Atopy *per se* has a poor predictive value in relation to pre-employment assessment	Applicants for jobs exposed to respiratory sensitizers should not be excluded on the basis of atopy alone
Defined questions on respiratory symptoms, e.g. wheeze and dyspnoea, improving when off work are a sensitive way of identifying occupational asthma	The first line of health surveillance of employees with significant exposure, e.g. to glutaraldehyde, should consist of a questionnaire with the appropriate items administered at intervals e.g. 6-monthly, and then yearly thereafter
Specificity of diagnosis can be achieved through means such as lung function tests before and after exposure	Positive respondents to the questionnaire should be followed up by work-exposure-related lung function tests, workplace reassessment and advice

compared were abstention from work (with or without bed rest), and early return to work. The intended outcome was a successful return to work and rehabilitation. A literature search suggested that the task (in terms of the quantity of relevant publications) was huge, although the quality and relevance of many of the papers was poor. Fortunately help was at hand because the topic was being reviewed by an expert group (Carter and Birrell 2000). One of the most important evidence-based recommendations was that 'Advice to continue ordinary activities of daily living as normally as possible despite the pain can give equivalent or faster symptomatic recovery from the acute symptoms, and leads to shorter periods of work loss, fewer recurrences and less work loss over the following year than "traditional" medical treatment (advice to rest and "let pain be your guide" for return to normal activity).' This was implemented as OHS policy and communicated to workers, their GPs and employers, resulting in a reduction in sickness absence.

There were other corollaries to this exercise; for example, better criteria were used to assess cases of back pain for the purposes of conducting diagnostic 'triage' and for assessing psychosocial risk factors. Moreover, having endorsed the evidence-based guidelines, these were later adapted to audit the observed practice through a peer review method as discussed later in this chapter.

COMMUNICATION

The doctor in industry needs to develop special skills in communication, probably even wider than those of the average medical practitioner. Skills at assessing workplace health risks, clinical acumen with patients and advice on management of problems are only of limited value if the doctor cannot 'get the message across'. The role of the physician may include communicating an assessment of, for example, a health effect as a consequence of work to a semi-literate unskilled worker, to a medical colleague (usually the GP) or to a professional manager. Although the underlying principle to be communicated may be the same, the detail of the content and the language used may vary. It is essential for the physician to be familiar with the language used by the employees and employers in describing their tasks, their raw materials and their products. There is no substitute for frequent workplace visits to achieve this two-way communication, although reading of relevant literature such as chemistry textbooks or process handbooks may help.

Case history 11.4

On commencing a new job in a manufacturing company, a physician was invited to lunch with the seven senior managers in their private dining room, adjoining but separate from the main canteen. He accepted and the meal was a useful way of introducing himself and of understanding their jobs. He was told that he was welcome to lunch with them every day when he was on site. However, he resolved instead to have lunch in the canteen on most days, either with the nurse or the safety officer or other staff. This meant that he learnt much more about the workers' jobs and concerns and could communicate with them better. Perhaps more importantly he could in an unspoken way reinforce the message of impartiality and confidentiality by not conveying the impression of being 'in the bosses' pockets' but of associating with all members of staff in a proportionate manner.

Although in the first instance many communications are verbal, there are many circumstances where the written word is essential. Thus, formal referrals from a manager to assess a worker should include an explicit written statement of the problem as perceived by the manager, the evidence for it, and the advice required from the physician. Principles such as this have been discussed in more detail in earlier chapters but are worth reinforcing. Another circumstance when written explicit advice is certainly warranted arises when a physician has evidence of a significant health risk as a consequence of work. The observations leading to this conclusion and specific remedial advice should be stated. If management procrastinates or prevaricates unduly in the face of a substantial risk, words to the effect that, in the physician's judgment, the risk warrants alerting the enforcement agency concerned and the firm's insurers can result in a flurry of activity where all else has failed. These trump cards should, however, be used judiciously because perseverance and persuasion are usually preferable tools.

Main channels and content of communication

The doctor in industry should make it clear from the time of his appointment that all employees as individuals have direct access to him (often through the medium of the occupational health nurse) and that he is available for confidential consultations. Communication with appropriate managers is important. Thus a physician who has access to the factory manager is more likely to influence a change for the better in working conditions for the employees than one who is relegated to communicating with a junior member of the personnel department. Where the quality of line management is good and effective, it is probably better to liaise with the appropriate manager, rather than the personnel officer, about working conditions in his department or the problems of an individual worker.

An increasing proportion of occupational physicians have a policy of providing the worker automatically with copies of their advice to the employer, while any letters of referral from the employer are correspondingly copied to the worker. In any case the physician should always confirm with the worker the reason for the referral and explain what questions are being posed and what advice will be given in response. By way of recapitulation, many or all of the following elements should feature in the information provided by the occupational physician to the employee after making a clinical assessment:

- the nature of the clinical problem (if there is one) and the occupational implications – in so far as attendance, safety, performance and fitness are concerned
- important causative or contributory factors
- the likely severity and duration of the above
- what steps should be taken by the worker and the employer, as appropriate, to reduce the adverse consequences
- how certain the physician is of this advice
- what the physician will be saying, why and to whom
- any other reasonable advice or information that the worker requests, either spontaneously or in response to an invitation from the physician.

Communication with the general practitioner

In the majority of cases in which an employee asks or is referred to consult with the occupational physician, there is no need for the GP to be consulted in advance. Some guidelines may be offered to exceptions to this. Thus, for example, if a worker has been off sick for a prolonged period and the GP's sickness certificates suggest a serious organic or mental illness that may affect the worker's physical or emotional fitness to come and be seen, then the two doctors should probably liaise first. Once the occupational physician has seen a worker in consultation, there are circumstances when advice to, or other communication with, the GP is usually warranted with the worker's consent. These **include** situations where the occupational physician's assessment and plan:

- have important implications for the worker's employment, such as a recommendation for retirement on grounds of ill-health
- require cooperation with the GP, for example, for the purposes of organizing a guided rehabilitation to work, or referral to another specialist or agency
- require further information that the worker might not be able to relate reliably, such as the result of relevant investigations, drug history, severity of past psychiatric illness
- could result in education or information for the GP relevant to the management of that worker/patient or to other workers, such as by identifying risks to health from work or circumstances in which recurrent problems may be expected.

Communication with the Safety Committee and others

An important forum for the doctor in industry to communicate with both employers and employees is the Safety Committee, or other equivalent body. In the United

Kingdom, the provision of a Safety Committee had been an explicit consequence of the Health and Safety, etc. at Work Act (1974) and the relevant guidelines also stated that the occupational physician should be an *ex officio* member. Unfortunately, many Safety Committees are anodyne and effete bodies, in which employers are represented by a junior member of management and employees by shop stewards, or union apprentices aspiring to this and with little training in health and safety matters. Nevertheless, the active contribution of an enthusiastic doctor can considerably improve the value of the Safety Committee, and its contribution to the health and safety of employees.

The physician's role on the Safety Committee should be that of an independent expert witness, not a representative of either party nor a chairman, adjudicator or arbitrator. It is up to the employer's and employees' representatives to reach agreement on how to control the risks to health from work. The physician's contribution should include formal reporting to the committee on relevant health problems within the workplace, summary accounts of the results of health surveillance of groups of workers, and responding to requests for specific advice from the committee. The doctor should advise the committee and assist it in its interpretation of current or proposed legislation (such as European Community proposals for directives). Important or controversial articles in the scientific or lay press that may be relevant to the firm in question should be explained to the committee. It may also be appropriate for the occupational physician to present a regular, perhaps yearly or 6-monthly, report of activities, plans and targets to the committee, highlighting the major, strategic issues rather than being drawn on trivial items like the siting of hand washbasins or fire extinguishers!

In summary, active contribution to the Safety Committee without fear or favour is an essential part of the responsibilities of the doctor in industry. Physicians who do not undertake this and who allow themselves merely to be summoned to attend Safety Committee meetings only at management's behest in order 'to reassure the workers' end up being treated by the workforce at best with misgivings and at worst with suspicion and contempt.

Finally, a physician who works for a large firm or one with the potential for special and serious risks to the health of its employees should make the effort of establishing links with the Health and Safety Executive, or other enforcement organization, relevant services and specialists at the local hospital and local GPs.

ETHICS

The professional and ethical responsibilities of the doctor in industry to the individual worker, especially with regard to confidentiality, consent and the duty of care are essentially no less than those applicable to other physicians. However, the doctor's duties to all employees within the workforce also entail a responsibility to give essential advice on fitness, safety and related health risks to the employer, and care must be taken to observe appropriate ethical principles in so doing. Particular attention should be paid to communication between the workplace doctor, professional colleagues and managers and employees. Thus the independent and politically neutral stance of the OHS should be understood by all and its role in providing a healthy and safe workplace facilitated. The booklet of the Faculty of Occupational Medicine (of the Royal College of Physicians of London) entitled *Guidance On Ethics For Occupational*

Physicians (sixth edition in preparation) is essential reading. The main tenet, namely that the physician's prime concern is the health of the patient, who is here defined as the employee for whom the doctor has responsibility, is paramount in occupational medicine.

Confidentiality and consent

The physician is normally bound to keep in confidence all that is disclosed in the course of his relationship with the patient. However, there may be rare exceptional circumstances, in occupational medicine as in other specialties, where this obligation is not absolute but after careful thought may have to be limited. The terms of consent that apply to a consultation between an employee and an occupational physician should be explicit. When an employee is referred by the employer to the occupational physician, the latter should confirm these terms along with the purpose and plan of the consultation. Thus, it should be pointed out that the employer will be advised impartially on matters of fitness to attend work, to perform it satisfactorily and safely, and on the risks to health from work. All other matters remain in confidence between the physician and the employee.

Case history 11.5

A worker whose job entailed driving goods within and between various sites of a firm was referred to the occupational physician on account of repeated multiple short absences, usually attributed to abdominal pain, dyspepsia, diarrhoea and vomiting. The worker's breath smelt of alcohol and after close questioning by the physician, it transpired that he had a serious alcohol problem and, not infrequently, drove at work while still under the influence of drink. He did not wish the physician to disclose this fact or the implications of it to his manager. The physician explained that his responsibility to the worker and his colleagues required him to advise the manager 'that the worker is temporarily unfit to drive for medical reasons. This unfitness is not necessarily permanent but will be reviewed after 4 weeks. He remains fit to carry out other portering duties.' The cause of this unfitness was not disclosed to the manager. A programme of alcohol counselling was commenced and after a further two reviews the physician advised the manager that the worker could resume vocational driving.

This example illustrates a common ethical problem in industry where an individual's abuse of alcohol can endanger himself and others. Many companies recognize this problem by having a written policy agreed by management and unions to deal with alcohol and drug abuse, providing appropriate opportunities for rehabilitation.

Case history 11.6

A foundry worker engaged in a non-ferrous foundry was being seen by an appointed doctor for the purposes of health surveillance in relation to his exposure to lead. His tasks in fettling included the use of handheld vibrating tools to remove excess metal from the castings. The occupational physician incidentally elicited symptoms of vibration white finger. He sought the employee's consent to advise the employer so that the employer could take appropriate remedial steps as well as reporting the occupational disease to the Health and Safety Executive. The worker asked whether the physician could guarantee his continuing employment without adverse changes in his status and earnings. Obviously the physician could not do this and the worker denied his consent for his employer to be informed.

Many workers fear, sometimes justifiably, that they will be discriminated against if they develop an industrial disease. They may therefore be very reluctant to allow a doctor to inform the employer of their condition. This may, in turn, lead to delays in preventive measures being implemented. Bearing in mind what you have read so far about the investigation and management of occupational diseases, what steps would you now have taken?

> The physician suggested that he could speak to a medical colleague in the Health and Safety Executive to present the problem in confidence and seek help discreetly. The worker agreed to this, and agreed to the occupational physician communicating his concerns to the GP. After an appropriate interval, an official of the Health and Safety Executive made a 'routine' visit to the foundry, assessed exposure to vibration and made appropriate recommendations to the employers.

If the physician had advised the employer of the diagnosis, then the employer would have been legally obliged to report this to the Health and Safety Executive [under the Reporting of Injuries, Diseases and Dangerous Occurrences Regulations (RIDDOR)]. As with industrial accidents, so also with disease there is evidence of underreporting. If the physician has reason to suspect that this may be happening, then he should discuss his suspicions with medical colleagues in the Employment Medical Advisory Service of the Health and Safety Executive.

Occupational health reports and records

The occupational physician is the custodian of clinical records and access to these is limited to clinical staff (physicians and nurses). Clerical staff in the OHS must have the confidential nature of these records stressed to them and give a commitment to respect this confidentiality when they join the service before being allowed the access that is necessary for them to perform their duties. It may bear repeating to managers and to workers that even though the employers may own the case notes, in the same way that they may own everything else in the firm, the notes are in the secure custody of the physician and nurse and their contents will not be disclosed to the employer without the individual worker's informed consent. Similar considerations apply to clinical data that are stored electronically. Statutory obligations must be complied with, specifically those under Data Protection and Freedom of Information legislation, such as the need for registration and the entitlement of individuals to access to data held about them. Security measures, limitation of access and explicit documents to confirm this are particularly important where systems are shared or accessible through means of electronic communication, or where linkage is required, for example, with environmental data monitored by an occupational hygienist.

The doctor in industry should generally be prepared to discuss the contents of the occupational health records with the worker they concern. However, for this and other reasons, it may be useful to have the record subdivided. Thus, for example, separate sections should be devoted to pre-employment assessments, consultations following self-referral or referral by management and statutory health surveillance. Even in the last mentioned, a distinction may need to be made between the purely clinical data such as symptoms questionnaires or lung function tests on the one hand and a record of exposure, physician's conclusion and other basic information that may constitute statutory 'health records'.

Legal disclosure of occupational health records can pose serious dilemmas – with or without consent. An important distinction must be drawn between a request for clinical records from a solicitor and a court order for disclosure of specified documents. The latter must be complied with or the physician may incur unlimited penalty if found to be in contempt of court. In the case of a request from a solicitor, the accompanying written consent of the worker concerned is essential. However, even with the worker's consent, there could be complications. Thus, some parts of the occupational health record of the individual may bear no relation to the occupational injury or illness in respect of which litigation is in progress. Rarely, the names of other employees involved in a particular incident or exposure may appear in the record of the index worker and might need to be masked in any copy made. One situation in which there does not yet appear to be a clear consensus arises when a worker's solicitor asks for release of the worker's clinical record with the worker's consent while this consent is denied to the employer's solicitor. Understandably, the employer and his legal advisers may feel unfairly frustrated in that they are denied the information they need to respond to the worker's solicitor in anticipation of a possible Industrial Tribunal hearing or a Civil Action in a Law Court. One possible solution is to point out that the employer technically owns the clinical record. While this does not confer the right of access to the clinical record, it can entitle him to deny it to others. A consent by the worker for the relevant parts of the clinical record to be made available to solicitors on both sides could then resolve the impasse.

There is one specific exception to the rule that the occupational physician must disclose a report to the court in response to a court order or to the worker's solicitor with his consent. This arises when the occupational physician is specifically asked to see the worker and advise solely for legal purposes. Usually this request arises from the firm's solicitor. The physician must explain the special nature of this request to the worker and that neither the worker nor the worker's solicitor will be entitled to see the report but that it will be a privileged communication to the firm's solicitor.

Ethical relations with the general practitioner and other physicians

The role of the doctor in industry does not ordinarily extend to treatment of disease, prevention of ill-health that is not work related nor the provision of a 'second opinion'. Thus the treatment that an occupational physician undertakes should be limited to emergency measures, whether specific to occupational medicine or otherwise. In any case the GP should be informed of this as soon as practical and reasonable. Although limited administration of non-prescription therapeutic agents, such as minor analgesic agents, emollient creams, etc., need not warrant special attempts at liaison with the GP, any other treatment of consequence should be agreed. Referral to a specialist in another discipline should ordinarily only be undertaken with the agreement of the GP, except in an emergency. The role of the occupational physician in the prevention of ill-health and the promotion of health in those respects that are not strictly work related is discussed in Chapter 10. Advice of proven merit such as exhorting the worker to stop smoking is not likely to be contentious between medical practitioners and indeed should be encouraged. However, the implementation of other steps, such as cervical screening, should await an opportunity for the GP to voice an opinion, or veto, especially as such matters may form part of the GP's contract of employment. Finally, it should be stressed that the ethical constraints in relation to consent apply just as much to ethical relations with the GP as with anyone else. Thus a worker might not wish his GP to be aware of aspects of his medical history that could prejudice his chances of obtaining life insurance cover.

Occasionally workers may have misgivings about the security and confidentiality of information disclosed to the GP. The occupational physician may discuss these concerns with the worker and even try to allay them or find a reasonable compromise. Eventually, though, the worker's wishes must be respected, however irrational they may appear. Similar considerations apply to ethical relations with other physicians.

Ethical dilemmas

There are bound to be situations where guidelines do not provide explicit answers to an ethical dilemma. Yet there are very few circumstances in occupational medicine where a doctor has to advise or act without the possibility of time to think. Therefore, an occupational physician who might be in some doubt as to the 'correct' action should seek the advice of a senior colleague known to them personally or within an appropriate academic or professional organization.

AUDIT IN OCCUPATIONAL MEDICINE

Audit has been defined as 'the systematic critical analysis of the quality of medical care. This may include, for example, the procedures used for diagnosis and treatment, the use of resources and the resulting outcome and quality of life for the patient.' However, one should not lose sight of the origin of the word (Latin: 'audire' – to hear or listen). Audit should therefore be primarily a dialogue aimed at improving quality and not a rigid 'accounting' exercise. It is relevant to all medical specialties and is gaining importance worldwide as part of the need to provide quality of service to the consumer. There are various reasons why audit is particularly relevant to the practice of occupational medicine. First, doctors in industry practise in isolation (as distinct from, say, hospital 'firms' or group general practices) and therefore formal attempts at convening for the purposes of audit are important to ensure quality of care. Second, such doctors may not be fully accredited specialists and some of them, especially part-timers, are not engaged in any formal training programme. Audit can serve a very useful educational role, particularly for these physicians, by guiding them in better ways of managing common problems.

Definition and taxonomy of audit

Several definitions, types and taxonomies of audit have been described, some of which require clarification for the reader. Thus, for example, some authorities prefer to use the term 'clinical audit' rather than 'medical audit' to highlight the need to involve other healthcare disciplines, notably occupational health nurses. On the other hand, the 'clinical' adjective may tend to restrict the audit to the quality of care for the individual client/worker within the narrow confines of his clinical (Greek: 'kline' = couch or bed) consultation. At this level, audit of the quality of assessments, communication and advice and of the individual outcome is very important for the purposes of continuing education of the healthcare professional as well as to ensure that quality of care for the individual is paramount before other quantitative performance indicators are embarked upon. At a higher and wider organizational level, audit should cover the effectiveness and efficiency of the service. **Effectiveness** is defined as the extent to which a specific intervention, procedure, regimen or service, when deployed in the field, does what it is intended to do for a defined population. **Efficiency** measures the effects or end-results achieved in relation to the effort expended in terms of money, resources and time.

When classified along another dimension, audit can be subdivided into audit of structure, process and outcome. Structure deals with the quantity, type of resources available and organizational framework. Process deals with what is carried out by way of assessment, advice and other intervention in relation to the worker. Outcome measures the results of the intervention by the occupational physician or OHS, such as reduction in morbidity or in health risks.

- **Audit of structure.** This can include auditing staff numbers and qualifications, physical resources such as essential office and consulting facilities with comfort and appropriate diagnostic tools. It also includes record storage and 'virtual' structures such as policies. Although auditing the quality of structures, by determining whether or not there is compliance with an agreed standard, is relatively cheap and easy it might have little bearing on the effectiveness and efficiency of OHS, and hence on the quality delivered to the workers or their employers.
- **Process.** This includes administrative processes such as the handling of requests for appointments and booking of appointments, scheduling of routine health surveillance, and workplace assessments. However, the most important processes are the workplace risk assessment processes and the clinical processes. It is essential to follow agreed, and, where possible, evidence-based protocols and guidelines including assessment at commencement of employment, health surveillance or other periodic medical surveillance, immunization and rehabilitation. Ensuring the quality of process is very valuable if it addresses important determinants of outcome, and has many advantages. Thus it can be cheaper, more sensitive and permit quicker remedial action than evaluating outcome.
- **Outcome.** A few outcomes of great importance to workers can be easily assessed directly, quantitatively and objectively; for example, post-immunization antibody titres. Assuring outcomes such as long-term morbidity and mortality intuitively appears more valuable than focusing on the quality of process but it may entail high expense, and certainly requires a longer time scale if a demonstrable reduction in health risk is taken as an outcome quality standard. Moreover, the work of the OHS itself does not often produce an outcome independent of other factors outside the OHS. Nevertheless, the advice or other activity of the OHS can be considered as an intermediate output, the quality of which can be assured; for example, the advice given by the OHS to managers.

Choosing topics for audit in occupational medicine

The product of the possible topics needing audit and the possible means of accomplishing this for each topic is legion. The following guidelines should help a reasonable initial choice to be made. The topic to be audited should be locally common, or of high health risk or high cost in other ways and timely in its relevance. A preliminary review of the reasons for referral to the OHS, problems identified at consultations, 'accident' rates, and sickness absence rates, all major resource commitments of the OHS, should reveal many possible topics for audit. Alternatively, a random review of consultation records as outlined below has the merit of being simple and of selecting common reasons for consultation.

It is essential to have a standard against which to compare the observed practice. Many activities undertaken in occupational medicine do not have a wide enough consensus or a solid scientific basis to serve as a 'gold standard' and it may not be rewarding to audit these in detail, especially if there is additional local divergence on, for example, the means of rehabilitating workers with musculoskeletal injury, or on the extent of counselling for psychological stress. Nevertheless, basic information relating to health records, nationally agreed protocols on vaccination, for example, or a sound evidence base as in Case history 11.3 can be useful starting points in comparing observed practice with a standard. Topics should be chosen in which there is likely to be the need and the means for improvement in practice following comparison with the standard, the implementation of change and where the audit itself is cheap and simple. Thus the audit should seek to be cost effective by improving outcome and efficiency by education and changes in practice, at least initially. In summary it is essential to audit what needs to be audited rather than what can be. Audit is an iterative process of cycles, which should result in an improvement and eventually sustained assurance of quality in particular areas while identifying needs and methods of audit in new areas (Fig. 11.1).

(a) Ideal cycle of audit

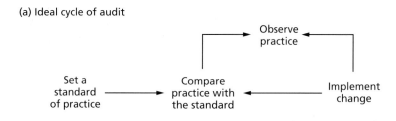

(b) Pragmatic cycle of audit

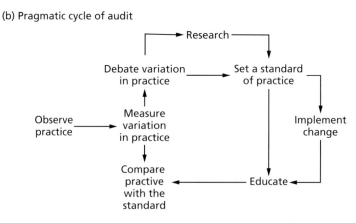

Fig. 11.1 *The cycle of audit and related activities in occupational medicine.*

Methods of audit

In certain situations, especially of an educational nature (trainer and trainee) or in a hierarchical context (chief physician and his juniors), occupational physicians meet to discuss and approve the conduct of their work. However, this is not an adequate system for audit because it involves only certain professional relationships and the subjects or case records covered are literally at the choice of either party. One means of more formal audit, especially of the process of occupational medical care, starts with the random selection of a small number of consultation records sampled from a serially kept daybook. These are then shared out between the participating physicians such that each acts in turn as auditor or has his consultation note audited. The auditor reviews, in private, the consultation record against a pro forma with key issues highlighted, perhaps assisted by a set of explicit criteria where these have been agreed. Subsequently, at an audit meeting, the auditor presents a brief verbal account of his assessment of the consultation record and this is usually followed by a short debate. A short summary of relevant points discussed and agreed actions is kept. These minutes are retained and can be used as confirmatory evidence of the audit and to assist the pursuit of remedial action. The detailed pro formas can then be destroyed. The benefits of this form of internal peer review audit can be illustrated by the following example:

Case history 11.7

A 36-year-old nurse was referred to the occupational physician with a history of multiple episodes of sickness absence and unacceptable behaviour at work. A previous hospital admission had suggested that her symptoms may have been related to alcohol abuse. The occupational physician had deemed her fit to return to her duties and had reviewed her once. The notes were sketchy and the results of the examination were not recorded. The peer group felt that more detailed assessment, record-keeping and further review was warranted when there was evidence of alcohol abuse. Guidelines for further management of such cases were agreed, including the policy that similar assessments should address the following points and be audited against them:

- current level of fitness for work
- likely date of return to work
- specific limitations in redeployment of the employee
- likelihood of the employee to render regular and efficient service in the future in terms of attendance, performance and safety
- likely duration of any residual disability
- advice on whether work could be affecting the employee's health
- specific advice on rehabilitation, including steps to be taken, targets to be set, and plan for monitoring progress.

To continue illustrating audit of process with the theme of respiratory health surveillance that started as a 'thread' at the beginning of this chapter, Table 11.3 shows how various aspects of the service can be audited.

The practically universal availability of computerized facilities in OHS assists considerably in the development of quantitative and ongoing methods of audit of process and of outcome. The data required must be collected accurately and prospectively, easily retrieved for the purposes of the audit but otherwise securely kept. Thus strategic objectives and specific targets may usefully be set, for example, for the

Table 11.3 *Possible steps in the audit of respiratory health surveillance*

Element to be audited	Method of audit
Identification of exposures significant enough to warrant action	Occupational hygiene professional review of sample of risk assessments completed by line managers, or by professional peers
Identification of target population	Review of sample of workplaces, and of tasks undertaken there, and comparison with lists of employees subjected to health surveillance
Health surveillance protocol	Review of sensitivity and specificity of the questionnaire, calibration of diagnostic tools
Health assessment of employees	Peer review audit of stratified random sample of records of health surveillance
Reporting of cases as required by statute or policy	Confidential comparison of random sample of positive cases from peer review audit of health surveillance against actual reports
Managerial response to results of health surveillance	Review of workplaces with high frequency of adverse effects for evidence of implementation of change
Trends in frequency of adverse health effect (e.g of respiratory or skin sensitization)	Review of validated frequency rates against time, classified by category of employees, workplace and task

uptake of a vaccination programme, and for acceptable time intervals for sickness absence or other referrals for specific problems to the occupational health department, as well as acceptable time intervals for the assessment and response by the occupational physician. However, caution needs to be applied in interpreting these data. Some research has shown no correlation between the response times of occupational physicians and the peer-reviewed quality of their response. It therefore follows that complementary approaches may be needed to assess both the quality and the timeliness of the assessment process. Both the quality of the OHS 'output', that is, the advice given, as well as the managerial response can be evaluated by comparing them with the subsequent experience of return to work in the time interval indicated, implementation of the OHS advice on redeployment and rehabilitation, as well as possible recurrence of the original reason for referral.

Whatever topics are audited or methods used, it is important for the audit to be non-threatening, educational and interesting for all participants as well as being objective, repeatable, effective and efficient in its aims.

CONCLUSION

Although different models of occupational healthcare delivery exist even within a community based on shared norms such as the European Union, fundamental concepts regarding quality and its delivery as well as ethics of practice still apply in all circumstances. Doctors in industry should aim to improve the quality of medical advice and the effectiveness and efficiency of the service through appropriate searches for and implementation of evidence-based practice. Evaluation through forms of audit is an important tool for ensuring that professional practice and service delivery conform to the predetermined needs and standards.

REFERENCES

Carter JT, Birrell LN (eds). *Occupational health guidelines for the management of low back pain at work – principal recommendations.* London, UK: Faculty of Occupational Medicine; 2000.

Sackett DL et al. *Evidence-Based Medicine: How to Practice and Teach EBM.* (Book with CD-ROM). London, UK: Churchill Livingstone; 2005.

Waddell G, Burton AK. *Occupational health guidelines for the management of low back pain at work* (leaflet for practitioners). London, UK: Faculty of Occupational Medicine, Royal College of Physicians of London; 2000.

Wright D et al. *Guidance On Ethics For Occupational Physicians*, 5th edn. London, UK: Faculty of Occupational Medicine, Royal College of Physicians of London; 1999.

Appendix 1

Reporting schemes and prescribed diseases

REPORTING SCHEMES

A number of reporting schemes have been introduced in an attempt to quantify the amount of harm caused by accidents and health risks at work. Within the UK the main scheme is the statutory requirement to report certain injuries and diseases under the RIDDOR regulations. It has been recognized, however, that there is considerable underreporting to this scheme and further sources of information are necessary better to estimate the prevalence of occupational ill-health. The Health and Safety Executive (HSE) has carried out four population surveys of self-reported work-related illness since 1990, and also funds a voluntary reporting programme for doctors, the Health and Occupation Reporting (THOR) network, which is run by the University of Manchester.

The situation in Europe is more complex, with each member state having its own list of occupational diseases carrying entitlement to compensation. While Spain has a modest list of 71 occupational diseases, France has 300! In order to try to introduce some standardization and improve the level of reporting, the European Commission in 1990 recommended the adoption of a European Schedule of Occupational Diseases. This lists five broad categories: diseases caused by chemicals; skin diseases; diseases caused by inhalation of substances; infectious and parasitic diseases; and diseases caused by physical agents. In addition it also lists diseases suspected of being occupational which should also be subject to notification. To date the recommendations have not been fully implemented within the European Union.

The Reporting of Injuries, Diseases and Dangerous Occurrences (RIDDOR) Regulations 1995

The RIDDOR regulations require employers to report certain accidents and diseases to the HSE, or, in certain cases, the Local Authority. The accidents and dangerous occurrences are described in Chapter 6. It should be noted, however, that a number of conditions that might be regarded as diseases are reportable under accidents if that is what caused them. For example, toxic pneumonitis following inhalation of irritant gases, or a slipped disc injury incurred while lifting a heavy weight would not be reportable under the list of diseases but should be reported under accidents if they result in over 3 days of absence from work.

Employers must report all cases of a defined list of diseases occurring among their employees *where they receive a doctor's written diagnosis and the affected employee's current job involves the work activity specifically associated with the disease.*

The responsibility for reporting rests with the employer but occupational physicians and other doctors have a role to play in advising the employer, usually through a sickness certificate, when a patient has been diagnosed with an occupational disease.

The following table lists the most commonly reported occupational diseases.

Disease	Numbers reported under RIDDOR 1993–1998
Occupational asthma	482
Other illness caused by a pathogen	324
Cramp of hand/forearm	431*
Decompression sickness	169
Occupational dermatitis	769*
Carpal tunnel syndrome	186*
Tenosynovitis	870*
Vibration white finger	1076

*Figures for 1996–1998 only.

It is only since 1996 that this list has included the more common diseases such as dermatitis and upper limb disorders, as well as some very rare ones. Because of the lack of awareness of employers (or doctors) to report incidences of oil folliculitis or barotrauma to the ear it is acknowledged that there is substantial underreporting of certain conditions.

The HSE has carried out a series of surveys of self-reported work-related illness, using supplementary questionnaires included in the Labour Force Survey, last repeated in 2003/2004. (This is an annual survey of households in the UK carried out by the Office of Population Censuses and Surveys (OPCS) on behalf of the Department of Employment.) The results suggested that the common work-related diseases in the UK are as listed in the following table.

Work-related disease	Approximate prevalence 2001–2002
Back disorders	470 000
Other musculoskeletal disorders	640 000
Stress/depression	560 000
Lower respiratory disease	180 000
Deafness	80 000
Skin disease	30 000

These figures are self-reported so they probably represent an overestimate but give some indication of the size of the problem. They also suggest that the most common work-related diseases present to general practitioners, orthopaedic surgeons and psychiatrists.

Voluntary reporting schemes

Other schemes for certain doctors to report cases of suspected occupational disease voluntarily exist. The main UK system, THOR (The Health and Occupation Network), is co-ordinated by the Centre for Occupational Health at the University of Manchester. Over more than a decade several schemes have been introduced, including:

- SWORD (Surveillance of Work-Related and Occupational Respiratory Disease)
- EPI-DERM (Occupational Skin Surveillance)
- OPRA (Occupational Physicians Reporting Activity)
- MOSS (Musculoskeletal Occupational Surveillance Scheme)
- OSSA (Occupational Surveillance Scheme for Audiological physicians)
- SIDAW (Surveillance of Infectious Diseases at Work)
- SOSMI (Surveillance of Occupational Stress and Mental Illness)
- THOR-GP (Surveillance of occupational disease and injury in general practice).

Under these schemes, specialists in respiratory medicine, dermatology, occupational medicine, rheumatology, ear, nose and throat, communicable diseases and psychiatry make regular returns giving brief details of new cases of established or suspected occupational disease. The intention behind these schemes is gradually to build up a realistic picture of the incidence of important occupational disease. Data comparing the incidence of various diseases reported to each scheme are published regularly by the HSE and the University of Manchester: www.coeh.man.ac.uk/thor.

PRESCRIBED DISEASES

The Prescribed Diseases are a list of conditions prescribed under the Industrial Injuries Scheme administered by the Department for Work and Pensions of the United Kingdom. The purpose of the list is to define those occupational diseases for which Industrial Injuries Benefit is payable. This compensates workers who have become disabled by a prescribed occupational disease. The self-employed are not covered by the scheme. In order for a disease to be prescribed an occupational cause must be well established. The list is kept under review by the Industrial Injuries Advisory Council, who make additions from time to time.

Prescribed Diseases are classified into four groups according to the nature of the causative agent for each disease:

A. physical agents
B. biological agents
C. chemical agents
D. miscellaneous.

Some examples of the most common Prescribed Diseases are listed in the following table.

Disease	Disease no.	Claims assessed 1996–1997 (n)
Cramp of hand or forearm	A4	98
Beat knee	A6	129
Tenosynovitis	A8	513
Occupational deafness	A10	413
Vibration white finger	A11	3288
Carpal tunnel syndrome	A12	297
Papilloma of bladder	C23	40
Allergic rhinitis	D4	352
Dermatitis	D5	336
Total claims for all prescribed diseases (n)	5535	

It should be noted these figures represent numbers of claimants, and only 1523 out of a total of 5535 claims for occupational diseases were awarded benefits.

Industrial Injuries Benefit

Of all those with work-related illness, only the most severely affected become sufficiently disabled to qualify for benefits. In the UK, approximately 35 000 people are currently receiving disablement benefits for a work-related disease. Deafness is the most common cause criterion for receiving benefits, followed by asbestos-related diseases and pneumoconioses. Other common conditions for which benefits are awarded are vibration white finger and upper limb disorders.

With regard to claiming for occupational disease:

- the claimant must have one of the diseases listed
- the claimant must have been employed, after 1948, in the type of work listed for the disease and
- the disease must have been caused by that work.

Independent adjudicating authorities decide claims. There are two chains of adjudication, one medical and one non-medical. The non-medical chain deals with exclusively lay questions, such as, did the claimant work in an occupation prescribed in relation to the disease claimed? The medical adjudication authorities, an insurance officer, the medical board and the medical appeal tribunal decide the strictly medical questions regarding diagnosis and degree of disablement, but the question of causation is decided solely by the insurance officer. The extent of a claimant's disablement as a result of loss of mental or physical faculty is assessed in comparison with a normal person of the same age and sex. The threshold for benefit is 14% disability, and the higher the percentage, the more benefit is payable. Less than 14% disability does not qualify for disablement benefit unless the patient has pneumoconiosis, byssinosis or diffuse mesothelioma. In the case of occupational deafness, the threshold for benefit is 20%.

Appendix 2

Sources of further information – the internet

INTRODUCTION

This appendix will deal in a summary form with some of the salient points regarding the use of the internet in Occupational Health. The internet is essentially a linked worldwide network of computers (and file servers). It can contribute to medical and health issues in a number of ways. Thus in its simplest form it can be used as a vehicle for electronic mail (e-mail). However, in the present context, it will probably be of greatest value through the World Wide Web (WWW). In order to gain maximum benefit from this account, it is strongly recommended that the 'Universal Resource Locators' (URLs) below are accessed. These are a sort of 'WWW internet address' that will tell your computer which file to obtain from another computer or server, perhaps on the other side of the planet, and how it should be accessed. The ones below start with 'http' meaning 'HyperText Transfer Protocol', that is, they essentially seek text files (or other data files such as images, rarely other types too) that have special attributes to permit linkage to other files and transfer these to your computer. Other protocols exist such as 'ftp' (File Transfer Protocol). One important interactive advantage exhibited by the WWW, and which cannot be matched by other information technology such as CD-ROMs, is the capacity to disseminate and access 'real-time' up-to-date opinion, information or data sets.

In order to support readers of this book, a website has been set up cross-referring to the book and designed to be used in conjunction with the text, to provide occasional complementary and supplementary information, especially to provide links to 'web pages' through URLs that might otherwise become out-dated in the text of the book. Readers should therefore access the following portal:
http://www.agius.com/pom

GENERAL INFORMATION SEARCHING AND LINKING

Many 'search engines' (such as 'Google'), if used uncritically, can be a very inefficient, and sometimes misleading, way of sourcing reliable occupational health information. There are a number of better ways of seeking information with some degree of validation or vetting, and these are often summarized within various 'directories' or 'gateways' or similar resources, for example:

http://www.ccohs.ca/resources/www.html
http://www.agius.com/hew/links/

Specialist resources

Specialist resources accessible via the internet broadly speaking fall into two categories: those in which the internet provides original peer-reviewed material, and those in which it provides digests or other compilations. The former category includes facilities for online literature searches such as through Medline and Embase. These yield citations and usually abstracts of peer-reviewed work but which are primarily still published in hard copy, although an ever-increasing proportion of journals are now publishing their full text on-line. A useful free starting point is Pub Med:

http://www.ncbi.nlm.nih.gov/entrez

The other category consists of resources on a range of issues such as toxicological databases, material safety/hazard data sheets, and accounts of occupational diseases, ergonomics, occupational hygiene, etc., which are becoming more widely available. Rather than providing lists of these, the reader may wish to pursue them through the hypertext links from the URLs given in the previous section, although two (one on toxicology and the second on 'Cochrane' evidence base) are particularly worthy of mention:

http://toxnet.nlm.nih.gov/
http://www.cohf.fi/

Official governmental or supra-governmental resources

The World Health Organization and several other international bodies publish material on the internet that is relevant to occupational health or cognate areas such as chemical safety. National governments and their agencies are increasingly publishing material in this manner. Dissemination of government policy, through media releases, laws and regulations and consultation documents, via the WWW is bound to increase. The main European Union portal through which information from each of its members can be accessed is:

http://europe.osha.eu.int/

Professional associations and learned societies

Several professional associations and learned societies now have their own WWW pages. A list of some of these can be found on:

http://www.agius.com/hew/links/ society.htm

These include the American College of Occupational and Environmental Medicine, the American Association of Occupational Health Nursing, the American Industrial Hygiene Association, the British Occupational Hygiene Society, the Society of Occupational Medicine, the Faculty of Occupational Medicine, the International Commission on Occupational Health, and an ever-growing number of many more all over the world. They often provide information regarding training in occupational medicine and allied disciplines.

Subscription services and continuing professional education

Various private and other websites offer subscription services online and these are likely eventually completely to replace CD databases for toxicological and other information. The WWW is likely to be an increasingly important vehicle for continuing professional development, through academic and other bodies to complement the resources provided by governmental bodies, private organizations and the learned societies/professional bodies. Links are provided through the aforementioned portal.

E-MAIL LISTS AND NEWSGROUPS

E-mail is not simply a quicker means of despatching letters and data-files. It can be a very efficient and effective way of soliciting or dispensing comment within one's professional peer-group, especially through moderated lists. Links are provided also through the aforementioned portal.

Newsgroups may tend to be more easily accessible, but the quality of their content may be somewhat more dubious.

QUALITY ON THE INTERNET

One of the advantages of the internet is that it provides a relatively cheap and easy means of publishing and publicizing one's own views worldwide in a freelance manner. In general this is a good thing as it fosters debate and dissemination of information. However, a side-effect is that a proportion of the material is produced by zealots and bigots and consumed by the ignorant or naïve, whether well-intentioned or not. Sometimes material which is very attractive in its presentation may be weak in the validity of its content. It has to be said that the internet is probably no more or no less susceptible to concerns about quality than the spoken word or that which is written on paper. Thus just as one would not necessarily accept as valid a conversation overheard at a bus stop or an article in some newspapers or magazines, one should have the same reservations about anything gleaned from 'surfing the net', from a 'newsgroup' or from an 'e-mail list'.

CONCLUSION

The internet is being increasingly used as a vehicle for professional information in a wide range of subjects including occupational health. As pressures in the workplace increase, it can provide an effective and efficient means for networking with peers, for obtaining information, keeping abreast of developments and for continuing professional development.

Appendix 3

Sources of further information – books and journals

INTRODUCTION

This appendix overlaps significantly with Appendix 2 because an increasing number of journals in particular now appear online. It lists sources of information that provide helpful information and guidance to the occupational physician who is seeking to solve a particular problem in clinical practice. Occupational health information is scattered throughout the literature in several subject areas. It is found in general as well as specialist medical journals and in a range of biomedical science journals.

TEXTBOOKS

General and encyclopaedic

Baxter PJ *et al.* (eds). *Hunter's Diseases of Occupations*, 9th edn. London, UK: Arnold; 1999.

Cox RAF, Edwards FC, Palmer K. *Fitness for Work: The medical aspects*, 3rd edn. Oxford, UK: Oxford University Press; 2000.

ILO Encyclopaedia of Occupational Safety. Geneva: International Labour Office; 1998. (This encyclopaedia remains a useful reference source. The articles are written by an international panel of experts and exhibit a variety of practice worldwide.)

Rom WN (ed.) *Environmental and Occupational Medicine*, 3rd edn. Boston, MA: Lippincott Williams & Wilkins; 1998.

Zenz C, Dickerson O, Horvath E Jr (eds). *Occupational Medicine*, 3rd edn. Philadelphia, PA: CV Mosby; 1994. (This is the major large American textbook that covers the whole range of occupational medicine, the wider aspects of occupational health and practical management issues.)

Specialist topics

Hendrick DJ *et al.* (eds). *Occupational Disorders of the Lung.* Philadelphia, PA: WB Saunders; 2002. (This book covers in some detail areas that commonly give rise to clinical problems associated with the lung in occupational medicine.)

Lewontin R. *It ain't necessarily so. The dream of the human genome and other illusions.* London, UK: Granta Books; 2000.

Lomborg B. *The sceptical environmentalist. Measuring the real state of the world.* Cambridge, UK: Cambridge University Press; 2001.

Margulis L. *The symbiotic planet. A new look at evolution.* London, UK: Weidenfeld and Nicolson; 1998.

Shrivastava P. *Bhopal. Anatomy of a crisis.* Cambridge, MA: Ballinger; 1987.

Zebrowski E. *Perils of a restless planet. Scientific perspectives on natural disasters.* Cambridge, UK: Cambridge University Press; 1997.

Occupational hygiene

Gill FS. *Monitoring for Health Hazards at Work*, 2nd edn. Oxford, UK: Blackwell Science; 1999. (This is a useful practical manual on monitoring hazards in the workplace. It is an essential book for anyone who occasionally has to undertake simple monitoring surveys in the absence of an occupational hygienist.)

CBI. *Counting the Costs: 2002 absence and labour turnover survey.* London, UK: Confederation of British Industry; 2001.

Davies NV, Teasdale P. *The costs to the British Economy of Work Accidents and Work-related Ill Health.* London, UK: HSE Publications; 1994.

Malcolm RM, Harrison J, Forster H. Effects of changing the pattern of sickness absence referrals in a local authority. *Occupational Medicine* 1993; 43:211–215.

Seccombe I. *Measuring and Monitoring Absence from Work*, Institute for Employment Studies Report 288. London, UK: Institute for Employment Studies; 1995.

Self-reported work-related illness in 1995: results from a household survey. London, UK: HSE; 1998.

Social Security Statistics. Government Statistical Service. London, UK: HMSO; 1992.

Toxicology

Bingham E, Cohrssen B, Powell CH (eds). *Patty's Toxicology*, 5th edn. 8 volume set. Philadelphia, PA: John Wiley and Sons Inc.; 2001. (This reference book provides detailed information on all aspects of worker and workplace health and safety. Whilst it is written for the American market, the principles are universally applicable. Previously combined into a single volume as *Patty's Industrial Hygiene and Toxicology*, for the fifth edition Industrial Hygiene and Toxicology are covered in separate publications.)

Klaassen CD (ed). *Casarett and Doull's Toxicology. The basic science of poisons*, 6th edn. London, UK: McGraw-Hill Education; 2001.

Patty FA, Harris RL (eds). *Patty's Industrial Hygiene*, 5th edn. Volume I: *Introduction to Industrial Hygiene; Recognition and Evaluation of Chemical Agents*; Volume 2:

Physical Agents; Biohazards; Engineering Control and Personal Protection; Volume 3: *Legal, Regulatory and Management*; Volume 4: *Specialized Topics and Allied Professions*. Philadelphia, PA: John Wiley and Sons Inc.; 2000.

Epidemiology

A basic knowledge of epidemiology is important when dealing with the health of groups of people as well as to allow critical appraisal of published papers. The selected book provides the necessary introduction to the subject.

Olsen J, Merletti F, Snashall D, Vuylsteek K. *Searching for Causes of Work-Related Diseases*. Oxford, UK: Oxford University Press; 1991.

PRIMARY JOURNALS

The following is a list of peer-reviewed journals that publish articles on occupational medicine. Articles appear in many other journals and so the list, which is in alphabetical order, should not be considered exhaustive.

American Industrial Hygiene Journal
Annals of Occupational Hygiene
Archives of Environmental Health
Occupational and Environmental Medicine
International Archives of Occupational and Environmental Health
Journal of Occupational Medicine
Journal of Toxicology
Occupational Medicine
Scandinavian Journal of Work, Environment and Health
The *British Medical Journal* and *The Lancet* publish leaders, review articles, original papers and case reports that are of relevance to occupational medicine.

Index

health surveillance of foundry workers
    125–6
pregnancy and fetus 43
lead dust sampling pump, 123 (fig)
lead poisoning 39 (table), 43–44, 58 (table)
    anaemia due to, 43 (fig)
    case history 6–7
    chelation therapy 95
    developed/developing world 44, 46
    misdiagnosed as acute appendicitis 95
    motor neuropathy 40
    suspension from work 188
lead refinery
    in India
        blood levels 44
        carbon monoxide-related fatality 45
learning difficulties
    definition of disabled 247
    local education authorities 247
    unemployment rate 243
    work placement 250
leather goods manufacture 38
legionnaire's disease (*Legionella* spp.) 17, 33, 46,
    177
legislation
    disability in EU
        Denmark 244
        Germany 245
        Spain 245–6
        United Kingdom 246–8
        variability 244
    health and safety, UK system as model 156
    international variation in health and safety
        156
    see also Acts of Parliament; Health and Safety,
        etc., at Work Act
leptospirosis (*Leptospira* spp.) 46, 95
leukaemia, 43 (fig)
light injury 82–3
    arc welding 37, 82–3
liver disease 42
locomotion 221–2
locomotor illnesses, prevalence 15
lost time rate 193
Lovelock, James 165–6
lower limb disorders
    beat knee 293 (table)
    below-knee amputation 221–2

chronic osteomyelitis of foot 221–2
degenerative joints and work fitness 114
fungal infections of coal mine workers 21
lumbar ache 35
lumbar spinal flexion 82
lung biopsy 56
lung cancer
    asbestos-related 98
    particulate pollution 172
    passive smoking 177, 259
    suspicion of occupational cause 26–7
    tobacco smoking and 2, 26, 178, 182–3
    vehicle exhausts and 175
lung disease
    asymptomatic with abnormal chest film 31–2
    breathlessness
        acute 27–30
        chronic 30–1
    chest pain 32
    dust-related, differential diagnosis, 54 (fig)
    investigations 53–7
        biopsy 56
        bronchoalveolar lavage 56
        chest radiography 52
        lung function 52–6
        skin tests 56, 73
    irritant chemicals 93–4
    mixed patterns 31
    obliterative bronchiolitis 145
    occupational causes, 23 (table)
    pneumonia 32–3
    pulmonary fibrosis 29–30
    reactive airways dysfunction syndrome 26
    smog exacerbating 167–8
    see also asbestos-related disease; asthma; lung
        cancer
lung function testing 53–6
Lyme disease (*Borrelia burgdorferi*) 46

machines
    accidental breakdown 105
    regular servicing 105
macular degeneration 232
malaise
    building-related 45, 46
    difficult to treat 45
'malingerers' 201
Malthus, Thomas 166